PATIENT
SAFETY

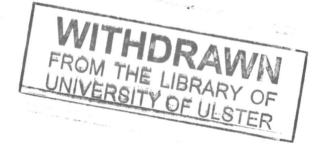

Commissioning Editor: Timothy Horne
Project Development Manager: Lulu Stader
Project Manager: Frances Affleck
Designer: Erik Bigland

PATIENT SAFETY

by

Charles Vincent

Smith & Nephew Foundation Professor of Clinical Safety Research
Imperial College of Science, Technology and Medicine London
Department of Surgical Oncology & Technology
St Mary's Hospital
London
UK

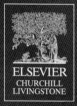

ELSEVIER
CHURCHILL
LIVINGSTONE

EDINBURGH LONDON NEW YORK OXFORD PHILADELPHIA ST LOUIS SYDNEY
TORONTO 2006

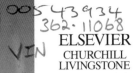

ELSEVIER
CHURCHILL
LIVINGSTONE

An imprint of Elsevier Science Limited

First published 2006

ISBN 0443101205

British Library Cataloguing in Publication Data
A catalogue record for this book is available from the British Library

Library of Congress Cataloging in Publication Data
A catalog record for this book is available from the Library of Congress

Notice
Medical knowledge is constantly changing. Standard safety precautions must be followed, but as new research and clinical experience broaden our knowledge, changes in treatment and drug therapy may become necessary or appropriate. Readers are advised to check the most current product information provided by the manufacturer of each drug to be administered to verify the recommended dose, the method and duration of administration, and contraindications. It is the responsibility of the practitioner, relying on experience and knowledge of the patient, to determine dosages and the best treatment for each individual patient. Neither the Publisher nor the author assumes any liability for any injury and/or damage to persons or property arising from this publication.

The Publisher

ELSEVIER your source for books, journals and multimedia in the health sciences

www.elsevierhealth.com

The Publisher's policy is to use paper manufactured from sustainable forests

Printed in China

PREFACE

Of the making of many books there is no end (Ecclesiastes)

Wants me to marry, get a home, settle down, write a book (Chuck Berry)

Ecclesiastes, the scourge of worldly pleasures, and Chuck Berry, the poet of rock-and-roll hedonism, had this much in common: they were both suspicious of the need and motives for writing books. Ecclesiastes warned that much study was a weariness of the flesh and Chuck Berry saw the writing of a book as the final, calamitous stage of the descent from youthful exuberance to quiescent middle age. In my case they were both right on the mark, showing both perceptiveness and prescience. More importantly though, their scepticism makes one think carefully about the reasons for writing a book. With books on medical error, clinical risk and patient safety appearing every year, why another book? As a student said to me, chiding me for the inclusion of a (no doubt fascinating) historical digression in a lecture: 'Professor, explain yourself'.

The first reason for the book is very simple: the importance of the topic. As you will see if you read on there is compelling evidence that, although healthcare brings enormous benefits to us all, errors are common and patients are frequently harmed. The nature and scale of this harm is hard to comprehend. It is made up, world wide, of hundreds of thousands of individual tragedies every year in which patients are traumatized, suffer unnecessary pain, are left disabled, or die. Many more people have their care interrupted or delayed by minor errors and problems that lead only to inconvenience, discomfort and perhaps some additional treatment or time in hospital. Although these incidents are not as serious for patients, they are a massive and relentless drain on scarce healthcare resources.

A second reason is that for all the books, reports, articles and websites devoted to patient safety, there is still no straightforward overview of the field. The books that are available are mostly multi-author, edited texts that, while they bring a rich diversity of perspective, are not primarily aimed at explaining the basic principles, characteristics and direction of the field. My aim has been to show the landscape of patient safety: how it evolved, the research that underpins the area, the key conceptual issues that have to be addressed, and the practical action needed to reduce error and harm and, when it does occur, to help those involved.

Third, patient safety is a meeting point for a multitude of other topics. The relevant literature is difficult to grasp, being scattered, diverse, and multidisciplinary in nature. Much of it is published in areas, such as cognitive psychology and ergonomics, which are unfamiliar to medicine. Worse still, many of the topics fundamental to progress in patient safety are themselves the subjects of huge literatures and much debate. For instance, a substantial amount of work has been carried out, from a number of different perspectives, on the factors that produce safe, high-performing teams. The same could be said of expertise, decision making, human error, human factors, information technology, leadership, organisational culture . . . the list goes on and on.

A fourth reason is to show that patient safety is, very simply, a tough problem. In healthcare, we are beginning to understand how difficult the safety problem is, in cultural, technical, clinical, and psychological terms, not to mention its massive scale and heterogeneity. Yet still, at safety conferences, you will hear people saying 'it's the culture', 'the key is strong leadership', 'team building is the answer', 'if we just had good professional standards all would be well', 'we know we've got a problem, lets just get on and fix it' and so on. Of course, all of these factors are important in some contexts, although none is sufficient, and there are some things that can and should be 'just fixed': removing dangerous drugs from wards when they don't need to be there seems a sensible precaution; scalding water temperatures in homes for old people certainly kill the bacteria but are also a serious hazard for the residents. These things just need action, although even solutions to problems of this kind might not be as straightforward as they seem. More often though, we are faced with hugely intractable, multifaceted problems that are deeply embedded within our healthcare systems. One of the greatest obstacles to progress on patient safety is, paradoxically, the attraction of neat solutions, whether political, organizational, or clinical. Is it likely that the problem of harm to healthcare is going to be simple to solve? Consider the nature of the problem.

Healthcare is the largest industry in the world, by far, larger then even the military in spending, numbers of people employed, use of resources and the wider impact on the population at large. It is, in addition, extraordinarily diverse in terms of the activities involved and the way it is delivered. Healthcare can be delivered in state-of-the-art facilities, across a bedside in a home or at a table set up in a field in rural India. Healthcare encompasses the mostly routine, but sometimes highly unpredictable and hazardous world of surgery; it also encompasses primary care, where patients can have relationships with their doctors over many years; some highly organized and ultra-safe processes, such as the management of blood products; and the inherently unpredictable, constantly changing environment of emergency medicine. To this list we can add mental health, care in the community, patients who monitor and treat their own condition and, by far the most important in poorer cultures, care given in people's homes. Most patient safety, taking its cue from high technology industries, has focused on relatively sophisticated hospital care; however, world wide most healthcare is given in the home, often self-administered or delivered by staff of widely differing levels of expertise and experience. In all these arenas both error and harm to patients are real possibilities and frequent actualities, although the nature of the harm, its causes, consequences and likely methods of prevention will differ widely according to context. Add into this the fact that not all harm is due to error in any simple sense, that most harm results from a chain of events and concatenation of circumstances, that human behaviour and liability to error is strongly affected by the inherent limitations of our brains, the environment in which we operate and the wider organisational context of the healthcare system. This is just the merest sketch of the arenas in which patient safety may be relevant and the many facets of risk and safety in healthcare. A straightforward problem? I don't think so.

The nature of the book

I hope that this book will be read by anyone either interested or involved in healthcare, as an introduction to patient safety. I have tried to write a clear, reasonably comprehensive overview of the major themes and topics. However, while I hope the book will be useful on the courses on patient safety that our now emerging, it is not a textbook. Such books tend to present a simplified version of a subject, eliminating complexity and dispute, leaving the reader with a tidy, sanitized version of events and a feeling that there is nothing challenging about the field. To my mind, the attempt in many papers and conferences to present all quality and safety issues in the simplest possible terms has been a disaster and a major obstacle both to progress generally and specifically to the engagement of clinicians. While trying to present the basic ideas clearly, I have also tried to show some of the difficulties, controversies and the intellectual challenge. In this sense I have tried to make the book a gateway into the field, rather than a self-contained introduction. Some truly wonderful books and papers have been written about patient safety, or topics relevant to it, and I have tried to show my own sources of inspiration and learning and direct people to them.

A book of this kind is inevitably highly selective and some decisions have to be made about what to cover and in how much detail. I have tried, as far as possible, to address generic issues that cross specialties and disciplinary boundaries, rather than examine specific clinical topics. Inevitably this produces a more abstract, theoretically driven book at times, but hopefully one with wider applicability and coverage. I have, however, included illustrations and specific clinical examples wherever possible, aiming to balance and illuminate the more general points. Patient safety is still largely confined to hospital medicine and to the developed world, and the book reflects this. Safety in primary care, mental health, care given in the home and patient safety in developing countries are vital issues but work on them has hardly begun. There is comparatively little discussion of the implementation of safety programmes or of organizational change, although many of the issues discussed, such as culture and leadership, bear directly on the practicalities of implementation. My intention, rather, has been to convey some of the essential understanding that must precede any such programmes, many of which are, to my mind, haphazard and without any defined direction or purpose.

The book is designed to be read straight through, although readers who wish to address particular themes and topics can select specific sections.

Broadly speaking, the book is divided into five main sections. The first two chapters address the history and evolution of patient safety. Patient safety emerged from a particular historical context and as a result of a number of different influences; understanding how it emerged is the best way, to my mind, to understand its character, strengths and limitations. The next two chapters address the nature and scale of harm, examining both the research evidence and the role of reporting systems. Chapters 5 and 6 form another section devoted to understanding why errors and accidents happen, reviewing the concept of human error, the nature of accidents, perspectives on safety and methods of analysing incidents. The next two chapters consider the impact of errors and harm on the people involved, patients and their families in Chapter 7 and clinical staff in Chapter 8. The final group of four chapters, the largest component of the book, all in one way or another concern the reduction of error and the ultimate aim of safe, reliable healthcare. Culture and leadership, standardization and process improvement and the role of information technology are the principal themes in Chapters 9, 10 and 11. The final chapter looks at how people create safety, in the sense of actively anticipating problems and negotiating the hazardous terrain of healthcare. These chapters also contain an ongoing discussion of the relative importance of these different approaches and the sometimes conflicting visions that underlie them.

ACKNOWLEDGEMENTS

Many people, whether they know it or not, have helped in the writing of this book. The list of references and sources is testament to the richness of the patient safety literature and I am certainly indebted to everyone named there. However, I particularly wish to thank people who through their actions, their writings or through conversation have expanded my view or changed the way I think about patient safety. This could be a very long list but I especially wish to single out Rene Amalberti, David Bates, Don Berwick, Richard Cook, Pat Croskerry, Jan Davis, Marc de Leval, Atul Gawande, Lucian Leape, Graham Neale, Tom Nolan, Jens Rasmussen, James Reason and Bob Wears. Two of these people, Lucian Leape and James Reason, require special mention both because of their influence on the field and the help they have given to me personally; both would be embarrassed by a too effusive encomium, but they will just have to put with it. Both have been an inspiration and unfailingly generous in their support and encouragement. Jim, in addition, has on many occasions managed to persuade my superiors that I was engaged in an enterprise of importance and farsightedness and not, as they sometimes suspected, an activity at best marginal and at worst disreputable.

Ros Jacklin, Graham Neale, Sisse Olsen, Jocelyn Potter and Bob Wears nobly read and commented on the entire manuscript resulting in many more apposite examples, much greater clarity and the removal of a variety of errors, infelicities and stupidities. I must particularly thank Graham, who provided a mass of incisive commentary and clinical understanding. To take just one example, the book would surely be the poorer without its brief account of the Rochdale Experiment, which led in the 1920s to a dramatic reduction in maternal mortality in a very poor area of England.

At the risk of sounding like a speech at the Oscars I also wish to thank the following people for in one way or another helping me over the years and so contributing to this book: my colleagues in the Clinical Risk Unit, Maria Woloshynowych and Sally Adams; my current colleagues in the Clinical Safety Research Unit for their enthusiasm for safety and their tolerance of my immersion in this project; Ara Darzi for seeing the potential of creating such a unit in a department of surgery, and for taking a chance on its director; Chris O'Donnell for backing the unit and giving me freedom of action; Liam Donaldson for bringing our group's work to a wider stage; Sue Osborne and Susan Williams for involving me in their pioneering work and Timothy Horne for pursuing his longstanding interest in the book. Anna Saunders not only handled all the tedious work of references with exemplary care and skill, but also read the early drafts, gently indicating areas of self-indulgence, incoherence and irrelevance. Most academic authors suffer from what a friend of mine called the benign neglect of academic editors; in complete contrast Lulu Stader has shown real interest in the book and its progress and given me unstinting expert help throughout.

The incomparable P.G. Wodehouse dedicated one of his books to his daughter Leonora, without whose never-failing sympathy and encouragement, as he said, it would have been finished in half the time. I must thank my wife Angela for her encouragement at a time of considerable difficulty for each of us; everything else I might thank her for is expressed in the dedication. I was also grateful for her confidence that I would, one day, actually finish the book. I hope that at least some readers will feel that something useful has emerged.

Acknowledgements

CONTENTS

For Angela

Medical harm: a brief history

The greatest benefit to mankind.
(Samuel Johnson's tribute to medicine)

It may seem a strange principle to enunciate as the very first requirement in a hospital that it should do the sick no harm.
(Nightingale 1863)

During the 1990s and the early years of the twenty-first century there was a deluge of statistics on medical error and harm to patients, a series of truly tragic cases of healthcare failure and a growing number of major government and professional reports on the need to make healthcare safer. There is now widespread acceptance and awareness of the problem of medical harm and a determination, in some quarters at least, to tackle it. It seems that we are only now waking up to the full scale of medical error and harm to patients. Yet awareness of medical harm and efforts to reduce it are as old as medicine itself, dating back to Hippocrates' classic dictum to 'abstain from harming or wronging any man'.

THE CURE CAN BE WORSE THAN THE DISEASE

Medicine has always been an inherently risky enterprise, the hopes of benefit and cure always linked to the possibility of harm. The word *pharmakos* means both remedy and poison; the words 'kill' and 'cure' were apparently closely linked in ancient Greece (Porter 1999). Throughout medical history there are instances of cures that proved worse than the disease, of terrible suffering inflicted on hapless patients in the name of medicine, and of well intentioned but deeply misguided interventions that did more harm than good. Think, for example, of the application of mercury and arsenic as medicines, the heroic bleeding cures of Benjamin Rush, the widespread use of lobotomy in the 1940s and the thalidomide disasters of the 1960s (Sharpe & Faden 1998). A history of medicine as harm, rather than benefit, could easily be written; a one-sided, incomplete history to be sure, but a feasible proposition nonetheless.

Looking back with all the smugness and wisdom of hindsight many of these so-called cures now seem to be absurd, even cruel. In all probability though, the doctors who inflicted these cures on their patients were intelligent, altruistic, committed physicians whose intention was to relieve suffering. The possibility of harm is inherent to the practice of medicine, especially at the frontiers of knowledge and experience. We might think that the advances of modern medicine mean that medical harm is now of only historical interest. However, for all its genuine and wonderful achievements, modern medicine too has the potential for considerable harm, perhaps even greater harm than in the past. As Chantler (1999) has observed, medicine used to be simple, ineffective and relatively safe; now it is complex, effective and potentially dangerous. New innovations bring new risks, greater power brings greater possibility of harm and new technology offers new possibilities for unforeseen outcomes and lethal hazards. The hazards associated with the delivery of simple, well-understood healthcare of course remain; consider, for example, the routine use of non-sterile injections in many developing countries. Before turning to the hazards of modern medicine, however, we will briefly review some important antecedents of our current concern with the safety of healthcare.

HEROIC MEDICINE AND NATURAL HEALING

The phrase 'first do no harm', a later twist on the original Hippocratic wording, can be traced to the 1849 treatise *Physician and patient* by Worthington Hooker, who in turn attributed it to an earlier source (Sharpe & Faden 1998). The background to this injunction, and its use at that point in the development of Western medicine, lay in a reaction to the 'heroic medicine' of the early nineteenth century.

Heroic medicine was, in essence, the willingness to intervene at all costs and put the saving of life above the immediate suffering of the patient. As Sharpe and Faden (1998) have pointed out, when reviewing the history of iatrogenic harm in American medicine, it is this period that stands out for the violence of its remedies. Heroism was certainly required of the patient in the mid-nineteenth century. For instance, in the treatment of cases of 'morbid excitement' such as yellow fever, Benjamin Rush, a leading exponent of heroic medicine, might drain over half the total blood volume from his patient. Yet Rush was heroic in his turn, staying in fever-ridden Philadelphia to care for his sick patients. Rush explicitly condemned the Hippocratic belief in the healing power of nature, stating that the first duty of a doctor was 'heroic action, to fight disease'.

Physicians more trusting of natural healing saw heroic medicine as dangerous, even murderous. Sharpe and Faden quote the assessment of J. Marion Sims, a famous gynaecological surgeon, writing in 1835 at the time of his graduation from medical school:

> I knew nothing about medicine, but I had sense enough to see that
> doctors were killing their patients, that medicine was not an exact
> science, that it was wholly empirical and that it would be better to trust
> entirely to Nature than to the hazardous skill of the doctors.
> **(Sharpe & Faden 1998 p 8)**

These extreme positions – of heroic intervention and natural healing – eventually gave way to a more conservative position, espoused by such leading physicians as Oliver Wendell Holmes, who attempted objectively to assess the balance of risk and benefit of any particular intervention. This recognizably modern approach puts patient outcome as the determining factor and explicitly broadens the physician's responsibility to the avoidance of pain and suffering, however induced – whether from the disease or the treatment.

Judgements about what constitutes harm are not straightforward and are irretrievably bound up with the personal philosophies of both physician and patient. To the sincere, if misguided, heroic practitioners, loss of life was the one overriding harm to be avoided and any action was justified in that pursuit. This was moderated by the more conservative position of striking a balance between intervening to achieve benefit and avoiding unnecessary suffering. Such dilemmas are, of course, common today when, for instance, a surgeon must consider whether an operation to remove a cancer in a terminally ill patient, which might prolong life, is worth the additional pain and suffering associated with the operation. The final decision nowadays might rest with the patient and family but they will be strongly influenced by medical advice. The patient too must decide whether to 'first do no harm' or whether to risk harm in the pursuit of other benefits.

HOSPITALISM AND HOSPITAL-ACQUIRED INFECTION

Dangerous treatments were one form of harm. However, hospitals could also be secondary sources of harm, in which patients acquired new diseases simply from being in hospital. By the mid-nineteenth century, anaesthesia had made surgery less traumatic and allowed surgeons time to operate in a careful and deliberate manner. Infection, however, was rife. Sepsis was so common, and gangrene so epidemic, that those entering hospital for surgery were 'exposed to more chance of death than the English soldier on the field of Waterloo' (Porter 1999 p 369). The term 'hospitalism' was coined to describe the disease-promoting qualities of hospitals, and some doctors believed that hospitals should be periodically burnt down. As late as 1863, Florence Nightingale introduced her *Notes on hospitals* as follows:

> It may seem a strange principle to enunciate as the very first requirement
> in a Hospital that it should do the sick no harm. It is quite necessary,
> nevertheless, to lay down such a principle, because the actual mortality
> in hospitals, especially in those of large crowded cities, is very much
> higher than any calculation founded on the mortality of the same class of
> diseases among patients treated out of hospital would lead us to expect.
> **(Nightingale, quoted in Sharpe & Faden 1998 p 157)**

Puerperal fever, striking mothers after childbirth, was particularly lethal and widely known to be more common in hospitals than after home deliveries. A small number of doctors in both England and America suspected that this was caused by transfer of 'germs' and argued that doctors should wash between autopsy and a birth. These claims of the contagious nature of puerperal fever, and the absurd possibility of it being transferred by doctors, were strongly rebutted by many, including the obstetrician Charles Meigs, who concluded his defence of his position with the marvellous assertion that 'a gentleman's hands are clean' (Sharpe & Faden 1998 p 154). Bacteria were apparently confined to the lower classes.

Dramatic evidence of the role of hygiene was provided by Ignaz Semmelweiss, in Vienna. Semmelweiss studied two obstetric wards: in ward one, mortality from infection hit a peak of 29%, with 600–800 women dying every year, whereas in ward two mortality was 3%. Semmelweiss noted that the only difference between wards was that patients on ward one were attended by medical students and those on ward two by midwifery students. When they changed places, the mortality rates reversed. Following the rapid death of a colleague who cut his finger during an autopsy, Semmelweiss concluded that his colleague had died of the same disease as the women and that puerperal fever was caused by the conveying of putrid particles to the pregnant woman during examinations. He instituted a policy of hand disinfection with chlorinated lime and mortality plummeted. Semmelweiss finally published his findings 1857, after similar findings in other hospitals, but found it difficult to persuade his fellow clinicians and his beliefs were still largely ignored when he died in 1865 (Jarvis 1994).

Lister faced similar battles to gain acceptance of the use of antiseptic techniques in surgery, partly because of scepticism about the existence of microorganisms capable of transmitting infection. However, by the end of the nineteenth century, with experimental support from the work of Pasteur and Koch, the principles of infection control and the new techniques of sterilization of instruments were fairly well established. Surgical gowns and masks, sterilization and rubber gloves were all in use and, most important, surgeons believed that safe surgery was both a possibility and a duty. However, 100 years later, with transmission of infection well understood and taught in every nursing and medical school, we face an epidemic of hospital-acquired infection. The causes of these infections are complex, with antibiotic-resistant organisms, hospital overcrowding, shortage of time and lack of easily available washing facilities all playing a part. However, as in Semmelweiss's time, a major factor is the difficulty of ensuring that staff, in the midst of all their other duties, do not forget to wash their hands between patients.

SURGICAL ERRORS AND SURGICAL OUTCOME

Ernest Codman, a Boston surgeon of the early twentieth century, was a pioneer in the scientific assessment of surgical outcome and in making patient outcome the guiding principle and justification of surgical intervention. Codman was so disgusted with the lack of evaluation at Massachusetts General Hospital that he resigned to set up his own 'End-Result' hospital. This was based on the, for Codman, common-sense notion that 'every hospital should follow every patient it treats, long enough to determine whether or not the treatment has been successful, and then to inquire "if not, why not" with a view to preventing similar failures in the future' (Sharpe & Faden 1998 p 29). Crucially, Codman was prepared to consider, and more remarkably make public, the occurrence of errors in treatment (Box 1.1) and to analyse their causes.

Medical harm: a brief history

> **Box 1.1 Codman's categories for the assessment of unsuccessful treatment**
>
> (from Sharpe & Faden 1998 p 30)
>
> - Errors due to lack of technical knowledge or skill
> - Errors due to lack of surgical judgement
> - Errors due to lack of care or equipment
> - Errors due to lack of diagnostic skill
> - The patient's unconquerable disease
> - The patient's refusal of treatment
> - The calamities of surgery or those accidents and complications over which we have no known control

In Box 1.2 Codman describes a case of apparently misdiagnosed appendicitis; the patient was followed up years after discharge to demonstrate the end result and the process error during care was linked to the end result. In this case, by the time of the follow-up the patient has a new problem of gallstones, which was not related to the original diagnostic error (Neuhauser 2002).

From 1911 to 1916, 337 patients were discharged from Codman's hospital, with 123 errors recorded. In addition to errors Codman recorded 'calamities of surgery' over which he had no control, but which he believed should be acknowledged and made known to the public. He was unsparing of himself noting, after ligating a patient's hepatic duct which led to their death, that he, 'had made an error of skill of the most gross character and even during the operation had failed to recognise it' (Neuhauser 2002).

Codman challenged his colleagues to demonstrate the efficacy of their procedures, and not rely solely on the prestige of their profession to justify their actions. Unless the methods of science were applied to the evaluation of outcomes, Codman contended, there was nothing to distinguish a surgeon from a genial charlatan. His denunciations of humbuggery, by which he meant putting income ahead of outcome, culminated in his presentation of a large cartoon at a meeting of the local Surgical Society. In the picture an ostrich is shown with its head beneath a pile of golden surgical eggs depicting the lucrative practices threatened by objective evaluation and publication of findings. This episode caused an uproar but, anticipating this, Codman had already resigned his post at Massachusetts General Hospital. Although Codman was ostracized and ridiculed by many, his proposals were nevertheless adopted by the American Surgical Society, although the eventual 'minimum standards for hospitals' instituted after World War I omitted two of the

> **Box 1.2 Codman's 'End Result' hospital report**
>
> (from Neuhauser 2002 p 104)
>
> **Case # 90 Jan 27 1913**
>
> Stout female – 36. Abdominal pain of 12 hours duration. Pre-op diagnosis sub acute appendicitis. Op (EAC & GWM) – Appendectomy. Appendix showed evidence of a previous attack but no sign of acute inflammation. Comp. none. [Error in diagnosis, Ed] Result August 13 well. August 18 1915. Now has symptoms of gallstones. Op advised, scar solid.

most crucial components: the analysis of outcomes and the classification of error. The minimum standard ran until 1952, when it was overtaken by the formation of the organization that eventually became the Joint Commission on Accreditation of Healthcare Organizations (JCAHO) the largest accrediting body in the United States (Sharpe & Faden 1998).

IATROGENIC DISEASE

In the early decades of the twentieth century, the scientific understanding of disease was well advanced and the excesses of heroic treatments had been curbed, but few effective treatments were available. Entering medical school in 1933, Lewis Thomas reflected that the purpose of the curriculum was:

> . . . to teach the recognition of disease entities, their classification, signs, symptoms, and laboratory manifestations and how to make an accurate diagnosis. The treatment of disease was the most minor part of the curriculum, almost left out altogether . . . nor do I remember much talk about treating disease at any time in the four years of medical school except by the surgeons, and most of their discussions dealt with the management of injuries, the drainage or removal of infected organs and tissues and, to a very limited extent, the excision of cancers.
> **(Thomas 1984 p 27–28)**

When medicine could achieve relatively little, it was hardly surprising that medical harm was far from people's minds, although Thomas does describe some fairly hair-raising treatments for delirium tremens involving massive doses of paraldehyde.

In the 1920s, however, the potential harm that could derive from medical treatment was explicitly recognized with the introduction of the term 'iatrogenic disease'. The word *iatrogenic* comes from the Greek words for physician– *iatros* – and *genesis*, meaning origin; iatrogenic disease is therefore an illness induced, in some way, by a physician. The first usage is credited to Bleuler's 1924 textbook of psychiatry and implied at that time a nervous problem induced as a result of a physician's diagnosis of a disease (Sharpe & Faden 1998). Thus a diagnosis of heart disease, for instance, could make the patient extremely anxious and induce an iatrogenic neurosis. Clinicians were therefore to be extremely careful when discussing diagnoses to avoid distressing or depressing the patient unduly. This well-intentioned paternalism is a far cry from today's insistence on disclosing risks of all kinds, which – as Bleuler and others recognized – carries its own hazards.

With the advances of medical science in the mid-twentieth century, the term iatrogenic disease broadened in scope to include harm due to the medical intervention itself. The particular stimulus for this was the increasing use of penicillin and other antibiotics. The post-war years saw a massive expansion in the number and types of medicine available, in the usage of drugs and in the availability of hospital beds and hospital treatments. By the mid-1950s, some doctors, notably David Barr and Robert Moser, were beginning to realize that potential hazards were associated with the enormous increase in drug use and availability. Barr's paper *The hazards of modern diagnosis and therapy* (Barr 1956) set out some of the major risks, but largely in the spirit of pointing out that there was an inevitable price to pay for therapeutic advance. Moser, however, went further in also considering the over-use of medical therapy, coining the phrase 'antibiotic abandon' to describe the use of penicillin for anything and everything. Moser's view of iatrogenic disease, at least by the time of his 1959 book *Diseases of medical progress*, was subtly different from Barr's in that he considered that these 'diseases of progress' would not have occurred if sound therapeutic practices had been employed. There is a suggestion at least in this view that harm is not entirely an unavoidable by-product of medical success but might also be due to unsound practice, in which treatments are given without clear indications and without due regard for the balance of risk and benefit. At that time, however, as Sharpe and Faden point out, questions of the balance of risk and benefit lay largely with the clinician, with little if any consideration of the patient's perspective.

SYSTEMATIC STUDIES OF THE HAZARDS OF HOSPITALIZATION

Although iatrogenic harm had been noted, it was seldom studied systematically. One of the first explicit, systematic prospective studies of iatrogenic complications was carried out in 1960–61 by Elihu Schimmel at Yale University Medical School. In retrospect, although it had limited impact at the time, this can be seen as a landmark study of the quality and safety of medical care. The study is of more than historical interest, first because it foreshadows many features of the major adverse event studies of the 1980s and 1990s and second because it achieved a rate of voluntary reporting of adverse events seldom seen before or since.

Schimmel, with the support of his departmental chairman, succeeded in mobilizing the junior doctors of three hospital wards to report and describe adverse episodes. Episodes were included if they resulted from acceptable diagnostic or therapeutic measures deliberately instituted in the hospital. The use of an explicit definition of harmful episodes was remarkably progressive in outlook but the study took care not to implicate the actions of clinical staff in any harm that might result from treatment; reactions due to error and reactions from previous treatment, and situations that were only potentially harmful were excluded. Even when errors were omitted the results were striking with 20% of patients experiencing one or more episodes and 16 fatalities resulting in part from diagnosis and treatment. Schimmel's summary (Box 1.3) bears a remarkable resemblance, in both content and tone, to the findings of the major record reviews of adverse events that are discussed in Chapters 2 and 3. His analysis clearly separated the impact of the disease from the negative impact of the procedure and determined the impact on the patients themselves (Tables 1.1 and 1.2). Schimmel remarked that the economic loss and emotional disturbance suffered by many patients were beyond the scope of the study, yet could not be considered insignificant complications of their medical care. Even today, we have still to assess the

Box 1.3 The hazards of hospitalization

(from Schimmel 1964 p 100)

The occurrence of hospital-induced complications in a university medical service was documented in the prospective investigation of over 1000 patients. The reported episodes were the untoward consequences of acceptable medical care in diagnosis and therapy. During the 8-month study, 240 episodes occurred in 198 patients. In 105 patients, hospitalization was either prolonged by an adverse episode or the manifestations were not resolved at the time of discharge. Thus, 20% of the patients admitted to the medical wards experienced one of more untoward episodes and 10% had a prolonged or unresolved episode. The severity of the 240 episodes was minor in 110, moderate in 82, and major in 48, of which 16 ended fatally. Patients encountering noxious episodes had a mean total hospitalization of 28.7 days compared with 11.4 days in other patients. The risk of having such episodes seemed directly related to the time spent in the hospital. The number and variety of these reactions emphasizes the magnitude and scope of hazards to which the hospitalized patient is exposed. A judicious selection of diagnostic and therapeutic measures can be made only with knowledge of these potential hazards as well as the proposed benefits.

full economic consequences of harm to patients and have barely addressed the emotional trauma.

In his conclusion, Schimmel both defends the practice of medicine and yet argues for much greater attention to risks. The difficulty of balancing potential benefit and potential harm, and the need for constant review and monitoring of that balance during a patient's treatment, is expressed with great clarity:

> The classical charge to the physician has always been *primum non nocere*. Modern medicine, however, has introduced procedures that cannot always be used harmlessly. To seek absolute safety is to advocate therapeutic nihilism at a time when the scope of medical care has grown

Table 1.1 Reactions to diagnostic procedures (adapted from Schimmel 1964)

Agent of procedure	Manifestation
Test drugs	
Histamine	Shock
Endotoxin	Fever and herpes
Endoscopy	
Oesophagoscopy	Perforation
Cystoscopy	Cardiac arrest
Cystoscopy	Pyelonephritis
Biopsy	
Liver	Haemorrhage
Stomach	Perforation
Lymph node	Paraesthesia
Radiography	
Barium enema	Cardiac arrest
Barium enema	Shock
Carotid angiogram	Haematoma

Table 1.2 Examples of fatal episodes (adapted from Schimmel 1964)

Agent or procedure	Manifestation of the episode	Age (years)	Underlying disease
Cystoscopy	Cardiac arrest	69	Chronic pyelonephritis
Thoracentesis	Ventricular fibrillation	76	Congestive heart failure
Oesophagoscopy	Perforation	50	Cirrhosis
Barium enema	Cardiac arrest	89	Tuberculous peritonitis
Heparin (i.v.)	Retroperitoneal haemorrhage	66	Hypernephroma
Blakemore tube	Asphyxia	59	Cirrhosis
Digoxin	Ventricular fibrillation	40	Rheumatic heart disease
Digitoxin and digoxin	Multifocal premature ventricular contractions	69	Arteriosclerotic heart disease
Penicillin	Staphylococcal enteritis	85	Pneumonia
Penicillin	Staphylococcal pneumonia	62	Myocardial infarction
Penicillin and streptomycin	Staphylococcal pneumonia	68	Tuberculous meningitis
Sedatives	Staphylococcal pneumonia	73	Parkinsonism

beyond previous imagination and power. The dangers of new measures must be accepted, are generally warranted by their benefits and should not preclude their useful employment. Until safer procedures evolve however, physicians will best serve their patients by weighing each measure according to its goals and risks, by choosing only those that have been justified, and by remaining prepared to alter the procedures when imminent or actual harm threatens to obliterate their good.

(Schimmel 1964 p 100)

In 1981, Steel et al set out to reassess Schimmel's findings in a medical service of a tertiary care hospital. They noted that in the preceding 15 years the number and complexity of diagnostic procedures had increased markedly, the number of drugs in use had increased and the patient population had aged. Of 815 patients in their study, an incredible 36% suffered an iatrogenic illness, with 9% being major in that they threatened life or produced a major disability. Exposure to drugs was the main factor leading to adverse effects, with nitrates, digoxin, lidocaine, aminophylline and heparin being the most dangerous. Cardiac catheterization, urinary catheterization and intravenous therapy were the principal procedures leading to problems, with falls also a serious issue. Staying longer in hospital was associated with a higher risk of iatrogenic illness. Steel et al's definition of iatrogenic included any illness resulting from a diagnostic procedure or treatment, either directly or indirectly, but they stressed that their definition did not imply culpability or that the problem was necessarily preventable. Nevertheless, by 1981, they were certainly willing to imply that many of the problems might be preventable. They called for monitoring of adverse occurrences, especially on medical wards, and educational programmes about iatrogenic disease. Twenty-five years on, iatrogenic disease and safety issues are still finding only a small corner in some medical and nursing curricula, although we at least now recognize incidents and adverse outcomes to a much greater extent.

MEDICAL NEMESIS

The medical profession has become a major threat to health. This arresting sentence begins Ivan Illich's polemic *Limits of medicine*, subtitled *Medical nemesis: the expropriation of health* (Illich 1977). Nemesis represents divine vengeance on mortals who behave in ways that the gods regard as their own prerogative. Medicine, argued Illich, had sought to move beyond its proper boundaries and by doing so was causing harm. Illich's broader argument, expressed in a number of books, was that many institutionalized activities had counterproductive effects. In *Deschooling society*, for instance, he argued that formal, institutionalized education robbed people of their own intellectual curiosity and abilities, just as medicine robbed people of their own capacities for self-care and autonomous living. Illich emphasized that medical harm was not just an unfortunate side effect of medical treatment that would eventually be resolved by technological and pharmacological advances; the only solution was for people themselves to resist unnecessary medical intervention and the medicalization of life.

Illich described three forms of iatrogenic effect:

- Clinical iatrogenesis: the direct harm done to patients.
- Social iatrogenesis: the excessive use of medicine to solve problems of living which encouraged people to become consumers of medicine rather than actively involved in shaping their own health and environment.
- Cultural iatrogenesis: an even deeper culturally mediated sapping of people's ability to deal with sickness and death. This is the tendency to make the ordinary suffering and experience of life and death into commodities, illnesses that required treatment, rather than life to be lived and experienced – the 'paralysis of healthy responses to illness and suffering' in Illich's memorable phrase.

In the early twenty-first century, the medicalization of life is a much less potent theme. Far from trying to medicalize life, doctors are now in retreat from the demands made on them and the unreasonable expectations thrust upon them. However, Illich's first theme of clinical iatrogenesis has proved remarkably far-sighted, although we might now see the causes of iatrogenic harm as different from those suggested by Illich. He assembled a powerful set of charges against medicine and the medical profession, encompassing a critique of the lack of evidence for high-technology medicine, evidence of useless or unnecessary treatment, and doctor-inflicted injuries. After reviewing the extant studies on the adverse effects of drugs, accidents in hospital and the hazards of hospitalization, Illich concluded that:

> The pain, dysfunction, disability, and anguish resulting from technical medical intervention now rival the morbidity due to traffic and industrial accidents and even war-related activities, and make the impact of medicine one of the most rapidly spreading epidemics of our time. Amongst murderous institutional torts, only modern malnutrition injures more people than iatrogenic disease in its various manifestations.
> (Illich 1977 p 35)

Illich's inflammatory language and wholesale attack on the enterprise of medicine hardly endeared him to the medical and nursing professions. Writing in 1997, John Bunker, who carried out some of the first studies on potentially unnecessary surgery, wrote that at the time he considered *Medical nemesis* to be an ill-informed and irresponsible attack on the medical profession. However, Bunker also acknowledged that doctors at the time had become so preoccupied with the problems of medical care that they failed to put them in the context of the good that medicine did, which they understandably took for granted. Bunker argued that Illich's more subtle, and more important, message about the dangers of social and cultural iatrogenesis was perhaps misunderstood at the time. Illich's belief in the healing powers of friendship, personal autonomy, social networks and relationships, and the importance of these factors in a fulfilled and healthy life, now seems particularly prescient. There is now, as there was not in the 1970s, a huge literature on the importance of psychological and social factors in health and an acceptance on all sides of the importance of personal responsibility for health.

Illich's particular contribution to the gradually growing literature on medical harm was in the ferocity of his argument and the challenge he posed to medicine and the medical profession. Others had recorded and written about the hazards of drugs and therapeutics, but Illich went much further to suggest that healthcare was actually a threat to health, comparable to that from traffic and industrial accidents. As we shall see in the next chapter this claim, outrageous and inflammatory at the time, reappears in sober government documents towards the end of the twentieth century.

REFERENCES

Barr DP 1956 Hazards of modern diagnosis and therapy – the price we pay. Journal of the American Medical Association 159:1452–1456

Bunker JP 1997 Ivan Illich and the pursuit of health. Journal of Health Services Research and Policy 2:56–59

Chantler C 1999 The role and education of doctors in the delivery of health care. Lancet 353:1178–1181

Illich I 1977 Limits to medicine. Medical nemesis: the expropriation of health. Pelican Books, London

Jarvis WR 1994 Handwashing – the Semmelweis lesson forgotten? The Lancet 144:1311

Moser RH 1959 Diseases of medical progress. C Thomas, Springfield, IL

Neuhauser D 2002 Ernest Amory Codman MD. Quality & Safety in Health Care 11:104–105

Nightingale F 1863 Notes on hospitals, 3rd edn. Longmans Green and Co, London

Porter R 1999 The greatest benefit to mankind. A medical history of humanity from antiquity to the present. Fontana Press, London

Schimmel EM 1964 The hazards of hospitalisation. Annals of Internal Medicine 60:100–110

Sharpe VA, Faden AI 1998 Medical harm. Historical, conceptual and ethical dimensions of iatrogenic illness. Cambridge University Press, Cambridge

Steel K, Gertman PM, Crescenzi C et al 1981 Iatrogenic illness on a general medical service at a university hospital. New England Journal of Medicine 304(11):638–642

Thomas L 1984 The youngest science. Oxford University Press, Oxford

The evolution of patient safety

2

The knowledgeable health reporter for the Boston Globe, Betsy Lehman, died from a drug overdose during chemotherapy. Willie King had the wrong leg amputated. Ben Kolb was eight years old when he died during 'minor' surgery during a drug mix up. These horrific cases that make of the headlines are just the tip of the iceberg.
(Kohn et al 1999 p 1)

Medical error and patient harm have been described and studied for well over a century. However, apart from a few isolated pioneers, the medical and nursing professions did not appear to recognize the extent and seriousness of the problem or, if they did, were not prepared to acknowledge it. Medical error was seldom acknowledged to patients, almost never mentioned in medical journals, not discussed publicly and not even considered by governments. The fact that thousands, probably millions, of people were being harmed unnecessarily, and that vast amounts of money were being wasted, seemed to have escaped everyone's attention. From our current understanding this seems a curious state of affairs. It is as if an epidemic were raging across a country without anybody noticing or troubling to investigate.

How then did patient safety evolve and emerge to assume its present importance? Understanding patient safety will be easier if we see how it emerged as a distinctive set of ideas and initiatives in a particular historical context. Understanding the origins and influences on patient safety is key to understanding its distinctive character and place in the general quality assurance and improvement armament. As we will see in this chapter, patient safety has been driven and shaped by a number of different influences. Some, such as the rising rate of litigation and some high-profile cases, have been negative in character but brought pressure for reform. Patients have become much more aware of medical error and are demanding action and a greater openness. Other influences are of a more positive character. There have always been doctors and nurses striving to improve the overall quality of care, and their efforts have been crucial to providing a landscape in which medical error and harm could finally be addressed. One of the great achievements of the last ten years is that medical error and patient harm are now acknowledged and discussed publicly by healthcare professionals, politicians and the general public. Other industries, with more visible and public accidents, have also had to give safety a much higher priority in recent years.

Healthcare has drawn some important lessons from them gaining a much more sophisticated understanding of the nature of error and accidents, and a more thoughtful and constructive approach to error prevention and the management of error. Before turning to a review of the various influences and drivers of patient safety, we will first consider the ways in which the term is defined.

DEFINITIONS OF PATIENT SAFETY

The term 'patient safety' is now widely used but seldom clearly defined. Those involved with patient safety are often also concerned with other quality of care issues and it is not easy, perhaps not possible or even desirable, to draw a sharp line between patient safety and related activities such as risk management and quality assurance. Patient safety can, at its simplest, be defined as:

> The avoidance, prevention and amelioration of adverse outcomes or injuries stemming from the process of healthcare.

This definition goes some way to differentiate patient safety from more general concerns about the quality of healthcare; the focus is on the 'dark side of quality' (Vincent 1997), care that is actually harmful rather than just not of a good standard. Healthcare is, in many cases at least, inherently hazardous and the definition implicitly acknowledges this. The definition also refers to the amelioration of adverse outcomes or injuries, which broadens the definition beyond traditional safety concerns towards an area that would, in many industries, be called disaster management. In healthcare, amelioration refers first to the need for rapid medical intervention to deal with the immediate crisis, and second to the need to care for injured patients and to support staff involved in a serious incident.

The short definition given above, however, does not really capture the defining characteristics of patient safety and its associated conceptual background. The US National Patient Safety Foundation sought to do this when setting out a research agenda for patient safety (Box 2.1). The Foundation

---

Box 2.1 Defining characteristics of patient safety

(adapted from US National Patient Safety Foundation 2000)

1. Patient safety is concerned primarily with the avoidance, prevention and amelioration of adverse outcomes or injuries stemming from healthcare itself. It should address events that span the continuum of 'errors' and 'deviations' to accidents.
2. Safety emerges from the interaction of the components of the system. It is more than the absence of adverse outcomes and it is more than avoidance of identifiable 'preventable' errors or occurrences. Safety does not reside in a person, device or department. Improving safety depends on learning how safety emerges from the interaction of components.
3. Patient safety is related to 'quality of care', but the two concepts are not synonymous. Safety is an important subset of quality. To date, activities to manage quality have not focused sufficiently on patient safety issues.

pointed particularly to the fact that traditional quality initiatives had not fully addressed error and harm, to the fact that safety resides in systems as well as people and to the fact that safety has to be actively pursued and promoted. Simply trying to avoid damage is not enough; rather, one must reduce errors of all kinds and pursue high reliability as an essential component of high-quality care.

Patient safety is sometimes equated with preventing error. This seems innocent enough, but is a potentially limiting assumption. There is no question that an understanding of error is fundamental to patient safety; however, there are differences of view as to whether the focus of patient safety research and practice should be on error or harm. Formulating an objective of a specific programme purely in terms of error reduction makes sense when you can define the errors in question and when you are sure that some at least are potential sources of harm. However, consider all the myriad forms of harm that can come from healthcare: complications of surgery, infection from unsafe injections, infection from over-crowded hospitals, adverse drug reactions, overdoses from badly designed infusion pumps and so on. Should we assume that all these are necessarily due to error? If we equate patient safety with error reduction we run the risk of not addressing forms of harm that are either not due to error or are only partly due to error. Furthermore, as we shall see later, error is a very slippery concept. Explanations of accidents and harm have evolved over the last few decades giving many different senses to the term error and to the different ways in which errors can be involved in the genesis of harm. In addition, many minor errors do not lead to harm and, indeed, might be necessary to learning and the maintenance of safety. For all these reasons, the reduction of harm should be the primary aim of patient safety, not the elimination of error.

LITIGATION AND RISK MANAGEMENT

Until relatively recently, litigation was seen as a financial and legal problem; patients who sued were seen as difficult or embittered, and lawyers who helped them as professionally and often personally suspect. Only gradually did those addressing the problem come to understand that litigation was a reflection of the much more serious underlying problem of harm to patients; for this reason litigation is part of the story of patient safety.

Litigation and medical malpractice crises have occurred on a regular basis for over 150 years, each time accompanied by worries about public trust in doctors and by much associated commentary and soul searching, some of it rather hysterical in nature. Litigation in medicine dates back to the middle of the nineteenth century, when the relaxation of professional regulation and the introduction of a free market in both medical and legal services simultaneously fuelled a decline in standards in medicine, dissatisfaction from patients and the availability of lawyers to initiate proceedings. Between 1840 and 1860 the rate of malpractice cases increased tenfold and medical journals, after more than 50 years of barely noticing malpractice, suddenly became all but obsessed with the problem (Mohr 2000).

A historical perspective on litigation tempers reaction to the latest media-driven litigation crisis but there is no doubt that litigation is a longstanding problem for healthcare. The most visible sign of increasing rates of litigation are the steadily rising malpractice premiums paid by doctors. In 1949 the average premium paid by New York doctors was just $65 a year, rising only to $250 in 1965, jumping to $3000 in 1975 and to $23,000 in 1985. By 1989, US malpractice premiums appeared to have reached a plateau, although that plateau was very high for some specialties (Hiatt et al 1989). Insurance premiums for Long Island neurosurgeons and obstetricians ranged from $160,000 to $200,000 per annum, although admittedly New York State premiums were among the highest in the US, and probably in the world. However, although larger and larger sums of money were being expended, injured patients seldom received large awards. Patients, as we shall see, sue relatively infrequently after adverse events and much of the money expended is swallowed up in fees and administration. The huge awards that hit the headlines for severely damaged babies are entirely untypical. Compensation for being condemned to a life of pain and suffering after hospital injury is not usually very generous in any country.

The UK followed a similar pattern, although a little later than the US. Given the interest in litigation in the UK it is surprising that there is in fact very little hard data about the total costs, partly because of continually changing compensation arrangements over the last two decades. Some of the best data available come from the Oxfordshire health region, which has kept a comprehensive claims database since 1974 (Fenn et al 2000). As Fig. 2.1 shows, there has been a steady rise in both new and closed claims, with rates of litigation doubling in between 1988 and 1998, although hospital activity increased by only about 30% in the same period. Only about 30% of the claims led to paid compensation, with the average claim in the period since 1990 being about £20,000. Most claims are much lower than this, as the average is greatly affected by a small number of very large claims; most compensation is very modest (Fenn et al 2000).

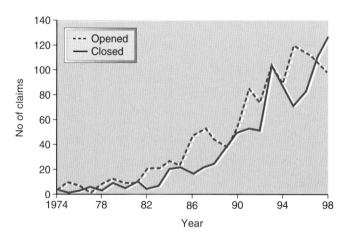

Fig. 2.1 Medical negligence claims, Oxfordshire Health Authority, UK 1974–98 (from Fenn et al 2000 British Medical Journal 320:1567–1571, amended and reproduced with permission from the BMJ Publishing Group).

In 1999–2000, the NHS Litigation Authority closed 3254 claims at a cost of £386 million, although this figure does not include all claims to the NHS or all costs (Fenn 2002). Even if we suppose an overall annual figure of about £500 million this is still only of the order of half of 1% of the NHS budget, a serious expenditure but hardly a threat to the overall system. The often-quoted figure of £4.4 billion in fact refers to the possible total cost of all outstanding claims if they were continued and if they were actually paid over a timescale of several decades. This not very helpful statistic is often quoted as the annual cost of claims, which is exceedingly misleading and grossly overestimates the financial impact of litigation.

The Harvard Medical Practice Study and the feasibility of no-fault compensation

The rising rate of litigation in the 1980s led some to consider whether compensation might be offered on a no-fault basis, bypassing the expense and unpleasantness of the adversarial legal process. The Harvard Medical Practice Study (HMPS), still the most famous study in the field of patient safety, was originally established to assess the number of potentially compensable cases in New York State, not primarily as a study of the quality and safety of care (Hiatt et al 1989). However, its major legacy has been to reveal the scale of harm to patients.

Both before and after the study New York State, and other jurisdictions, had tried a wide range of legal and financial measures to stem the rise in litigation and associated rise in malpractice premiums. These included caps on fees and damages, changes to the way doctors were insured, changes to the way damages were calculated and prior screening of claims. The main report summarizes these and notes that they seemed to have had relatively little effect on litigation, although by the time of the publication of the report (in 1989) the authors noted a calmer malpractice atmosphere. The subsequent publication of the clinical aspects of the study in the *New England Journal of Medicine* made it clear that the issue of no-fault compensation had become secondary; the authors viewed the findings as reflecting major problems in the quality of care (Brennan et al 1991, Leape et al 1991). The study found that patients were unintentionally harmed by treatment in almost 4% of admissions in New York, and about 1% of patients were seriously harmed. These findings were later to receive massive publicity with the release of the Institute of Medicine report in 1999 (Kohn et al 1999).

Litigation as a means of compensating injured patients is expensive and, in many cases, a rather inefficient means of awarding compensation. Although compensation is important in some cases, patients often turn to litigation for entirely other reasons, often being driven in despair to litigation through a failure to receive the apologies, explanations and support that they both deserve and need (Vincent 2001). The process of litigation in serious cases can be traumatic for all concerned, even with sympathetic and efficient lawyers on both sides. The threat of litigation is also often cited as a deterrent to the open reporting and investigation of adverse events, and as a major barrier to patient safety. However, for all this, litigation has undoubtedly been a powerful driver of patient safety. Litigation raised public and professional awareness of adverse outcomes, and ultimately led to the development of clinical risk management. In the US, risk management has had a primarily legal and financial orientation, and risk managers are only now becoming involved in safety issues. In the UK and other countries, however, risk management had a clinical orientation from its inception, as well as a concern with legal and financial issues. Clinical risk management in this wider sense is therefore roughly equivalent to patient safety; the terminology varies from country to country but the aims of clinical risk management and patient safety are the same – to reduce or eliminate harm to patients (Vincent 1995, 2001).

HIGH-PROFILE CASES

Certain 'celebrated' cases attain particular prominence and evoke complicated reactions. Richard Cook, David Woods and Charlotte Miller (1998) describe some particularly sad cases in their introduction to the report *A tale of two stories: contrasting views of patient safety* and make some important comments about the public perception of these cases:

> The case of Willie King in Florida, in becoming the 'wrong leg' case, captures our collective dread of wrong site surgery. The death of Libby Zion has come to represent not just the danger of drug–drug interaction but also the issues of work hours and supervision of residents – capturing symbolically our fear of medical care at the hands of overworked, tired or novice practitioners without adequate supervision. Celebrated cases such as these serve as markers in the discussion of the healthcare system and patient safety. As such, the reactions to these tragic losses become the obstacles and opportunities to enhance safety.
> **(Cook et al 1998 p 7)**

Cook et al go on to argue that the public account of these stories is usually a gross over-simplification of what actually occurred and that it is equally important to investigate run-of-the-mill cases and success stories to understand the complex, dynamic process of healthcare. Such disastrous cases, however, came to symbolize fear of a more widespread failure of the healthcare system, provoking more general concerns about medical error. Perhaps it wasn't just a question of finding a good, reliable doctor; perhaps the system was unsafe? Such concerns are magnified a hundred-fold when there is hard evidence of longstanding problems in a service and a series of tragic losses. This is well illustrated by the events that led to in the UK to the inquiry into cardiac surgery at the Bristol Royal Infirmary (Box 2.2).

The impact in the UK of the events at Bristol on healthcare professionals and the general public is hard to understate. The editor of the *British Medical Journal* wrote in an editorial entitled *All changed, changed utterly* that 'British medicine will be transformed by the Bristol case' (Smith 1998). He highlighted a number of important issues but particularly the impact the Bristol case had on the faith and trust which people have in their doctors. The subsequent inquiry could have been recriminatory and divisive but, in fact, achieved the remarkable feat of bringing positive, forward-looking change from disaster and tragedy. The changes it recommended are still being absorbed and acted on.

Box 2.2 Events leading up to the Bristol Inquiry

(adapted from Walshe & Offen 2001)

In the late 1980s some clinical staff at the Bristol Royal Infirmary began to raise concerns about the quality of paediatric cardiac surgery by two surgeons. In essence, it was suggested that the results of paediatric cardiac surgery were less good than at other specialist units and that mortality was substantially higher than in comparable units. Between 1989 and 1994 there was a continuing conflict at the hospital about the issue between surgeons, anaesthetists, cardiologists and managers. Agreement was eventually reached that a specialist paediatric cardiac surgeon should be appointed and that in the meantime a moratorium on certain procedures should be observed. In January 1995, before the surgeon was appointed, a child called Joshua Loveday was scheduled for surgery against the advice of anaesthetists, some surgeons and the Department of Health. He died, and this led to further surgery being halted, an external inquiry being commissioned, and to extensive local and national media attention.

Parents of some of the children complained to the General Medical Council, which, in 1997, examined the cases of 53 children, 29 of whom had died and four of whom suffered severe brain damage. Three doctors were found guilty of serious professional misconduct and two were struck off the medical register.

The Secretary of State for Health immediately established an inquiry, costing £14 million, chaired by Professor Ian Kennedy. This began in October 1998 and the subsequent report, published in July 2001, made almost 200 recommendations.

The inquiry report is massive and we can make only a few general points here about the relevance of the Bristol affair to patient safety. The tragedy for all concerned was undeniable, the media attention relentless and long running. The fact that routine, although highly skilled and complex, healthcare could be substandard to the point of being dangerous was abundantly clear. The impetus for open scrutiny of surgical performance, and indeed the outcomes of healthcare generally, was huge and the subject of error and human fallibility in healthcare was out in the open (Treasure 1998). The inquiry was also noteworthy in, from the outset, adopting a systems approach to analysing what had happened, by which poor performance and errors were seen as the product of systems that were not working well, as much as the result of any particular individual's conduct (Department of Health (DoH) 2001). In practice, this meant that whereas most inquiries would have started by grilling the surgeons involved, Professor Kennedy's team began by examining the wider context, and moved only gradually towards specific events and individuals. This approach revealed the role of contextual and system factors much more powerfully and showed how the actions of individuals were influenced and constrained by the wider organization and environment. Bristol, therefore, came to exemplify wider problems within the NHS and the conclusions of the inquiry were therefore widely applicable. Recommendations were made on open risk communication to patients, the manner of communication and support, the process of informed consent, the need for a proper response to tragic events, the vital role of team work, the monitoring of the quality of care, the role of regulation and a host of other issues.

Other countries have had their Bristols. Canada, for instance, experienced a similar high-profile tragedy in the paediatric cardiac service at Winnipeg. Jan Davies, the leading clinical advisor to that inquiry, drew explicit parallels between Winnipeg and a major aviation disaster at Dryden (Davies 1994), holding out the hope that both events would provoke enduring system wide changes:

> The Inquest [on the children who died] has the potential to do for medicine what Dryden did for aviation. And I say medicine and not just paediatric cardiac surgery because the lessons that can be learned have relevance to every type of medical and surgical practice. From the outset there should be a system of quality assurance: regular monitoring and documenting of processes and outcomes, with links back to the structural and procedural elements of the programme. There should also be a system of ad hoc review, which can be set in place if there is a sudden and unexpected problem with the process or outcome of care. All this should be set in an organisational and regulatory culture which recognises that human errors will occur but attempts to proactively manage them. If the inquest in Winnipeg can show how to do this, the deaths of passengers in Dryden and patients in Winnipeg will not have been in vain.
>
> **(Davies, from Helmreich & Merrit 1998 p 199)**

LEARNING FROM ERROR

Litigation and high-profile cases have driven patient safety through the horror of the cases involved, the personal pain and the determination on all sides to prevent such incidents in the future. However, more positive influences and events have also played a major role. In examining these we will begin with a call for reappraisal of attitudes to medical error.

In 1983, Neil McIntyre, Professor of Medicine, and the philosopher Sir Karl Popper, published a paper *The critical attitude in medicine: the need for a new ethics*, which called on doctors and others to actively seek out errors and use them to advance both their personal knowledge and medical knowledge generally. This paper is densely, almost unbelievably, rich in ideas and embraces ethics, philosophy of science, the doctor–patient relationship, attitudes to fallibility and uncertainty, professional regulation and methods for enhancing the quality of care. Summarizing all the arguments is not feasible, but two extracts illustrate some of the main themes:

> To learn only from one's own mistakes would be a slow and painful process and unnecessarily costly to one's patients. Experiences need to be pooled so that doctors may also learn from the errors of others. This requires a willingness to admit one has erred and to discuss the factors that may have been responsible. It calls for a critical attitude to one's own work and that of others.
>
> **(McIntyre & Popper 1983 p 1919)**

> No species of fallibility is more important or less understood than fallibility in medical practice. The physician's propensity for damaging error is widely denied, perhaps because it is so intensely feared. Physicians and surgeons often flinch from even identifying error in clinical practice, let alone recording it, presumably because they

themselves hold that error arises either from their or their colleagues ignorance or ineptitude. But errors need to be recorded and analysed if we are to discover why they occurred and how they could have been prevented
(McIntyre & Popper 1983 p 1919)

According to this view, error becomes something of value, a resource and clue to progress, both scientifically and clinically. The call to learn from mistakes has close links with Popper's philosophy of science, in which he argued that scientific knowledge is inherently provisional and that progress in science depends, at least in part, on the recognition of flaws and problems in accepted theories. Popper argues that whereas there is truth in the traditional view that knowledge grows through the accumulation of facts, advances often come about through the recognition of error, by the overthrow of old knowledge and mistaken theories. Many famous scientists, such as Sir Peter Medawar, have been profoundly influenced by Popper in their approach to fundamental scientific problems, finding the emphasis on hypothesis and conjecture both creative and liberating (Medawar 1969).

McIntyre and Popper (1983) argue that being an authority, in the sense of a wise and reliable fount of knowledge, is often seen as a professional ideal in both science and medicine. However, this view has terrible consequences. Authority tends to become important in its own right; an authority is not expected to err and, if it does, its errors tend to be covered up to uphold the idea of authority. So mistakes are hidden, and the consequences of this tendency can be worse than the mistakes themselves.

It is not only scientific authority that is questioned here, but professional authority of all kinds. In medicine this means that, whereas one should respect the knowledge and experience of senior clinicians, one should not regard them as 'authorities' in the sense of inevitably being correct. An environment in which junior staff feel unable to question senior staff about their decisions and actions is profoundly dangerous to patients. There are, of course, many obstacles to more open communication and the spirit of Karl Popper might be no help to the hapless junior doctor when her authoritarian consultant turns his baleful eye on her. Popper's view of error is, however, a constant reminder that error and uncertainty are no respecters of status.

Reminding oneself that one might be wrong, and being aware of that in daily life, is not something that comes easily to us. Gerd Gigerenzer, after reviewing many instances in which a sense of certainty was completely unwarranted, has advised us to always remember what he terms 'Franklin's law', so-called because of Benjamin Franklin's statement that nothing is certain in life except death and taxes (Gigerenzer 2002). Franklin's law makes us mindful of fallibility and uncertainty, enabling us to constantly reappraise apparent certainties in the certainty that some of them will turn out to be wrong!

QUALITY PAVES THE WAY FOR SAFETY

Unless substantial progress had been made in the understanding and practice of quality improvement, it is highly unlikely that the tougher issues underlying patient safety would ever have emerged. Summarizing the history of attempts to measure and improve the quality of healthcare would require a book in its own right, so this will necessarily be a brief overview. Progress on quality, although dramatic in many industrial settings, was slow, uneven and subject to much resistance in healthcare. The basic assumption for many was that quality was a natural outcome of conscientious work by highly motivated clinicians, with quality problems being due to the occasional 'bad apple'. In 1984, Maxwell still had to argue that an honest concern about quality, however genuine, is not the same as methodical assessment based on reliable evidence. There was also little understanding that poor quality might not be due to bad apples, but inherent in the very structures and processes of the healthcare system itself.

Dimensions of quality

Avedis Donabedian, the first great theorist of healthcare quality, made the now classic distinction between the structure, process and outcome of healthcare. This was fundamental to understanding that quality depended on the relationship between many components and that process and outcome could be assessed separately (Donabedian 1968). Donabedian also emphasized that quality of care encompassed not only the technical excellence of the care but also the manner and humanity with which it was delivered, a commonplace distinction nowadays but not in the 1960s. This is not to say that clinicians were not caring and compassionate, only that this was not viewed as a component of quality of care, still less that such subtle, human features of healthcare might be measured. Maxwell (1984) took this idea further, identifying six core dimensions of quality: technical excellence, social acceptability, humanity, cost, equity and relevance to need.

Safety does not feature at all in Maxwell's list of quality dimensions, although it is certainly related to technical excellence and acceptability. Why is this? It seems the most basic requirement of any public or privately delivered service where risk is involved. If we travel by road or train, if we fly, stay in hotels, or live near nuclear power plants, we want above all to be safe. It is easy now, with the benefit of hindsight, to see that safety is an essential part of quality, but at that time the language of error and harm had not entered healthcare discourse. By 1999, however, the Institute of Medicine report *To err is human* put safety to the fore, describing it as the first dimension of quality (Kohn et al 1999).

The relationship between safety and quality in healthcare has not been properly examined, probably because it is a rather thorny issue. Many people are content to describe the relationship between safety and quality as a continuum, with safety issues simply being the 'hard edge' of more general quality concerns. However, this does little more than sidestep the issue, and tends to suggest that safety and quality concerns are necessarily complementary. There is, however, often a trade-off between safety and some dimensions of quality. Care that maximizes access and reduces cost for instance, highly desirable in a publicly funded system like the British NHS, can run the risk of degrading safety.

Improving the quality of healthcare

Although Ernest Codman was one of the few clinicians to explicitly address error, there are many other examples of pioneering quality initiatives early in the twentieth century. For instance, in 1928 the British Ministry of Health set up a committee to examine maternal morbidity and mortality, instigating confidential enquiries on 5800 cases (Kerr 1932). This spurred Andrew Topping, a remarkable medical officer for health, to set up his own programme, which became known as the Rochdale experiment. At that time Rochdale, an industrial town in the North West of England, had a maternal mortality of nine deaths per 1000 deliveries. Topping instituted antenatal clinics, meetings between midwives and family doctors, established a puerperal fever ward, established a specialist consultant post and backed it all by education and public meetings. Within 5 years, mortality had reduced to 1.7 per 1000 (Oxley et al 1935).

National reports on maternal mortality were produced intermittently in subsequent years, but progress was rather haphazard. Finally, the Confidential Enquiry into Maternal Deaths was established which, since 1952, has produced triennial reports on all maternal deaths and endeavoured to establish why they had occurred and how they might be prevented (Sharpe & Faden 1998). Similar enquiries are now conducted into deaths after surgery, stillbirth and homicide and suicide (Vincent 1993). Quality problems in routine care were also being examined. By the early 1970s, for instance, it was clear that there were widespread variations in rates of surgery for similar conditions in different geographical areas in ways that could not be accounted for by medical need (Wennberg & Gittlesohn 1973). Quality problems were inferred from these variations but much of the imperative for examining variation, particularly in the US, stemmed from economic considerations rather than the harm caused by unnecessary surgery. Regulatory agencies and professional societies investigated and acted on complaints made about healthcare professionals although, in Britain at least, this seldom extended to assessment of clinical competence. Amazingly, it was only in 1995 that the General Medical Council was finally empowered, by the Medical (Professional Performance) Act 1995 (HMSO 1995), to investigate the clinical abilities of doctors as well as their general conduct. Prior to that, sexual misdemeanours might bring down the wrath of the Council but competence did not fall within its remit.

Attempts were also being made to improve the processes and organization of healthcare by drawing on the practice and methodology of quality assurance approaches in manufacturing industry, such as continuous quality improvement, total quality management, business process re-engineering and quality circles. Such methods had been particularly influential in Japan, and were sometimes credited for the emergence of high quality and reliability in the Japanese motor industry. These approaches combine a respect for and reliance on data as a basis for quality improvement, together with an attempt to harness the ideas and creativity of the workforce to create change, test the effects and sustain them. For example, in American industries in the early 1980s the emphasis was on continuous quality improvement of processes throughout the organization. The idea was that everyone should have an opportunity to improve his or her own particular part of the work process.

This led to many small-scale improvements but a lack of attention to large systems, which was the emphasis of the subsequent focus on re-engineering (redesign of large systems). Recent approaches stress the need to combine both these perspectives to achieve sustained quality improvement (Langley et al 1996).

By the mid-1980s, therefore, there had been some progress in understanding and applying the methods of quality improvement and important studies and initiatives by a number of organizations. However, for clinicians, quality of the system overall was really someone else's business; they wanted to be left to get on with treating their patients. Progress over the next decade in the UK has been well summarized by Kieran Walshe and Nigel Offen in their description of their report of the background to the events of the Bristol Inquiry (2001):

> Between 1984 and 1995 the place of quality improvement in the British NHS was transformed. At the start of that period, clinicians took part in a range of informal and quasi-educational activities aimed at improving the quality of practice, but there were few, if any, healthcare organisations who could claim to have a systematic approach to measuring or improving quality. Moreover many clinicians and professional organisations had a record of being disinterested, sceptical, or even actively hostile towards the idea that systematic or formal quality improvement activities had much to offer in healthcare.
>
> Ten years later much had changed. A raft of national and local quality initiatives, had generated a great deal of activity, virtually all healthcare organisations had established clinical audit or quality improvement systems and structures, and the culture had been changed substantially. It had become common to question clinical practices and to seek to improve them, activities which might have been difficult or even impossible a decade earlier.
> **(Walshe & Offen 2001 p 251)**

The developments described by Walshe and Offen in Britain were paralleled in other healthcare systems, although with different emphases and timescales. This section can sketch only a very rough outline of the evolution of quality assurance in healthcare. The main thrust should, however, be clear. In the 1980s and early 1990s, before the full emergence of patient safety, there was a massive growth in awareness of the importance of systematic quality improvement, variously effective action on the ground and an understanding that quality was not just another headline-capturing government initiative to be endured while it was flavour of the month, but was here to stay. This was an essential support and background to the hard look at the damage done by healthcare that was to follow.

HUMAN FACTORS AND SAFETY IN HIGH-RISK INDUSTRIES

Patient safety has rather different intellectual origins from quality improvement. Whereas practitioners of quality improvement in healthcare tended to look to industrial process improvement as their model, patient safety researchers and practitioners have looked to high-risk industries, such as aviation and the chemical and nuclear industries, which have an explicit focus on safety that is usually reinforced by a powerful external regulator. These industries have invested heavily in human factors, a hybrid discipline drawing on ergonomics, psychology and practical experience in safety critical industries. Many of the important developments in the psychology of error have their origins in studies of major accidents in these complex industries. These issues will be addressed in more detail in later chapters. For the moment, we will simply set the scene and demonstrate the importance of this line of work to patient safety.

One of the true pioneers in this area is Jeffrey Cooper. Cooper trained originally as a bioengineer. In 1972 he was employed by the Massachusetts General Hospital to work on developing machines for anaesthesiology researchers (Cooper et al 1978, 1984, Gawande 2002). Observing anaesthetists in the operating room, he noticed how poorly anaesthetic machines were designed and how conducive they were to error. For example, a clockwise turn of a dial decreased the concentration of a powerful anaesthetic in some machines but increased the concentration in others – a real recipe for disaster. Cooper's work extended well beyond the more traditional approach to anaesthetic misadventure, in that he examined anaesthetic errors and incidents from an explicitly psychological perspective, exploring both the clinical aspects and the psychological and environmental sources of error.

Cooper et al's 1984 paper provides a remarkably sophisticated analysis of the many factors that contribute to errors and adverse outcomes and is the foundation of much later work on safety in anaesthesia. Contrary to the prevailing assumption that the initial stages of the anaesthesia were the most dangerous, Cooper and his colleagues discovered that most incidents occurred during the operation, when the anaesthetist's vigilance was most likely to ebb. The most important problems involved errors in managing the patient's breathing, such as undetected disconnections and mistakes in managing the airway or the anaesthetic machine. Cooper also discussed factors that might have contributed to an error, such as fatigue and inadequate experience.

Cooper (1994), reflecting on the impact of the studies, noted that they seem to have stirred the anaesthesia community into recognizing the frequency of human error in the specialty and generated great interest in reducing the rate of mistakes by instituting many different preventive strategies. Cooper's work in the 1970s had provoked much debate but little action until Ellison Pierce was elected President of the American Society of Anesthesiologists in 1982. The daughter of one of Pierce's friends had died under anaesthetic while having wisdom teeth extracted and this case in particular galvanized Pierce to persuade the profession that it was possible to reduce the then 1 in 10,000 death rate from anaesthesia (Gawande 2002) to the extremely low rate seen today. Anaesthesia, together with obstetrics, led the way in a systematic approach to the reduction of harm, foreshadowing the wider patient safety movement a decade later (Gaba 2000).

The evolution of patient safety

25

ERROR IN MEDICINE: PSYCHOLOGY ENTERS THE ARENA

In 1994 the subject of error in medicine was, with some notable exceptions, largely confined to anaesthesia. A prescient and seminal paper (Leape 1994), still widely cited, addressed the question of error in medicine head on and brought some entirely new perspectives to bear. Lucian Leape, one of the authors of the Harvard Medical Practice Study, began by noting that a number of studies suggested that error rates in medicine were particularly high, that error was an emotionally fraught subject and that medicine had yet to seriously address error in the way that other safety critical industries had. As regards prevention, Leape argued that:

> Error prevention in medicine had characteristically followed what might be called the perfectibility model: if physicians and nurses could be properly trained and motivated, then they would make no mistakes. The methods used to achieve this goal are training and punishment. Training is directed towards teaching people to do the right thing. In nursing, rigid adherence to protocols is emphasised. In medicine the emphasis is less on rules and more on knowledge. Punishment is through social opprobrium or peer disapproval. The professional cultures of medicine and nursing typically use blame to encourage proper performance. Errors are caused by a lack of sufficient attention or, worse, lack of caring enough to make sure you are correct.
> **(Leape 1994 p 1852)**

Leape, drawing on the psychology of error and human performance, rejected this formulation on several counts. Many errors are often beyond the individual's conscious control; they are precipitated by a wide range of factors, which are often also beyond the individual's control; systems that rely on error-free performance are doomed to failure, as are reactive attempts to prevent errors that rely on discipline and training. He went on to argue that if physicians, nurses, pharmacists and administrators were to succeed in reducing errors in hospital care, they would need to fundamentally change the way they think about errors (Leape 1994)

Leape went on to outline some central tenets of cognitive psychology, in particular the work of Jens Rasmussen and James Reason (discussed in detail in Chapter 4). Although Reason had made some forays into the question of error in medicine (Eagle et al 1992, Reason 1993), Leape's paper brought his work to the attention of healthcare professionals in a leading medical journal. Leape explicitly stated that the solutions to the problem of medical error did not lie primarily within medicine but in the disciplines of psychology and human factors, and he set out proposals for error reduction that acknowledged human limitations and fallibility and relied more on changing the conditions of work than on training.

Cooper and Leape are not the only authors to understand the importance of human factors and psychology to medical harm and medical error at an early stage. For instance, Marilyn Bogner's 1994 book *Human error in medicine* contained many insightful and important chapters by David Woods, Richard Cook, Neville Moray and others; and James Reason articulated his theory of accidents and discussed its application in medicine in *Medical accidents* (Vincent 1993). Cooper and Leape were, however, particularly important influences and they illustrate the more general point that some of the defining characteristics of patient safety are its acceptance of the importance of psychology and the lessons to be learnt from other safety critical industries.

PROFESSIONAL AND GOVERNMENT REPORTS: PATIENT SAFETY HITS THE HEADLINES

The US Institute of Medicine's 1999 report *To err is human* (Kohn et al 1999) is a stark, lucid and unarguable plea for action on patient safety at all levels of the healthcare system. Without doubt, the publication of this report was the single most important spur to the development of patient safety, catapulting it into public and political awareness and galvanizing political and professional will at the highest levels in the US. Leape described the impact of the report as follows:

> Few publications in recent memory have received as much notice or stimulated as swift a response among policy makers as the Institute of Medicine (IOM) report. Within 2 weeks of the report's release in November 1999, Congress began hearings and the President ordered a government-wide study of the feasibility of implementing the report's recommendations. The Institute of Medicine called for a national effort to include establishment of a Centre for Patient Safety within the Agency for Healthcare Research and Quality, expanded reporting of adverse events and errors, development of safety programmes in health care organisations, and intensified efforts by regulators, health care purchasers, and professional societies. However, while the objective of the report, and the thrust of its recommendations, was to stimulate a national effort to improve patient safety, what initially grabbed public attention was the declaration that between 44,000 and 98,000 people die in US hospitals annually as a result of medical errors.
>
> **(Leape 2000 p 95)**

To err is human – the first of a series of reports on safety and quality from the Institute – was far more wide ranging than the headline figures suggest. A large number of studies of error and harm were reviewed; the causes of harm, the nature of safe and unsafe systems and the role of leadership and regulation were all examined, themes we will return to in later chapters. The principal aim of the report was to establish patient safety as a major requirement and activity of modern healthcare, by establishing national centres and programmes, expanding and improving reporting systems and driving safety in clinical practice through the involvement of clinicians, purchasers of healthcare, regulatory agencies and the public (Box 2.3).

An organization with a memory: learning from adverse events in the NHS

The British equivalent of the Institute of Medicine report was prepared by a group led by Professor Liam Donaldson, the UK's Chief Medical Officer, and

---

Box 2.3 *To err is human*: principal recommendations of the IOM report

(adapted from Kohn et al 1999)

- Congress should create a Centre for Patient Safety.
- A nationwide mandatory reporting system should be established.
- The development of voluntary reporting should be encouraged.
- Congress should pass legislation to extend peer review protection to patient safety data.
- Performance standards and expectations for healthcare organizations and healthcare professionals should focus greater attention on patient safety.
- The Food and Drug Administration should increase attention to the safe use of drugs in both the pre- and post-marketing processes.
- Healthcare organizations and the professionals affiliated with them should make continually improved patient safety a declared and serious aim by establishing patient safety programmes with defined executive responsibility.
- Healthcare organizations should implement proven medication safety practices.

---

released with a foreword by the then Minister for Health, Alan Milburn. Unlike the Institute of Medicine report, it emanated from government and was authorized for release by the Secretary of State for Health (Box 2.4).

In comparison with *To err is human*, *An organisation with a memory* (DoH 2000) has a much stronger focus on learning from other high-risk industries, systems thinking and the need for cultural change. The report's primary emphasis, however, was – as the title suggests – on learning. Reviewing the systems of learning from errors in the NHS, the report identified numerous weaknesses with the processes and contrasted this unfavourably with other high-risk industries. Great stress was also laid on understanding the underlying causes of adverse events and on the potential parallels between healthcare and other environments, although the parallels between healthcare and other industries should not be over-stated, as we will discuss later. The arguments of the report were more that human beings working in complex systems of all kinds are prone to similar errors and subject to similar pressures, as shown in the examples in Box 2.5.

Understanding the causes of failure is, of course, not sufficient to ensure learning and action, particularly in an organization as large as the NHS. The report DH referred to the 'patchwork of systems' that exist to monitor and learn from adverse events in the UK, and to the need to improve the cover-

---

Box 2.4 Adverse events in the UK NHS (per annum)

(adapted from DoH 2000, Vincent et al 2001)

- 400 people die or are seriously injured each year in incidents involving medical devices.
- Nearly 10,000 people are reported as experiencing serious adverse drug reactions.
- Around 1150 people who have been in recent contact with mental health services commit suicide.
- Hospital-acquired infections, about 15% of which are thought to be avoidable, cost the NHS nearly £1 billion.
- Adverse events occur in around 10% of admissions, at a rate in excess of 850,000.
- Adverse events cost the service an estimated £2 billion in additional hospital stays alone, without taking any account of the human or wider economic costs.

Box 2.5 Parallels between healthcare and aviation

(from DoH 2000 p 40–41, 43)

Misinterpretation of instruments

Aviation

Two aircraft came close to colliding over London when an air traffic controller instructed the wrong pilot to descend. The two aircraft were circling, waiting to land, but they were so close to each other on the controller's radar screen that their identity tags were difficult to read. The controller wanted the lower of the two aircraft to descend but mistakenly instructed the higher aircraft to do so. The aircraft were within approximately 400 feet of each other when the pilot of the higher aircraft spotted the danger and climbed to safety.

Healthcare

Machines called cardiotocographs (CTGs) are used to monitor and display fetal heart rate during labour. They rely on ultrasonic detection of fetal heart movements. Reports to the Medical Devices Agency revealed that several incidents occurred when, despite the monitors showing a heart trace, babies were delivered stillborn. In all probability the CTG was recording the mother's heartbeat rather than that of the fetus. A safety notice issued in March 1998 advised users of CTG monitors to confirm that the CTG is displaying the fetal heart rate, to use monitors in accordance with manufacturers' instructions and not to place reliance on a single monitoring system.

Dangerous omissions

Aviation

An aircraft of the Royal Flight was forced to make an emergency landing when the aircrew noticed that all four of the aircraft's engines were experiencing a significant drop in oil pressure. Before landing, the pilot had to shut down two of the engines, and a third as they taxied on the runway. Upon investigation, the cause of the problem was found to be that none of the engine oil seals had been replaced during routine maintenance and so when the engines were running they were all losing oil.

Healthcare

Two patients died in separate incidents when partially used containers of intravenous fluid were reconnected to administration sets. Both patients suffered fatal air embolisms (air bubbles in the bloodstream). A subsequent safety notice emphasized that partially used intravenous fluid containers should always be discarded because re-use increases the risk of both air embolism and infection.

---

age, consistency and immediacy of reporting and learning. Reporting of incidents was extremely patchy and reporting of near misses almost non-existent. *An organisation with a memory* has led, among other things, to the creation of the National Patient Safety Agency (NPSA), which has established a national reporting system. The remit of the NPSA, however, is not simply to collate incident reports, but also to learn from them and to develop solutions to safety problems. Above all, the Agency is endeavouring to change the culture of the NHS from one of blame, focus on individual error and short-term fixes to proactive safety management. Table 2.1 summarizes some of the problems that currently exist and the aspirations for the future.

PATIENT SAFETY RESEARCH COMES OF AGE

As we saw in Chapter 1, research on error and harm has a long history, but only comparatively recently has a sustained body of research emerged. Before that, research on safety in medicine was viewed as at best a fringe topic and at worst

Table 2.1 A new approach to responding to adverse events in the NHS (adapted from DoH 2000)

Past	Future
Fear of reprisals common	Generally blame-free reporting
Individuals scapegoated	Individuals held to account when justified
Disparate adverse event databases	All databases coordinated
Staff do not always hear the outcome of an investigation	Regular feedback to front-line staff
Individual training dominant	Team-based training more common
Attention focuses on individual error	Systems approach to hazards and prevention
Short-term fixing of problems	Emphasis on sustained risk reduction
Many adverse events regarded as isolated 'one-offs'	Potential for replication of similar adverse events recognized
Lessons from adverse events seen as primarily for the team concerned	Recognition that lessons might be relevant to others
Individual learning	Team based learning and developing of non-technical skills

disreputable. In the 1980s, there was so little research available that, when reviewing the extant literature, I suggested in the title of a paper that the lack of research attention given to medical accidents and medical negligence was itself negligent (Vincent 1989). Although there was considerable, if scattered, evidence of harm, the topic of errors and accidents in medicine was almost invisible in research terms. In 1990 the editor of the *British Medical Journal* argued for a study of the incidence of adverse events and was roundly criticized by the president of a medical royal college for drawing the attention of the mass media to medical error (Smith 2000). In 1990, Medline – one of the main medical research databases – did not even have a subject heading for medical error. Since the mid-1990s, however, the number of papers on error and safety-related topics has increased exponentially, with several hundred a year listed under medical error. In 2000, the *British Medical Journal* devoted an entire issue to the subject of medical error (Leape & Berwick 2000) in a determined effort to move the subject to the mainstream of academic and clinical enquiry. Many other leading medical journals have now followed suit, with major articles and series on patient safety. Some of the results of this research, particularly studies of the nature and scale of harm, are addressed in the next chapter.

REFERENCES

Bogner MS 1994 Human error in medicine. Lawrence Erlbaum Associates, Hillsdale, NJ

Brennan TA, Leape LL, Laird NM et al 1991 Incidence of adverse events and negligence in hospitalized patients; results from the Harvard Medical Practice Study I. New England Journal of Medicine 324:370–376

Cook RI, Woods DD, Miller CA 1998 A tale of two stories: contrasting views of patient safety. US National Patient Safety Foundation, North Adams, MA. Online. Available at: http://www.npsf.org/exec/front.html

Cooper JB 1994 Towards patient safety in anaesthesia. Annals Academy of Medicine 23:552–557

Cooper JB, Newbower RS, Long CD et al 1978 Preventable anesthesia mishaps: a study of human factors. Anesthesiology 49:399–406

Cooper JB, Newbower RS, Kitz RJ 1984 An analysis of major errors and equipment failures in anesthesia management: considerations for prevention and detection. Anesthesiology 60:34–42

Davies JM 1994 From Dryden to Winnipeg. In Helmreich RL, Merrit AC. Culture at work in aviation and medicine, Ashgate, Aldershot.

Department of Health (DoH) 2000 An organisation with a memory: learning from adverse events in the NHS. The Stationery Office, London

Department of Health (DoH) 2001 Learning from Bristol: the report of the public inquiry into children's heart surgery at the Bristol Royal Infirmary 1984–1995. HMSO, London

Donabedian A 1968 Promoting quality through evaluating the process of patient care. Medical Care 6:181–201

Eagle CJ, Davies JM, Reason J 1992 Accident analysis of large-scale technological disasters applied to an anaesthetic complication. Canadian Journal of Anaesthesia 39:118–122

Fenn P 2002 Counting the cost of medical negligence. British Medical Journal 325:233–234

Fenn P, Diacon S, Gray A et al 2000 Current cost of medical negligence in NHS hospitals: analysis of claims database. British Medical Journal 320:1567–1571

Gaba DM 2000 Anaesthesiology as a model for patient safety in health care. British Medical Journal 320: 785–788

Gawande A 2002 Complications: a surgeon's notes on an imperfect science. Picador, New York

Gigerenzer G 2002 Reckoning with risk. Learning to live with uncertainty. Penguin Books, London

Helmreich RL, Merrit AC 1998 Culture at work in aviation and medicine: national, organisational and professional influences. Ashgate, Aldershot

Hiatt HH, Barnes BA, Brennan TA et al 1989 A study of medical injury and medical malpractice: an overview. New England Journal of Medicine 321:480–484

HMSO 1995 Medical (Professional Performance) Act 1995. The Stationery Office, London

Kerr JM 1932 Maternal mortality and morbidity. E & S Livingstone, Edinburgh

Kohn L, Corrigan J, Donaldson ME 1999 To err is human. National Academy Press, Washington, DC

Langley GJ, Nolan KM, Nolan TW et al 1996 The improvement guide: a practical approach to enhancing organizational performance. Jossey-Bass Publishers, San Francisco

Leape LL 1994 Error in medicine. Journal of the American Medical Association 272:1851–1857

Leape LL 2000 Institute of Medicine figures are not exaggerated. Journal of the American Medical Association 284: 95–97

Leape LL, Berwick DM 2000 Safe health care: are we up to it? British Medical Journal 320:725–726

Leape LL, Brennan TA, Laird N et al 1991 The nature of adverse events in hospitalized patients. Results of the Harvard Medical Practice Study II. New England Journal of Medicine 324:377–384

Maxwell R 1984 Quality assessment in health. British Medical Journal 288:1470–1472

McIntyre N, Popper K 1983 The critical attitude in medicine: the need for a new ethics. British Medical Journal 287:1919–1923

Medawar P 1969 The art of the soluble. Creativity and originality in science. Pelican Books, London

Mohr JC 2000 American medical malpractice litigation in historical perspective. Journal of the American Medical Association 283:1731–1737

Oxley WHF, Philips MH, Young J 1935 Maternal mortality in Rochdale. British Medical Journal 1:304–307

Reason JT 1993 The human factor in medical accidents. In: Vincent C, Ennis M, Audley RJ (eds) Medical accidents. Oxford University Press, Oxford

Sharpe VA, Faden AI 1998 Medical harm. Historical, conceptual and ethical dimensions of iatrogenic illness. Cambridge University Press, Cambridge

Smith R 1998 All changed, utterly changed. British Medical Journal 316:1917–1918

Smith R 2000 Facing up to medical error. British Medical Journal 320 (18 March)

Treasure T 1998 Lessons from the Bristol case. More openness – on risks and an individual surgeons' performance. British Medical Journal 316:1685–1686

US National Patient Safety Foundation 2000 Agenda for research and development in patient safety. Online. Available at: http://www.npsf.org/download/researchagenda.pdf

Vincent C 1989 Research into medical accidents: a case of negligence? British Medical Journal 299:1150–1153

Vincent C 1993 The study of errors and accidents in medicine. In: Vincent CA, Ennis E, Audley RJ (eds) Medical accidents. Oxford University Press, Oxford

Vincent C 1995 Clinical risk management, 1st edn. BMJ Publications, London

Vincent C 1997 Risk, safety and the dark side of quality. British Medical Journal 314:1775–1776

Vincent C 2001 Caring for patients harmed by treatment. In: Vincent CA (ed) Clinical risk management. Enhancing patient safety, 2nd edn. BMJ Publications, London

Vincent C, Neale G, Woloshynowych M 2001 Adverse events in British hospitals: preliminary retrospective record review. British Medical Journal 322:517–519

Walshe K, Offen N 2001 A very public failure: lessons for quality improvement in healthcare organisations from the Bristol Royal Infirmary. Quality and Safety in Health Care 10:250–256

Wennberg J, Gittlesohn A 1973 Small area variations in health care delivery. Science 182:1102–1108

Studies of errors and adverse events in healthcare: the nature and scale of the problem

Of the top 20 risk factors that account for nearly three quarters of all deaths annually, adverse in-hospital events come in at number 11 above air pollution, alcohol and drugs, violence and road traffic injury.
(Davis 2004; on the findings of the New Zealand Adverse Events Study)

Reuse of injection equipment in the absence of sterilisation occurs in almost one third of injections in developing and transitional countries.
(Hutin et al 2003)

How safe is healthcare? How often do errors occur? Are the high-profile cases rare, isolated accidents in an otherwise safe system or are they, in the time-honoured phrase, just the tip of the iceberg? These apparently straightforward questions are, for various reasons, not easy to answer. Defining error and harm is not as simple as it might seem, different types of study illuminate different aspects of the problem and comparing findings from different settings is not always feasible. However, the number of studies assessing the incidence of error and harm has increased exponentially in the last few years and, although we cannot hope to cover them all, it is now possible to gain an understanding of the overall scale of the problem. As we shall see, although rates of error and harm vary in different settings, there is now substantial evidence of very high rates of error in many contexts and considerable evidence of harm to patients. First though, we must consider the main methods available for studying error and harm because, without this, it will be very difficult to make sense of the findings.

STUDYING ERRORS AND ADVERSE EVENTS

There are a number of methods of studying errors and adverse events, each of which has evolved over time and been adapted to different contexts. Each of the methods has particular strengths and advantages, and also weaknesses and limitations. Well, what's the best method you might reasonably ask? The answer is, as so often in research, that it depends on what you are trying to do and what questions you are trying to answer. Some methods are useful for identifying how often adverse events occur, others are stronger on why they happen; some are warning systems, rather than methods of counting, and so on. Failing to understand that different methods have different purposes has led to considerable confusion and much fruitless debate over the years. For instance, the major retrospective record reviews have sometimes been criticized for not providing data on human factors and other issues not identified in medical records. In fact, such studies are not intended to provide such information. Their primary purpose is to assess the nature and scale of harm, although recent review techniques also suggest that valuable information on cause and prevention can be extracted. In all cases, the methodology of a study will depend on the questions being addressed, the resources available and the context of the study.

Methods of study

Eric Thomas and Laura Petersen (2003) classified methods of studying errors and adverse events into eight broad groups and reviewed the respective advantages and disadvantages of each method. In their paper they use the term 'error' to include mistakes, close calls, near misses and factors that contribute to error. In a later chapter we will discuss the difficulties of defining and classifying errors, but in this section 'error' is used as a catch-all for any incident that does not involve patient harm. Adverse events imply harm or, at the very least, additional days in hospital. One has to be wary of patient safety terminology because the terms are sometimes used in different ways. For instance, a study by Andrews et al (1997) in the US showed a 17.7% rate of serious adverse events in a surgical unit, much higher than most other studies. However, the definition of 'adverse event' that Andrews et al used was different from that usually employed; and unlike most other studies, they used observation rather than record review. These are not flaws; the study is a good one. The point is that one has to be careful about definitions when interpreting findings and comparing studies.

Table 3.1 summarizes the main types of study of errors and adverse events, and their respective advantages and limitations. The language and content of the table has been adjusted from Thomas and Petersen's original source version; in particular a section on case analysis has been added. Case analyses, usually referred to as root cause analysis or systems analysis, share some of the features of morbidity and mortality meetings, but are generally more focused and follow a particular method of analysis (C Vincent 2003).

Methods differ in several respects. For instance, the various methods rely on different sources of data: medical records, observations, claims data, voluntary reports and so on. Some focus on single cases or small numbers of cases with particular characteristics, such as claims, whereas others attempt to randomly sample a defined population. Some methods are oriented towards detecting the incidence of errors and adverse events (i.e. how many), whereas others address their causes and contributory factors (i.e. why things go wrong). Thomas and Petersen suggest that the methods can be placed along a continuum with active clinical surveillance of specific types of adverse event (e.g. surgical complications) being the ideal method for assessing incidence and methods such as claims analysis and morbidity and mortality meetings being more oriented towards causes. There is no perfect way of

Table 3.1 Methods of studying errors and adverse (adapted from Thomas & Petersen 2003)

Study method	Advantages	Disadvantages
Morbidity and mortality conferences and autopsy	Can suggest contributory factors Familiar to healthcare providers	Hindsight bias Reporting bias Focused on diagnostic errors Infrequently used
Case analysis/root cause analysis	Can suggest contributory factors Structured systems approach Includes recent data from interviews	Hindsight bias Tends to focus on severe events Insufficiently standardized in practice
Claims analysis	Provides multiple perspectives (patients, providers, lawyers)	Hindsight bias Reporting bias Non-standardized source of data
Error reporting systems	Provide multiple perspectives over time Can be a part of routine operations	Reporting bias Hindsight bias
Administrative data analysis	Uses readily available data Inexpensive	Might rely on incomplete and inaccurate data The data are divorced from clinical context
Record review/ chart review	Uses readily available data Commonly used	Judgements about adverse events not reliable Medical records are incomplete Hindsight bias
Review of electronic medical record	Inexpensive after initial investment Monitors in real time Integrates multiple data sources	Susceptible to programming and/or data entry errors Expensive to implement
Observation of patient care	Potentially accurate and precise Provides data otherwise unavailable Detects more active errors than other methods	Time consuming and expensive Difficult to train reliable observers Potential concerns about confidentiality Possible to be overwhelmed with information
Active clinical surveillance	Potentially accurate and precise for adverse events	Time consuming and expensive

estimating the incidence of adverse events or of errors. For various reasons, all of them give a partial picture. Record review is comprehensive and systematic but, by definition, restricted to matters noted in the medical record. Reporting systems are strongly dependent on the willingness of staff to report and are a very imperfect reflection of the underlying rate of errors or adverse events (although they have other uses).

Hindsight bias

Hindsight bias is mentioned several times in Table 3.1. What is hindsight bias? The term derives from the psychological literature and in particular from experimental studies showing that people exaggerate in retrospect what they knew before an incident occurred – the 'knew it all along' effect. It is marvellously illustrated in Richard Cook's depiction (Fig. 3.1) of, on the left-hand side, a clinician faced with a difficult clinical decision and a bewildering array of alternatives. On the right-hand side, the 'expert' is reviewing the case after the event. Afterwards, with the benefit of hindsight, it all looks so simple and the 'expert' wonders why the clinician involved could not see the obvious connections. Looking back, the situation actually faced by the clinician is inevitably grossly simplified. We cannot capture the multiple pathways open to the clinician at the time, still less the dynamic, unfolding story of a clinical encounter, the fact that the clinician needs a break, and that he is simultaneously being harassed by a nurse about another patient and paged to resolve a discrepancy in a medication order.

Hindsight bias has another facet, perhaps better termed 'outcome bias', which is particularly relevant in healthcare. When an outcome is bad, those looking back are much more likely to be critical of care that has been given and more likely to detect errors. For instance, Caplan et al (1991) asked two groups of physicians to review two sets of notes. The sets of notes were identical but one group was told that the outcomes for the patients were satisfactory and the other group was told that the outcome was poor for the patient. The group who believed the outcomes were poor made much stronger criticisms of the care, even though the care described was exactly the same. So, we

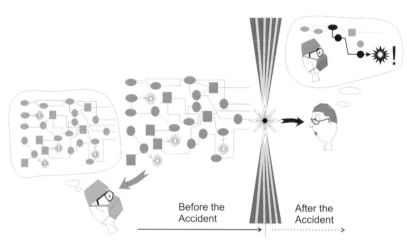

Fig. 3.1 Hindsight bias in clinical practice (from Cook et al 1998).

Studies of errors and adverse events in healthcare

simplify things in retrospect and tend to be more critical when the outcome is bad.

STUDIES OF THE QUALITY OF CARE

Evidence is accumulating that failing to provide standard treatment is a problem of epidemic proportions, which itself poses a serious threat to health. For instance, failing to give medication, such as not administering prophylactic antithrombotic agents before surgery, can result in harm to patients in the sense of leading to some potentially preventable thromboembolisms. Whether one classes this as a safety issue or a more general quality issue is a moot point and primarily a matter of terminology; either way, patients suffer.

Elizabeth McGlynn and colleagues carried out a study of 6712 adults in the US, examining their medical records and conducting telephone interviews (McGlynn et al 2003). Whereas most studies of the quality of care delivered have focused on a particular disease or a particular type of treatment, McGlynn and her colleagues wanted to make a general assessment of the quality of care delivered to adult Americans with significant health problems. Quality-of-care indicators were developed for a range of both acute and chronic conditions, which reflected the standard care that should have been delivered according to national guidelines (Table 3.2).

Incredibly, even in the US, with its legendarily high health costs (albeit mainly spent on 80% of the population), patients received only 55% of recommended care overall. Both over-use of care, unnecessary tests and treatment, and under-use were assessed, but under-use of healthcare was the more frequent problem. The proportion did not vary much between acute, chronic and preventive but did vary greatly between different medical conditions, ranging from almost 80% of correct care provided for senile cataract and breast cancer, down to below 25% for atrial fibrillation, hip fracture and alcohol dependence. Although the researchers acknowledge that more care could have been given than was recorded or remembered by patients, previous studies suggest that this would at most add a few percentage points to the indicator scores. They concluded soberly that:

> Our results indicate that on average, Americans receive about half of recommended medical care processes. Although this point estimate of the size of the quality problem may continue to be debated, the gap between what we know works and what is actually done is substantial enough to warrant attention. These deficits, which pose serious threats to the health and well-being of the U.S. public, persist despite initiatives by both the federal government and private health care delivery systems to improve care.

(McGlynn et al 2003 p 2644)

McGlynn and her colleagues argue that these findings have important implications for the general health of the population implying, in a sense, avoidable harm. For example, only 24% of people with diabetes in the study had regular blood tests, a requirement for close blood glucose control and the avoidance of complications. People with hypertension received 65% of the recommended

Table 3.2 Selected quality indicators and conditions (adapted from McGlynn et al 2003)

Condition (number of indicators)	Description of selected indicator	Type of care	Function	Mode	Problem with quality
Asthma (25)	Long-acting agents for patients with frequent use of short-acting beta antagonists	Chronic	Treatment	Medication	Under-use
Colorectal cancer (12)	Appropriate surgical treatment	Chronic	Treatment	Surgery	Under-use
Congestive heart failure (36)	Ejection fraction assessed before medical therapy	Chronic	Diagnosis	Laboratory testing or radiography	Under-use
Coronary artery disease (37)	Avoidance of nifedipine for patients with an acute myocardial infarction	Chronic	Treatment	Medication	Over-use
Diabetes (13)	Diet and exercise counselling	Chronic	Treatment	Counselling or education	Under-use
Hip fracture (9)	Prophylactic antibiotics given on day of surgery	Acute	Treatment	Medication	Under-use
Headache (21)	Use of appropriate first-line agents for patients with acute migraine	Acute	Treatment	Medication	Over-use
Hypertension (27)	Change in treatment when blood pressure is persistently under-controlled	Chronic	Follow-up	Medication	Under-use
Preventive care (38)	Screening for cervical cancer	Preventive	Screening	Laboratory testing or radiography	Under-use

care, and yet uncontrolled hypertension increases risk for heart disease, stroke and death. Studies of this kind do not directly assess harm but provide important information about the conditions in which patients can be harmed. As we will see in later chapters, serious incidents emerge from a background of much more frequent minor failures and problems in the delivery of care. As this particular study is set in the US, it is difficult to predict whether the results would be similar in different kinds of health system. In a publicly funded and more tightly controlled system, such as the British NHS, one might expect a closer adherence to procedure and protocol; on the other hand, most US physicians have financial incentives to investigate and treat, so one might expect higher rates of intervention.

STUDIES OF CLOSED CLAIMS

From studies of the process and overall quality of care, we now turn to studies of incidents defined by the outcome of care. Systematic record reviews are the most important outcome-based studies but claims for malpractice and medical negligence are also a potentially important source of information on the causes of harm to patients (Vincent 1993). Claims have an additional importance because of the profound impact of the litigation process on all those involved, whether patients, families or clinicians. Today, with many additional sources of information and methods of analysis, the role of claims data is being reappraised (DoH 2000), but the analysis of claims can still be instructive.

The Anaesthesia Closed Claims Project

The most important series of studies of claims is undoubtedly the ongoing Closed Claims Project of the American Society of Anesthetists (ASA) (Cheney 1999). In this project, a standard report form is completed by an anaesthetic reviewer for every claim where there is enough information to reconstruct the sequence of events and determine the nature and cause of the injury. By 1999, there were more than 4000 claims in the database. Respiratory events accounted for a large share of claims, especially for brain damage and death (Cheney 1999). The most common events leading to injury were inadequate ventilation, oesophageal intubation and difficult tracheal intubation. Findings from reviews of these claims contributed to the recommendation by the ASA Committee on Standards in the formulation of standards requiring pulse oximetry intraoperatively, the use of end-tidal CO_2 for the verification of endotracheal intubation and the use of pulse oximetry in the postanaesthesia care unit. Since then, further reports have appeared on ulnar nerve injury, spinal cord injury, airway trauma and postoperative visual loss.

Although the analyses of claims have highlighted important issues, the authors are assiduous in pointing out the limitations of the database as well as the potential for learning. For instance, Caplan et al (1990) found that although reviewers could identify that a problem had occurred, they could discern the mechanism of injury and the reasons for the problems in only about 10% of cases of respiratory episodes. The principal problems are that claims are an unrepresentative sample of errors and adverse events, that there is often a long time lag between the incident and the review and that judgements of the quality of care can be unduly influenced by a known poor outcome (Lee & Domino 2002). Cheney (1999), in a thoughtful review of the past successes and future prospects, provided an optimistic assessment of the ASA Closed Claims Project, although hedged with some cautions. He argued that closed claims review was still an important element of quality assurance and had revealed important and previously unappreciated aspects of adverse anaesthetic outcomes. Insights gained from these reviews can be used to formulate hypotheses aimed at improving the quality of anaesthetic care, thus providing a tool for advancing patient safety (Cheney 1999).

Other claims reviews

Although anaesthesia-related claims have dominated the research literature, reviews in several other specialties have been carried out. For instance, Ennis and Vincent (1990), in a review of serious obstetric claims, identified three major areas of concern: inadequate fetal monitoring, mismanagement of forceps and lack of involvement of senior staff. In a review of claims stemming from the practice of gastroenterology, Graham Neale (1998) showed that insufficient attention was paid to the risk:benefit ratio of invasive procedures and to the aftercare of patients who suffered an adverse event during a procedure. Gawande and colleagues (2003) carried out a particularly sophisticated study of claims, employing a case-control design to examine instances of retained instruments and sponges after an operative procedure. The main risk factors that predicted the occurrence of a retained foreign body were: undergoing emergency surgery, an unplanned change in operation and body mass index. By setting the analysed claims within a representative cohort, this design overcomes some of the limitations that occur in traditional methods of closed claims analysis.

STUDYING ADVERSE EVENTS USING CASE RECORD REVIEW

Retrospective reviews of medical records aim to assess the nature, incidence and economic impact of adverse events and to provide some information on their causes. Adverse events are defined as an unintended injury caused by medical management rather than the disease process; the full definition is provided in Box 3.1. The classic, pioneering study in this area is the Harvard Medical Practice Study, still hugely influential and much debated 20 years after it was carried out (Box 3.2).

The basic record review process is as follows. In phase I, nurses or experienced record clerks are trained to identify case records that satisfy one or more of 18 well-defined screening criteria, such as death, transfer to a special care unit or re-admission to hospital within 12 months. These have been shown to be associated with an increased likelihood of an adverse event (Neale & Woloshynowych 2003). In phase II, trained doctors analyse positively screened records in detail to determine whether they contain evidence of an adverse event

Box 3.1 Defining adverse events

(adapted from Brennan et al 1991)

- An adverse event is an unintended injury caused by medical management rather than by the disease process and which is sufficiently serious to lead to prolongation of hospitalization or to temporary or permanent impairment or disability to the patient at time of discharge or both.
- Medical management includes both the actions of an individual member of staff and the overall healthcare system.
- Medical management includes acts of omission (e.g. failure to diagnose or treat) and commission (e.g. incorrect treatment).
- Causation of adverse event by medical management is judged on a 6-point scale, where 1 indicates 'virtually no evidence for causation' and 6 indicates 'virtually certain evidence for causation'. Only adverse events with a score of '4' or higher, requiring evidence that causation is more likely than not, are reported in the results.
- Adverse events might or might not be preventable, a separate judgement from that of causation. Preventability is also judged on a 6-point scale, with only those adverse events scoring '4' or higher being considered preventable.
- Injury can result from intervention or from failure to intervene. Injuries that come about from failure to arrest the disease process are also included, provided that standard care would clearly have prevented the injury.
- The injury has to be unintended because injury can occur deliberately and with good reason (e.g. amputation).
- Adverse events include recognized complications, which will be judged as leading to harm but being of low preventability.

using a standard set of questions. The basic method has been followed in all the major national studies, although modifications of the review form and data capture have been developed (Woloshynowych et al 2003). The forthcoming French study (Michel et al 2004) has used prospective review, in the sense that record review is carried out close to the time of discharge on a previously defined set of patients and, in some cases, combined with interviews with staff.

Box 3.2 The Harvard Medical Practice Study

(adapted from Brennan et al 1991, Leape et al 1991)

The Harvard Medical Practice Study reviewed patient records of 30,121 randomly chosen hospitalizations from 51 randomly chosen acute care, non-psychiatric hospitals in New York State in 1984. The goal was to better understand the epidemiology of patient injury and to inform efforts to reform systems of patient compensation. The focus was therefore on injuries that might eventually lead to legal action. Minor errors and those causing only minor discomfort or inconvenience were not addressed.

Adverse events occurred in 3.7% of hospitalizations; 27.6% of these were due to negligence (defined as care that fell below the standard expected of physicians in that community, and which might therefore lead to legal action). Almost half (47.7%) of adverse events were associated with an operation. The most common non-operative adverse events were adverse drug events, followed by diagnostic mishaps, therapeutic mishaps, procedure-related events and others. Permanent disability resulted from 6.5% of adverse events and 13.6% involved the death of a patient.

Extrapolations from these data suggested that approximately 100,000 Americans die each year from adverse events. Later analyses indicated that 69.6% of adverse events were potentially preventable.

The original Harvard study, itself developed from a 1974 California study of over 20,000 hospitalizations (Harper Mills & von Bolschwing 1995), has been replicated in a number of other settings. The next major study was the Quality in Australian Health Care Study (Wilson et al 1995), which reviewed 14,179 randomly sampled records from 31 hospitals and found a 16.6% adverse event rate, about half of which were preventable. Permanent disability resulted from 13.7% of adverse events and 4.9% were associated with a death. The pattern of adverse events was similar, the largest number being operative, followed by diagnostic errors, therapeutic errors and adverse drug reactions. The higher rate in Australia, over four times that found in the US, is partly accounted for by the wider range of adverse events (for instance, adverse events occurring outside hospital were included), the focus on quality of care rather than negligence, and the inclusion of many more minor events in the class of adverse events. In a careful comparison of specific types of adverse events, Eric Thomas and colleagues also found that Australian reviewers reported many more minor expected or anticipated complications, such as wound infection, skin injury, and urinary tract infection. These are adverse events by the strict definition of the term but were not included by the American reviewers, who were focusing on more serious injuries (Thomas et al 2000).

Similar studies have been conducted in Utah and Colorado (Gawande et al 1999), in the UK (Vincent et al 2001), Denmark (Schioler et al 2001), New Zealand (Davis et al 2002), Canada (Baker et al 2004) and France (Michel et al 2004). The results of these studies are summarized in Table 3.3. Findings from the more recent studies show an adverse event rate per admission of around 10%, with about half the adverse events being judged preventable. The rate per

Study	Number of acute care hospitals	Date of admissions	Number of hospital admissions	Adverse event rate (% admissions)
California Insurance Feasibility Study	23	1974	20864	4.65*
Harvard Medical Practice Study (HMPS)	51	1984	30195	3.7
Utah–Colorado Study (UTCOS)	28	1992	14052	2.9
Quality in Australian Health Care Study (QAHCS)	28	1992	14179	16.6
United Kingdom	2	1999	1014	10.8
Denmark	17	1998	1097	9.0
New Zealand	13	1998	6579	11.2
France**	7	2002	778	14.5
Canada	20	2000	3745	7.5

Table 3.3 Adverse events in acute hospitals in seven countries

*The California study assessed 'potentially compensable events'.
**Figures from France are from the pilot study not the full study.

patient is always slightly higher, as some patients suffer more than one event. Examples of adverse events from the British study are shown in Box 3.3. Some, such as the reaction to anaesthetic, are not serious for the patient but are classed as an adverse event because there was an increased stay in hospital of 1 day; it was probably not preventable in that it would have been hard to predict such an idiosyncratic reaction. Many adverse events – about 70% in most studies – have no important consequences for the patient; their effects are more economic (in the sense of wasted time and resources) than clinical. Others, however, as the remaining examples show, have important consequences for the patients, both in terms of unnecessary suffering and extended time in hospital.

The impact and cost of adverse events

As the examples show, many patients suffer increased pain and disability from adverse events. Many also suffer psychological trauma and can experience failures in their treatment as a terrible betrayal of trust. Staff can experience shame, guilt and depression after making a mistake, with litigation and complaints imposing an additional burden (Vincent 1997). These profoundly important aspects of patient safety, generally given far too little attention, are considered in Chapters 7 and 8.

The financial cost of adverse events, in terms of additional treatment and extra days in hospital, are considerable and vastly greater than the costs of litigation. One of the most consistent findings from the record reviews is that, on average, a patient suffering an adverse event stays an extra 6 to 8 days in hospital. An extra few days in hospital is, clinically speaking, an unremarkable event and it is not necessarily particularly traumatic or unpleasant for the patient. However, when the sums are done and the findings extrapolated nation-

---

Box 3.3 Examples of adverse events of varying severity

(adapted from the UK study by Vincent et al 2001 and Neale et al 2001)

An 18-year-old girl was admitted as a day-surgery case for examination of the ears under anaesthetic. During recovery the patient suffered three fits related to the anaesthetic and required intravenous medication to control fits and an extended stay for overnight observation.

A 65-year-old woman was admitted to hospital for repair of a strangulated incisional hernia. Postoperatively, the wound site failed to heal. The patient was sent home with a discharging and offensive wound. She returned 3 days later with a gaping and infected wound, which required cleansing and re-suturing under a general anaesthetic, antibiotics and an extended hospital stay of 15 days.

A 24-year-old woman with spina bifida presented to the emergency department feeling unwell. Her ankles were swollen and she was noted to have recently had a urinary tract infection. She was treated with antibiotics and discharged home. A week later she was admitted to hospital with very swollen lower limbs, high blood pressure and raised central venous pressure. A diagnosis of hypertensive congestive cardiac failure was made, delayed a week because of an incomplete initial assessment in the emergency department.

A 53-year-old man with a history of stroke, MRSA infection, leg ulcers and heart failure was admitted for treatment of venous ulceration and cellulitis of both legs. Postoperatively, the patient had a urinary catheter in place, incorrect management of the catheter resulted in necrosis of the tip of the penis. He underwent a suprapubic catheterization and developed an infection. The patient's hospital stay was extended by 26 days.

ally, the costs are staggering. In Britain the cost of preventable adverse events is £1 billion per annum in lost bed days alone (Vincent et al 2001). The wider costs of lost working time, disability benefits and the wider economic consequences would be greater still. The Institute of Medicine report (Kohn et al 1999) estimated that, in the US, total annual national costs (lost income, lost household production, disability, healthcare costs) were between $17 billion and $29 billion for preventable adverse events and about double that for all adverse events. Healthcare costs accounted for over one-half of the total costs incurred. Even when using the lower estimates, the total national costs associated with adverse events and preventable adverse events represent approximately 4% and 2%, respectively, of national health expenditure in 1996. When considering this figure we should remember that the estimated adverse event rate in the US is much lower than in most other countries, so costs per head of population in other countries would probably be judged to be higher. Additionally, recall that these estimates are confined to the hospital sector; we have no idea of the additional costs of adverse events in primary care or mental health.

Can we compare rates in different countries?

Rates in the later adverse event studies from UK, Denmark and New Zealand are remarkably similar, all being around 10%; US rates are much lower, with Australia seemingly much higher. The lower rates in the US might reflect better quality care, but could also reflect the narrower focus on negligent injury rather than the broader quality improvement focus of most other studies (Thomas et al 2000). Do the figures really reflect the underlying standard of healthcare in these countries?

Although differences in adverse event rates between countries attract a great deal of media attention, much debate and occasional recrimination, the whole issue needs to be set in a broader context. Other attempts to compare health systems have produced a completely different picture. For example, the recent World Health Organization report (2000) on the health systems of 191 countries, ranked using an aggregate measure based on several dimensions (such as population health, health inequalities, responsiveness to need and financial fairness), provoked an intense debate on the validity of measuring and comparing healthcare systems (Walshe 2003). The US, despite its huge expenditure, was ranked 37th – bottom of the industrialized countries and below Greece, Portugal and Ireland.

Kieran Walshe (2003) has argued that all these discussions leave a fundamental question unanswered. What are international comparisons for? He suggests that they are too often driven by a desire for measurement for measurement's sake, and points out that what is needed is not so much international comparison, but international learning. Similarly, with patient safety, the precise differences in adverse event rates in different countries are of relatively little account. All countries have found a substantial and deeply worrying level of error and harm that constitutes a substantial public health problem. All involved agree that the methodology is not precise enough to permit formal comparisons or conclusions about the safety of the underlying healthcare systems. We can, however, learn a great deal from other countries' attempts to address the problem, examining different regulatory approaches for instance and reviewing what has worked well and which initiatives have not been fruitful.

DEATHS FROM ADVERSE EVENTS: CAN WE BELIEVE THE FINDINGS OF RETROSPECTIVE RECORD REVIEW?

Retrospective review, like any other research method, has its limitations and the findings of the studies have to be interpreted with due regard to the methodological limitations. Graham Neale, the lead clinician in the British study, has summarized the principal problems, while acknowledging the importance of the essential clinical findings. Neale and Woloshynowych (2003) pointed out, for instance, that the review process relies on the implicit judgements of doctors. Great efforts have been made to strengthen the accuracy and reproducibility of these judgements by training, by the use of structured data collection, by duplicate review with re-review and by resolution of disagreements, but their reliability remains no better than moderate. In a careful study, Kieran Walshe (2000) concluded that the recognition of adverse events by record review had moderate to good face, content and construct validity with respect to quality of care in a hospital setting.

These and other methodological issues have come to the fore in debates about the number of deaths due to adverse events, particularly after the headline-capturing claims that up to 98,000 Americans were dying each year from adverse events in hospital. The methodological arguments are too complex to summarize in their entirety here but it is important to note that the figures have been challenged, and to give a flavour of the arguments. For instance, one research team argued, following estimates of the death rate in hospital at the time of the study, that the patients who reportedly died from adverse events in the Harvard study were already severely ill and likely to die anyway (McDonald et al 2000). In a further challenge to the figures, Hayward and Hofer (2001) compared the findings with their own review of the standard of care of patients who died in hospital while having active, as opposed to palliative, care. They found that only 0.5% of patients would have lived longer than 3 months even if they had all had optimal care. So, yes, some deaths were perhaps preventable but the great majority of these people were already very ill and would have died anyway. How important an extra few months of life is would no doubt vary from person to person according to their disease and circumstances.

In a reply to McDonald and colleagues, Lucian Leape (2000) noted that:

> Some seem to have the impression that many of the deaths attributed to adverse events were minor incidents in severely ill people. This is not so. First . . . terminally ill patients were excluded from the study. Review of the cases . . . in which the care was most deficient reveals two groups of patients: a small group, 14%, who were severely ill and in whom the adverse event tipped the balance; and a larger group, 86%, for whom the error was not a superimposed event, but a major factor leading to the patient's death. Examples of the latter include a cerebrovascular accident

in a patient with atrial flutter who was not treated with anticoagulants, overwhelming sepsis due to spontaneous rupture of the intestine in a patient with signs of intestinal obstruction that was untreated for 24 hours, and brain damage from hypotension due to blood loss from unrecognized rupture of the spleen.

(Leape 2000 p 96)

The methods and arguments of those challenging the interpretation of the deaths in the Harvard study can in turn be challenged and the debate could run on and on. The Harvard study did not, in any case, specifically set out to examine the preventability of deaths in hospital and there is a limit to what can be achieved by arguing over 20-year-old data. All the authors in these disputes acknowledge the importance of the overall findings and the vital task of reducing errors and adverse events. Although it is right that methodological issues are aired, particularly in relation to the design of future studies, there is a danger that in arguing about the precise numbers the real work of documenting, understanding and preventing adverse events is neglected.

DO PHYSICIANS AND THE GENERAL PUBLIC BELIEVE THE FINDINGS?

The arcane, but important, arguments of methodologists do not hit the headlines; claims of 44,000–98,000 deaths do. But are these figures believed? Do they accord with the daily experience of physicians and the public? These questions have been addressed in a postal survey of 1000 doctors in Colorado, 1000 doctors across the US and telephone interviews with 500 members of the general public (Robinson et al 2002). As Table 3.4 shows, the general public

Table 3.4 Colorado physicians and public agreement with statements in the Institute of Medicine report (adapted from Robinson et al 2002)

Statement	Physicians (n = 594) (%) agreement	Public (n = 500) (%) agreement
The quality of healthcare in the US is a significant problem	29.1	67.6
Our healthcare system does not match the safety record attained in other industries	21.2	36.2
Error reduction in medicine should be a national priority	69.7	86.6
We need a national agency to provide leadership and research in reducing medical errors	24.1	59.8
We should implement a system of mandatory reporting of serious medical errors	54.7	90.2
A recent estimate that medical errors kill 44,000 to 98,000 Americans yearly is accurate	13.8	19.0

were more likely than doctors to believe that the quality and safety of health-care was a problem, that error reduction should be a priority and to support mandatory reporting of serious errors.

It appears, therefore, that a much higher proportion of the general public than of doctors is concerned about the safety of healthcare. Although the authors did not ascertain the reasons for this in their survey, they speculate that the public is unduly influenced by isolated but horrific accounts in the media. Alternatively, they suggest, physicians are not as concerned about errors as they should be. It might be that the difficulty of defining and measuring errors and of determining their preventability has led physicians to underestimate their frequency or not to recognize them at all. More surprisingly, only 21% of physicians surveyed thought that healthcare had not matched the safety records of other industries. From the evidence gathered in this chapter, even allowing for the methodological debates, this belief does seem hard to sustain. If healthcare was an airline, only dedicated risk takers, thrill seekers and those tired of living would fly on it. Members of the medical profession, in the US at least, seem curiously unaware of the hazards of the system they work in.

STUDIES OF ADVERSE EVENTS WITHIN SPECIALTIES AND IN OTHER SETTINGS

The adverse events studies considered so far have been aggregate studies, in the sense that they have assessed the nature and incidence of all types of adverse events across a whole sector of care. As patient safety evolves, however, more information is emerging on specific types of adverse event or from studies of particular settings. In addition, studies of complications of treatment are being re-examined more critically as we begin to appreciate that some complications might be due not to the inherent risk of treatment but to error and system problems. To illustrate these more specific studies we will briefly review surgical adverse events and cardiac arrests that happen within the hospital setting, before turning to consider the incidence of adverse events outside hospital.

Complications and adverse events in surgery

A significant percentage of adverse events are associated with a surgical procedure. For instance, in the Utah–Colorado Medical Practice Study the annual incidence rate of adverse events among hospitalized patients who received an operation was 3.0%, of which half were preventable. Some operations, such as extremity bypass graft, abdominal aortic aneurysm repair and colon resection, were at particularly high risk of preventable adverse events (Thomas & Brennan 2001).

In the UK, complication rates for some of the major operations are 20–25%, with an acceptable mortality of 5–10% (Vincent et al 2004). However, at least 30–50% of major complications occurring in patients undergoing general surgical procedures are thought to be avoidable. Many adverse events classified as operative are, on closer examination, found to be due to problems in ward management rather than intra-operative care. For instance, Neale et al (2001) identified preventable pressure ulcers, chest infections, falls and poor care of urethral catheters in their study of adverse events, together with a variety of problems with the administration of drugs and intravenous fluids.

Whereas the major record reviews have been enormously important in drawing attention to patient safety issues, future studies might move to the examination of defined adverse events in a prospective manner. For instance, in Canada, Wanzel and colleagues (2000) prospectively monitored the presence and documentation of complications for all 192 patients admitted over a 2-month period to a general surgical ward; 75 (39%) of the patients suffered a total of 144 complications, two of which were fatal, 10 life threatening and 90 of moderate severity. Almost all the complications were documented in the patient's notes, but two-thirds of them were not documented on the front sheet of the patient's final medical record and only 20% were reviewed at the weekly morbidity and mortality rounds. Nearly one-fifth of the complications were due, in part, to error.

In-hospital cardiac arrests

The majority of treated in-hospital cardiac arrests are potentially avoidable according to a recent study in one British hospital. Hodgetts et al (2002) reviewed 118 in-hospital cardiac arrests, excluding DNAR (do not attempt resuscitation) cases. An expert review panel unanimously agreed that over 60% of these arrests were potentially avoidable. Cardiac arrests were more likely at the weekend than during the week and avoidable cardiac arrests were five times more likely to happen on general wards than in critical care areas, and even more likely to occur in areas judged 'inappropriate' for the care of cardiac patients. In about half the avoidable cases clinical signs of deterioration in the preceding 24 hours were not acted on. The authors cite multiple system failures, including delays and errors in diagnosis, inadequate interpretation of symptoms and investigations, inexperienced doctors and management in inappropriate clinical areas as the primary causes of these arrests.

Adverse events after discharge from hospital

Forster et al (2003) have examined adverse events that occur after discharge from hospital. Reviewing 400 consecutive patients from a tertiary care hospital they found that a total of 76 patients (19%) suffered an adverse event, 23 (6%) a preventable adverse event and 24 (6%) an ameliorable adverse event. Adverse drug events were the most common followed by procedure related injuries that only became apparent after discharge. The authors point to the importance of the vulnerable transition between hospital and home.

Primary care

Even in advanced healthcare systems, most healthcare is provided in the community or in people's homes and there is clearly potential for errors and harm in both settings. Primary care differs from hospital care in many respects, providing long-term, individualized care to the full population across a very broad spectrum of health and illness. Doctors working in this setting, like emergency medicine practitioners, work with high levels of uncertainty and often incomplete information.

Primary care is more or less virgin territory in patient safety terms, in that systematic studies are still few and far between. Wilson and Sheikh could identify only 31 directly relevant articles over a 20-year period. Most concerned prescribing errors, although some attention had been given to diagnostic error. The overall frequency of diagnostic error is unknown. However, conditions that seem to be particularly problematic (at least with hindsight) include asthma, cancer, dermatological conditions, substance misuse and depression (Wilson & Sheikh 2002). The study of error and adverse events in primary care is likely to be an increasingly important area in the next few years.

STUDIES OF MEDICATION ERRORS AND ADVERSE DRUG EVENTS

Studies of medical error have been conducted in many areas of clinical practice encompassing, for instance, diagnostic errors, studies of autopsies, histopathology and the interpretation of X-rays, as well as an extensive literature on medical decision making and decision-making biases of various kinds (Croskerry 2002, Leape 1994). Studies of error are one way of examining the process of care and assessing whether it is meeting certain specified standards. Are diagnostic X-rays being read correctly? Are drugs being prescribed and administered correctly? Studies of errors therefore have a different orientation to studies of adverse events, which are focused on the outcomes of care. The most extensively studied area, which we will use as an exemplar of error studies, is medication error.

Medication errors

Medication errors can occur at any stage of the process of prescribing, preparation of the order and administration to the patient. Examples of the basic types of medication error include prescribing errors, omitting to give the drug, giving the wrong drug, giving too much or too little of the drug, failing to order the drug, preparing it incorrectly and giving it by the wrong route or the wrong rate of administration. With so many small steps in the chain from prescribing to the patient receiving the drug, there is plenty of scope for error. Studies of medication error have sometimes addressed the whole sequence of medication, from prescribing to administration, but most focus on one particular area. Writing in 1994, Lucian Leape summarized current knowledge of medication error by stating that studies suggested that they occurred in 2–14% of patients admitted to hospital (Leape 1994). Since then, many hospitals in the US, and to a lesser extent elsewhere, have introduced computerized order entry systems, which have greatly reduced the possibilities of some types of error, particularly because they often incorporate warning systems and flags of possible contraindications and allergic reactions.

Most hospitals worldwide, however, are still using written orders and inter-pretation. Bryony Dean and colleagues examined the rate of clinically mean-ingful prescribing error in one British hospital still using written orders, using pharmacists to prospectively check prescription details of a sample of patients over a 4-week period (Dean et al 2002). About 36,200 orders were written, 1.5% of which contained a prescribing error, a quarter of which were potentially serious. For instance, an elderly patient was prescribed five times the intended 10-mg dose of diazepam, because the order was written up as 10 ml (equivalent to 50 mg). These figures equated to about 150 prescribing errors per week in that hospital, and about 35 serious errors. Dean and colleagues commented that a medication order was written about every 20 seconds during the daytime, so the rate of error did not seem that high. However – annually – hundreds of patients were experiencing potentially serious errors.

Intravenous drug administration, requiring some technical skill and the use of equipment, offers additional hazards and possibilities for error over oral medication. Katja Taxis and Nick Barber (2003) observed 430 intravenous drug doses and found that almost half involved an error, either of the preparation of the drug or its administration. Some examples of more serious errors are shown in Box 3.4. Most preparation errors were associated with multiple-step preparations, such as drugs that required reconstitution with a solvent and addition of a dilutent. Typical errors were preparing the wrong dose or select-ing the wrong solvent. The more complex the procedure, the more chance of error occurring, a theme we will return to in later chapters.

Medication error rates are not always so high. In some settings, perhaps those with more routine use of specific drugs or those where a more procedu-ralized approach is possible, rates are lower. For instance, in one study the rate of major errors in 30,000 cytotoxic preparations was only 0.19% (Limat et al 2001). These rates seem impressively low, but might still equate to substantial numbers of patients being affected each year across a hospital and still more across a country.

Box 3.4 Examples of potentially serious intravenous drug errors
(adapted from Taxis & Barber 2003)

- The whole content of a vial containing 125,000 international units of heparin was prepared as a continuous infusion, resulting in a five times overdose to a patient on a general medical ward in a teaching hospital.

Comment: haemorrhage is one of the serious, potentially life-threatening complications of an overdose of heparin.

- A nurse injected 750 mg vancomycin into an infusion bag of 0.9% sodium chloride (already connected to the patient's cannula) without mixing the solution. The patient probably received a concentrated solution of vancomycin as a bolus.

Comment: rapid infusions of vancomycin carry the risk of reactions such as severe hypotension (including shock and cardiac arrest) and flushing of the upper body.

- An intensive care patient's continuous infusion of adrenaline (epinephrine) was interrupted for about 10 minutes because the new infusion had not been prepared in advance.

Comment: this patient's blood pressure dropped to a dangerously low level. A bolus dose of adrenaline was given to stabilize him until the adrenaline infusion was restarted.

Adverse drug events

Studies of medication errors assess whether a drug was prescribed and administered correctly; there might or might not have been any actual or potential harm to the patient. Studies of adverse drug events, by contrast, focus on the harm that might or might not have been caused by an error. For instance, if a patient suffers an allergic reaction that could not have been predicted then this is unfortunate, but not an error. If the patient's medical record specifies the allergy and he or she is still given the drug, then it is certainly classed as an error, although investigation might reveal a quite complex net of causes.

In the US, Bates et al (1995) found that adverse drug events (ADE; defined as an injury resulting from medical intervention related to a drug) occurred in 6.5% of hospitalizations. In a more recent review of 10 studies from four different countries, Kanjanarat and colleagues (Kanjanarat et al 2003) found that the median rate of ADEs in hospitalized patients was 1.8%, with about a third being judged preventable. Examples of frequent ADEs were overdoses of antihypertensive drugs leading to bradycardia or hypertension, penicillin prescribed with a known history of allergic reactions to the drug, warfarin overdoses and inadequate monitoring leading to haemorrhages, and opioid over-dose or under-dose associated with respiratory depression and poor pain control, respectively. The under-use of a drug is a slightly wider than usual definition of ADE but there is no doubt that the erroneous under-use of a drug for pain does cause avoidable suffering.

Evidence is accumulating that many adverse drug events occur outside hospital, often leading to hospital admission. For instance, in Boston, Tejal Gandhi and colleagues reviewed 661 out-patients on a variety of drug regimens in a careful study that involved both record review and telephone interviews with the patients over a 3-month period (Gandhi et al 2003). Incredibly, almost a quarter of these people were assessed as suffering ADEs and about 6% of the patients were suffering serious reactions. Serious ADEs included bradycardia, hypotension and gastrointestinal bleeding, many of which were clearly preventable.

Other consequences were less serious, in that they did not present immediate threat to life but were certainly serious for the patient. For instance, one patient suffered prolonged sexual dysfunction after his doctor failed to stop a selective serotonin uptake inhibitor; another had continued sleep disturbance due to taking an antidepressant that his doctor was not aware of. Such reactions represent prolonged, avoidable suffering over many months, to say nothing of the waste of time and resources. If these findings were replicated across the US, the cost implications would be staggering.

Many patients experiencing drug-related problems outside hospital end up in hospital because of them; treatment aimed at keeping people well has the opposite effect and puts them into hospital. In a review of 15 studies, Winterstein and colleagues (2002) found that an average of 4.3% of all hospital admissions were drug related, concluding that drug-related morbidity is a significant healthcare problem and that much of it is preventable. The following drug groups are most likely to lead to drug-related admissions: antibiotics, anticoagulants, beta-blockers, digoxin, diuretics, hypoglycaemics and non-steroidal anti-inflammatories (Howard et al 2003, Wiffen et al 2002).

HOSPITAL-ACQUIRED INFECTION

Nosocomial, or hospital-acquired, infection (more properly called healthcare-associated infection) is the most common complication affecting hospitalized patients. In the Harvard Medical Practice Study a single type of hospital-acquired infection, surgical wound infection, was the second largest category of adverse events (Burke 2003). Currently, 5–10% of patients admitted to hospital in Britain and the US acquire one or more infections; millions of people each year are affected. In the US, 90,000 deaths a year are attributed to these infections, which add an estimated $5 billion to the costs of care. Intensive care units sustain even higher rates, approximately 30% of patients being affected, with an impact on both morbidity and mortality (J Vincent 2003).

Four types account for about 80% of nosocomial infections: urinary tract infections, often associated with catheter use; bloodstream infections, often due to intravascular devices; surgical site infection and pneumonia. Each of these four types can arise in more than one way and might be due to one or more different bacterial species. Intravenous lines are a particularly potent source of infection and the chance of infection is increased the longer the line remains in place. This is particularly disturbing because a recent study suggested that the lines inserted into patients are often not being used. At any one time, a third of patients in a general hospital setting had intravenous lines or catheters inserted: one-third of these lines were not in active use; 20% of the cannulae inserted were never used at all and, overall, 5% of the lines in use led to an unpleasant complication (Baker et al 2002).

Not all infections are necessarily preventable by any means but there is a consensus that many could be avoided by interventions such as the proper use of prophylactic antibiotics before surgery and hand hygiene campaigns among staff. Despite many studies, and massive campaigns, there is still widespread failure to adhere to basic standards of hand hygiene and it is hugely difficult to bring about change.

Infection control has for decades been seen as a public health problem and tackled by specialist doctors and infection control nurses, rather than linked with general quality-improvement work. The emergence of the patient safety movement has energized and supported infection control, leading to those involved widening their remit to monitor antibiotic use as well as infection and to associate themselves with the broader drive to make healthcare safer (Burke 2003). Patient safety, in turn, might be able to learn much from the techniques of infection control, particularly the methods of surveillance, rapid response to problems and epidemiological analyses. Infection control requires, among other things, careful specification of the types of infection coupled with both a rapid response to outbreaks and systematic, routine surveillance and monitoring. As Thomas and Petersen (2003) note, potentially the most precise and accurate method of measuring adverse events is to specify in advance the type of event and actively search for them. For example, the measurement of postoperative myocardial infarctions, rather than simply relying on reporting or record review, might include administration of electrocardiogram and measurement of cardiac enzymes in a planned, prospective cohort study or even, if resources allow, on an ongoing basis.

PATIENT SAFETY IN DEVELOPING COUNTRIES: THE CASE OF INJECTION SAFETY

Patient safety, in the form described in this book, has developed primarily in advanced, relatively well-resourced healthcare systems. However, the safety of healthcare is of huge concern in poorer countries. The World Health Organization (WHO) has established a number of safety-related programmes targeted mainly at developing countries and concerning such matters as the safety of blood products, chemical safety, vaccine and immunization safety, drug safety and medical device safety. Currently, these tend to be run as separate programmes but the WHO resolution on patient safety and the work of the World Alliance on Patient Safety should bring some integration of these projects with patient safety acting as an umbrella concept. To get a sense of the scale of problems facing developing healthcare systems, we will look briefly at the question of injection safety, drawing on a comprehensive review by Yvan Hutin and colleagues (Hutin et al 2003).

During the twentieth century, injection use increased tremendously and injections are now probably the most common healthcare procedure. Many injections given to provide treatment in developing countries are in fact unnecessary, as oral drug treatment would be equally or more effective. The belief in the power of injections, as opposed to pills, is one reason for the continuation of this practice. The dangers come from the reuse of syringes without sterilization, with syringes often just being rinsed in water between injections. This should not be seen as simply due to poor training or low standards; in a poor country everything is reused because there is no alternative. Although lack of knowledge and poor standards play a part, the danger is hugely compounded by the basic lack of resources and the need to reuse any item of equipment if at all possible.

A huge proportion of injections are given unsafely and the numbers of people affected are staggering (Fig. 3.2). In some countries in South-east Asia as many as 75% of injections are unsafe, leading to massive risk of hepatitis, HIV infection and other blood-borne pathogens. Hutin and colleagues call for the risks of unsafe injections to be highlighted in all HIV programmes, better management of sharps waste and the increased use of single-use syringes, which are unusable after the first injection has been given. They suggest that donors funding programmes of drug delivery should ensure that they include the cost of these syringes, or they will do more harm than good. WHO programmes, particularly in Burkina Faso, have demonstrated that major change can be achieved.

The extent of harm to patients from healthcare systems in the developing world is largely unknown but the potential for error and harm in fragile, under-funded systems is proportionately greater still. The poor state of infrastructure and equipment, unreliable supply and quality of drugs, shortcomings in waste management and infection control and severe under-financing of essential operating costs make the probability of error and harm much greater than in industrialized countries.

We might think that aiming for safety in healthcare is the prerogative of rich countries and advanced healthcare systems – that safety is a luxury poor people cannot afford. In fact the reverse may be true. When you have few

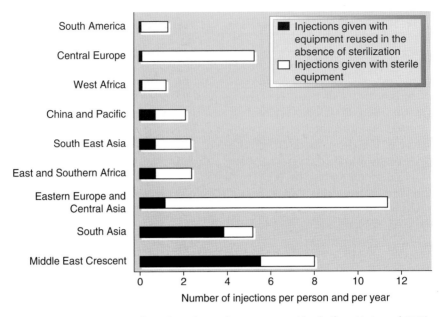

Fig. 3.2 Injections given with sterile and reused equipment worldwide (from Hutin et al 2003 British Medical Journal 327:1075, amended and reproduced with permission from the BMJ Publishing Group).

resources it is all the more important that you do not cause harm or waste those resources with poor-quality care. Those living in poverty with little healthcare available can least afford unsafe, low-quality care.

REFERENCES

Andrews LB, Stocking C, Krizek T et al 1997 An alternative strategy for studying adverse events in medical care. Lancet 349:309–313

Baker N, Tweedale C, Ellis CJ 2002 Adverse events with medical devices may go unreported. British Medical Journal 325:905

Baker GR, Norton PG, Flintoff V et al 2004 The Canadian adverse events study: the incidence of adverse events among hospital patients in Canada. Canadian Medical Association Journal 170:1678–1686

Bates DW, Cullen DJ, Laird N et al 1995 Incidence of adverse drug events and potential adverse drug events. Journal of the American Medical Association 274:29–34

Brennan TA, Leape LL, Laird NM et al 1991 Incidence of adverse events and negligence in hospitalized patients; results from the Harvard Medical Practice Study I. New England Journal of Medicine 324:370–376

Burke JP 2003 Infection control – a problem for patient safety. New England Journal of Medicine 348:651

Caplan RA, Posner KL, Ward RJ et al 1990 Adverse respiratory events in anesthesia: a closed claims analysis. Anesthesiology 72:828–833

Caplan RA, Posner KL, Cheney FW 1991 Effect of outcome on physicians' judgements of appropriateness of care. Journal of the American Medical Association 265, 1957–1960

Cheney FW 1999 The American Society of Anesthesiologists Closed Claims Project: what have we learned, how has it affected practice, and how will it affect practice in the future? Anesthesiology 91:552–556

Cook RI, Woods DD, Miller CA 1998 A tale of two stories: contrasting views of patient safety. US National Patient Safety Foundation, North Adams, MA. Online. Available at: http://www.npsf.org/exec/front.html

Croskerry P 2002 Achieving quality in clinical decision making: cognitive strategies and detection of bias. Academic Emergency Medicine 9:1184–1204

Davis P 2004 Health care as a risk factor. Canadian Medical Association Journal 170: 1688–1689

Davis P, Lay-Yee R, Briant R et al 2002 Adverse events in New Zealand public hospitals I: occurrence and impact. New Zealand Medical Journal 115:U271

Dean B, Schachter M, Vincent C et al 2002 Prescribing errors in hospital inpatients: their incidence and clinical significance. Quality and Safety in Health Care 11:340–344

Department of Health (DoH) 2000 An organisation with a memory: learning from adverse events in the NHS. The Stationery Office, London

Ennis M, Vincent CA 1990 Obstetric accidents: a review of 64 cases. British Medical Journal 300:1365–1367

Forster AJ, Murff HJ, Peterson JF et al 2003 The incidence and severity of adverse events affecting patients after discharge from the hospital. Annals of Internal Medicine 138:161–167

Gandhi TK, Weingart SN, Borus J et al 2003 Adverse drug events in ambulatory care. New England Journal of Medicine 348:1556–1564

Gawande A, Thomas EJ, Zinner MJ et al 1999 The incidence and nature of surgical adverse events in Utah and Colorado in 1992. Surgery 126:66–75

Gawande A, Studdert DM, Orav EJ et al 2003 Risk factors for retained instruments and sponges after surgery. New England Journal of Medicine 348:229–235

Harper Mills D, von Bolschwing GE 1995 Clinical risk management. Experiences from the United States. In: Vincent C (ed) Clinical risk management, 1st edn. BMJ Publications, London

Hayward RA Hofer TP 2001 Estimating hospital deaths due to medical errors. Journal of the American Medical Association 286:415–420

Hodgetts TJ, Kenward G, Vlackonikolis I et al 2002 Incidence, location and reasons for avoidable in-hospital cardiac arrest in a district general hospital. Resuscitation 54:115–123

Howard RL, Avery AJ, Howard PD et al 2003 Investigation into the reasons for preventable drug related admissions to a medical admissions unit: observational study. Quality and Safety in Healthcare 12:280–285

Hutin YJF, Hauri AM, Armstrong GL 2003 Use of injections in healthcare settings world-wide, 2000: literature review and regional estimates. British Medical Journal 327:1075

Kanjanarat P, Winterstein AG, Johns TE et al 2003 Nature of preventable adverse drug events in hospitals: a literature review. American Journal of Health System Pharmacy 60: 1750–1759

Kohn L, Corrigan J, Donaldson ME 1999 To err is human. National Academy Press, Washington DC

Leape LL 1994 Error in medicine. Journal of the American Medical Association 272:1851–1857

Leape LL 2000 Institute of Medicine medical error figures are not exaggerated. Journal of the American Medical Association 284: 95–97

Leape LL, Brennan TA, Laird N et al 1991 The nature of adverse events in hospitalized patients. Results of the Harvard Medical Practice Study II. The New England Journal of Medicine 324:377–384

Lee LA, Domino KB 2002 The Closed Claims Project. Has it influenced anesthetic practice and outcome? Anesthesiology Clinics of North America 20:247–263

Limat S, Drouhin JP, Demesmay K et al 2001 Incidence and risk factors of preparation errors in a centralized cytotoxic preparation unit. Pharmacy World and Science 23:102–106

McDonald CJ, Weiner M, Hui SL 2000 Deaths due to medical errors are exaggerated in Institute of Medicine report. Journal of the American Medical Association 284:93–95

McGlynn EA, Asch SM, Adams J et al 2003 The quality of health care delivered to adults in the United States. New England Journal of Medicine 348:2635–2645

Michel P, Quenon JL, de Sarasqueta AM et al 2004 Comparison of three methods for estimating rates of adverse events and rates of preventable adverse events in acute care hospitals. British Medical Journal 328:199

Neale G 1998 Reducing risks in gastroenterological practice. Gut 42: 139–142

Neale G, Woloshynowych M 2003 Retrospective case record review: a blunt instrument that needs sharpening. Quality and Safety in Health Care 12:2–3

Neale G, Woloshynowych M, Vincent CA 2001 Exploring the causes of adverse events in NHS hospital practice. Journal of the Royal Society of Medicine 94:322–330

Robinson AR, Hohmann KB, Rifkin JI et al 2002 Physician and public opinions on quality of health care and the problem of medical errors. Archives of Internal Medicine 162:2186–2190

Schioler T, Lipczak H, Pedersen BL et al 2001 Danish adverse event study. Incidence of adverse events in hospitals. A retrospective study of medical records. Ugeskr Laeger 163:1585–1586

Taxis K, Barber N 2003 Ethnographic study of incidence and severity of intravenous drug errors. British Medical Journal 326:684

Thomas EJ, Brennan T 2001 Errors and adverse events in medicine: an overview. In: Vincent C (ed) Clinical risk management. Enhancing patient safety, 2nd edn. BMJ Publications, London

Thomas EJ, Petersen LA 2003 Measuring errors and adverse events in health care. Journal of General Internal Medicine 18:61–67

Thomas EJ, Studdert DM, Runciman WB et al 2000 A comparison of iatrogenic injury studies in Australia and the USA 1: context, methods, case mix, population, patient and hospital characteristics. International Journal for Quality in Health Care 12:371–378

Vincent C 1993 The study of errors and accidents in medicine. In: Vincent C, Ennis E (eds) Medical accidents. Oxford University Press, Oxford

Vincent C 1997 Risk, safety and the dark side of quality. British Medical Journal 314:1775–1776

Vincent C 2003 Understanding and responding to adverse events. New England Journal of Medicine 348:1051–1056

Vincent C, Neale G, Woloshynowych M 2001 Adverse events in British hospitals: preliminary retrospective record review. British Medical Journal 322:517–519

Vincent C, Moorthy K, Sarker SK et al 2004 Systems approaches to surgical quality and safety: from concept to measurement. Annals of Surgery 239:475–482

Vincent J 2003 Nosocomial infections in adult intensive-care units. Lancet 361:2068–2077

Walshe K 2000 Adverse events in health care: issues in measurement. Quality in Health Care 9: 47–52

Walshe K 2003 International comparisons of the quality of health care: what do they tell us? Quality and Safety in Health Care 12:4–5

Wanzel KR, Jamieson CG, Bohnen JM 2000 Complications on a general surgery service: incidence and reporting. Canadian Journal of Surgery 4:113–117

Wiffen P, Gill M, Edwards J et al 2002 Adverse drug reactions in hospital patients. A systematic review of the prospective and retrospective studies. Bandolier Extra. Online. Available at: http://www.jr2.ox.ac.uk/bandolier/Extraforbando/ADRPM.pdf

Wilson T, Sheikh A 2002 Enhancing public safety in primary care. British Medical Journal 324:584–587

Wilson RM, Runciman WB, Gibber RW et al 1995 The Quality in Australian Health Care Study. Medical Journal of Australia 163:458–471

Winterstein AG, Sauer BC, Hepler CD et al 2002 Preventable drug-related hospital admissions. Annals of Pharmacotherapy 36:1238–1248

Woloshynowych M, Neale G, Vincent C 2003 Case record review of adverse events: a new approach. Quality and Safety in Health Care 12:411–415

World Health Organization (WHO) 2000 The World health report 2000: health systems, improving performance. WHO, Geneva

Reporting and learning systems

4

I never checked the pump setting. I just whacked the thing in when I was doing a few other things and I suddenly looked at this guy's blood pressure and went 'Holy God' and that was it. The sweat was pouring off me. He was absolutely fine, laying flat for a while but . . . I remember this battle-axe of a nursing officer coming up to me and she said to me 'Every nurse has made a mistake; how you feel is how everyone will feel when they've done it, but what have you learned from it?'

Reporting. A word with many shades of meaning and associations that range from the innocuous to the sinister. The school report, dreaded by many of us, prepared by an authority that, depending on your school days, might be benevolent, indifferent or malign. In the darker reaches of its meaning reporting has overtones of Big Brother, treachery and betrayal. Yet reporting is also communication; positive, informative and necessary: the reporting of events around the world in the news, the reports produced by organizations and governments to inform (or to obscure) and the simple telling of stories and recounting of events. The many types of reporting in healthcare have associations with all these meanings, which leads to much confusion and considerable suspicion of attempts to encourage reporting of errors, clinical incidents and safety issues.

Reporting in patient safety is, ideally, the communication of safety-relevant information. However, patient safety reporting is often confused, or at least tainted, with other forms of reporting and there are circumstances in which different forms of reporting might be invoked simultaneously. Confused? It's hardly surprising. Reporting systems in most healthcare systems lack cohesion and integration: there is frequent duplication of function, multiple systems in operation within any one institution and many different activities are lumped together under the general term 'reporting'. As a first step we will examine some of the different types of reporting as a necessary prelude to examining safety-reporting systems.

VARIETIES OF HEALTHCARE REPORTING SYSTEMS

Every healthcare system uses reporting systems of various kinds, and these have different purposes. To illustrate the principal types we will examine reporting systems in the British National Health Service (NHS) and some of the problems of the existing abundance of poorly integrated systems. As a national system, the NHS should, in principle, be able to develop a more rational system than, say, the US, with its hugely heterogeneous system of public and privately funded healthcare providers. However, reporting systems have mushroomed and, with the new interest in patient safety, no professional speciality or organization is complete without a reporting system (Box 4.1).

The agencies listed in the box have many responsibilities and in most cases receiving reports of one kind or another is only a small part of their function. Nevertheless, for the NHS to respond, or even remember, the agencies who might require reports is, to say the least, burdensome. In addition to the external agencies listed in the box, there are also a number of specialty reporting systems, such as that run by the Royal College of Anaesthetists and the local incident reporting and risk management systems run by most hospitals and healthcare organizations.

Investigation of serious incidents is a core function of some of the agencies, such as the coroner or the police. When circumstances are unusual or suspicious, perhaps criminal, the coroner might carry out an investigation, although the depth and sophistication of the investigation of healthcare incidents is variable. Investigations can also be carried out by Health Authorities or regulatory agencies such the Healthcare Commission. The Health and Safety Executive in the UK also acts as a regulator on safety matters, although

---

Box 4.1 Agencies requiring some form of report from NHS organizations

- Chief Medical Officer
- Coroner
- Counter-fraud and Security Agency
- Environmental Health Agency
- General Dental Council
- General Medical Council
- Health and Safety Executive
- Health Professions Council
- Health Protection Agency
- Healthcare Commission
- Medicines Healthcare Products Regulatory Agency
- National Clinical Assessment Authority
- National Patient Safety Agency
- NHS Estates
- NHS Information Authority
- NHS Litigation Authority
- Nursing and Midwifery Council
- Police
- Prison Health Service
- Purchasing and Supply Agency
- Royal Pharmaceutical Society
- Royal College of Nursing
- Sterilization and Embryology Authority
- Strategic Health Authorities

---

its focus is on the safety of staff, buildings and equipment; it has not yet extended its remit to the safety of clinical interventions. In the US, regulatory agencies also require reporting of certain types of events. For instance, the Joint Commission on Accreditation of Healthcare Organizations (JCAHO) both investigates and receives reports on serious 'sentinel events'. JCAHO, commendably, tries to extract as much learning as possible from these events but the comparatively low reporting rates suggest that this is perceived as primarily a regulatory exercise rather than an opportunity for learning.

Reporting is also relevant when there are doubts about the competence or behaviour of individual clinicians. Doctors in the UK have a duty to report any colleague who is endangering patients to the General Medical Council, and other professions have similar responsibilities. A small number of clinicians are indeed a danger, sometimes through recklessness or criminality, but more often because of lapsing skills, ill health or personal problems. Healthcare organizations are often slow to act on such problems, and slow to report, from loyalty to colleagues and an often misplaced confidence that 'things will sort themselves out'.

REPORTING FOR LEARNING

Some reporting systems have an explicit focus on learning. For instance, the British Yellow Card scheme, in operation since 1964, acts as a means for doctors, dentists, coroners and hospital pharmacists to report adverse drug reactions. Since 1964 more than 350,000 UK reports of suspected adverse reactions have been received. Reporting levels are quite consistent and there is good cooperation from health professionals. Facilities for electronic reporting are being introduced to improve the speed and ease of the process and help reduce under-reporting (DoH 2000).

The systems for learning in the British NHS, and indeed in many other countries, are fragmentary and unsystematic (Box 4.2). The establishment of the UK National Patient Safety Agency (NPSA) has brought more coordination of information about safety issues and harm and wider dissemination of the lessons from serious incidents, such as deaths from spinal injections. The NPSA was charged with setting up a national reporting and learning system; note the inclusion of the word learning, and the implication that reporting by itself is not sufficient to improve safety. Reporting for learning is also the

---

Box 4.2 Weaknesses in current NHS incident reporting systems

(from DoH 2000 p 54)

- No standardized, operational definition of incident.
- Coverage and sophistication of local incident reporting systems varies widely.
- Incident reporting in primary care is largely ignored.
- Regional incident reporting systems undoubtedly miss some serious incidents and take hardly any account of less serious incidents.
- No standardized approach to investigating serious incidents at any level.
- Current systems do not facilitate learning across the NHS as a whole.

rationale for many other reporting systems, particularly those run within clinical specialties. Local risk management systems can also have a learning focus but still primarily act as warnings of impending complaints and litigation, functions that often sit uneasily with patient safety initiatives. Before describing these systems, however, we will examine reporting systems outside healthcare to see how incident reporting and analysis is approached and what lessons have been learned over the years.

AVIATION, AEROSPACE AND NUCLEAR REPORTING AND LEARNING SYSTEMS

Safety-reporting systems that are learning oriented are well developed in some other industries, particularly aviation and the nuclear industry, although this has not always been the case. Captain Mike Holton describes the situation that led to the establishment of the British Airways Safety Information System (BASIS), a state of affairs that might be strangely familiar to many clinicians and managers in healthcare:

> In 1989 British Airways possessed 47 four-drawer filing cabinets full of the results of past investigations. Most of this paperwork had only historic value. An army of personnel would have been required if the files were to be comprehensively examined for trends or to produce useful analyses.
> **(DoH 2000 p 45)**

However, in the last 15 years there have been major advances in the way safety issues are reported and monitored. The Aviation Safety System (Box 4.3) operates internationally, linking regulatory oversight with company information systems. The system has five principal components, which combine to

---

Box 4.3 Components of the aviation safety system

(from DoH 2000 p 44)

- **Accident and serious incident investigations**, governed by the International Convention on International Civil Aviation (ICAO) Accident/Incident Data Reporting Programme (ADREP). ADREP includes provision for the international dissemination of investigation reports.
- **The Mandatory Occurrence Reporting Scheme (MORS)**, which provides a mechanism for notifying and reporting a range of adverse occurrences regardless of whether they result in an accident. MORS feeds into a database at national level for trend analysis and feedback to the industry.
- **The Confidential Human Factors Incident Reporting Programme (CHIRP)**, which is administered by an independent body and which provides sensitive follow-up and feedback on reports of human errors that have been rendered anonymous.
- **Company safety information systems**, such as British Airways' BASIS system, which record all levels of safety-related incidents. Information is shared on a peer basis within systems and staff report with an explicit reassurance that no individual will be pursued for an honest mistake.
- **Operational monitoring systems**, which proactively monitor crew competency through regular checks and review Flight Data Recorder information from every flight. There is management/union agreement on handling of any incidents or failures detected.

provide a means of detecting, analysing and acting on actual incidents and 'near misses' or other errors, along with proactive identification of issues that have the potential to pose a safety risk if left unchecked. These systems can respond very rapidly when the occasion demands.

The comparisons between healthcare and aviation are often over-stated but the experience of large-scale reporting systems in aviation has proved extremely instructive. Whereas the content of reports in aviation and health-care will obviously be very different, there is much common ground in respect of the principles of reporting and the culture, attitudes and behaviour that must be fostered if they are to be trusted and effective. Paul Barach and Stephen Small (2000) carried out a comprehensive review of systems outside medicine, including interviews with experts and directors of reporting sys-tems, to see what lessons they held for healthcare. Table 4.1 shows the main reporting systems they identified.

Most industrial reporting systems have a broad remit in that reporting of near misses, general safety issues and anything that worries the pilots or operators is encouraged. As can be seen from Fig. 4.1, the US National Aeronautics and Space Administration (NASA) is absolutely explicit that every member of staff has a responsibility to report a safety issue and equal-ly explicit about the responsibility of the person receiving the report to do something about it; every member of staff is empowered to go higher up the chain until he or she gets a response. (Ask yourself how this compares with your own working environment.) All the reporting systems give feedback in the form of regular reports on recent incidents and, crucially, actions taken to enhance safety; they might also give feedback to individuals who make reports. Near-miss reporting is vital because such incidents give warnings of potential catastrophes and enable proactive, preventive approaches to safety, while also bringing a constant reminder of the ever-present dangers in indus-tries that by any standard, are already very safe.

Mandatory or voluntary?

Some reporting systems are mandatory, in that reporting is compulsory, but many operate on a voluntary basis. This might seem odd when the lives of so many people are at stake. Surely, people should be compelled to report inci-dents? Charles Billings, who designed, tested and managed the Aviation Safety Reporting System over a period of 20 years, takes the view that how-ever you start, reporting always becomes voluntary in the end. This might be because of inertia on the part of the reporters, constraints such as shortage of time or because the hospital or staff decide that this particular incident falls outside the requirements because it is unusual in some respect or because of the fine print in the manual (Billings 1998). This is not simply cynicism. The point is that reporting systems, whether mandatory or voluntary, only really work if the people reporting are committed to the system. If they can see it is worthwhile, they will report, if not, then there are always reasons why this or that incident does not need to be reported.

In healthcare, there might be a case for mandatory reporting of some kinds of incidents, although the reasons for this concern accountability rather than

Table 4.1 Reporting systems in aviation and the nuclear industry

Industry	Reporting system	Ownership	Regu-latory	Mandatory/ voluntary	Anony-mous	Confi-dential	Narrative	Industry Immunity	Thres-hold	Feed-back
Aviation	Aviation safety reporting system	Federal. Administered by NASA	Yes	Voluntary	After filed	Yes	Yes	Yes	All non-accidents	Yes
Aviation	Aviation safety airways programme	American Airlines	No	Voluntary	No	Yes	Yes	No	All non-crashes	Yes
Aviation	Airline Pilots Association	Federal Aviation Authority with Pilot Association	No	Voluntary	No	Yes	Yes	No	All incidents	Yes
Aviation	Air safety report	British Airways	No	Mandatory	No	Yes	Yes	No	Safety related events	Yes

Aviation	Confidential human factors reporting programme	British Airways	No	Voluntary	Yes	Yes	No, but can expand	No	Human factors data	Yes
Aviation	Special event search and master analysis	British Airways	Yes	Mandatory	No	Yes	N/A	Yes	Monitors flight data recorder	Yes
Aerospace	NASA	Federal	Yes	Mandatory	No	Yes	Yes	No	All safety events	Yes
Nuclear	Human factors information system	Federal with private input	Yes	Voluntary	No	Yes	Yes	Yes	Human factors safety issues	Yes
Nuclear	NRC Allegations systems process	Federal	Yes	Voluntary	No	Yes	Yes	Yes	All safety concerns	Yes

(Adapted from Barach & Small 2000 British Medical Journal 320:759–763; amended and reproduced with permission from the BMJ Publishing Group).

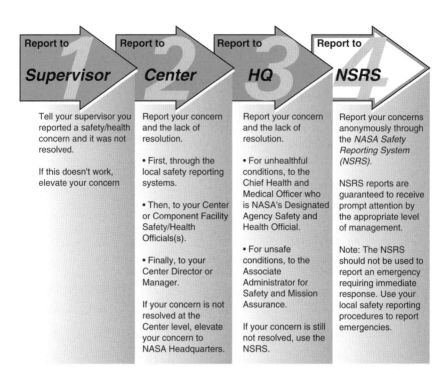

Fig. 4.1 The US National Aeronautics and Space Administration (NASA) hazard safety report (from NASA at: http://www.nasa.gov).

learning. The Institute of Medicine report (Kohn et al 1999), for instance, recommended that a nationwide mandatory reporting system be established for adverse events that involve death or serious harm. This is intended to parallel the mandatory system for reporting serious aviation accidents, which runs alongside the voluntary reporting of incidents where no harm is done. However, the report does stress that mandatory reporting to a regulatory body has other purposes apart from learning: such systems demonstrate the accountability of organizations for serious incidents, offer a minimum level of protection to the public and provide assurance that serious incidents are fully investigated. Most important such bodies have the power to impose changes across healthcare organizations where necessary.

Confidentiality and anonymity

Confidentiality is common to all the reporting systems and some care is taken, even in systems run by regulators, to separate reporting systems from disciplinary and performance management functions. Very few of the systems offer anonymous reporting though, which would seem to be an easy way of ensuring confidentiality. Why is this? Professionalism and accountability play a part. A professional ethic demands that pilots report safety-critical issues not only because they are obliged to but because it is seen as important and a core professional responsibility; seen from this perspective anonymity is not required. Anonymity of the reporter in any case carries a major disadvantage, which is that those running the system cannot go back for further information to clarify the story. As Table 4.1 shows, almost all systems encourage the reporting of a narrative – a story of what happened. Reporting that is restricted to basic factual details, as is often the case in healthcare, is not that useful because it reveals little about the causes of the incident. The narrative, the pilot's reflections and the subsequent review by an expert, often a retired pilot, bring a richness to reporting data that is its real value.

Counting, classification and getting the story

In healthcare, many risk managers submit monthly reports of numbers of incidents to various committees, clinicians and managers. Billings suggests (Box 4.4) that this, by itself, is largely a waste of time because reporting systems never capture the actual rate of incidents on the ground and it is as well to understand that from the start. The monthly graphs of incident counts produced by healthcare risk managers are largely uninformative, except as an index of the staff's willingness to report. Does that mean reporting is of no value? Not at all. It has a difference purpose, which is to alert people to the existence of a problem.

Much effort is also devoted in healthcare to defining the incidents that should be reported and devising classification systems to capture them. Of course, careful definition of some aspects of incidents is both feasible and desirable. But Billings cautions us that the real meaning of the incidents is apparent only in the narrative and will never be captured by classification alone. To make real sense of an incident you must have the story and, furthermore, the story must be interpreted by someone who knows the work and knows the context. The implication of this is that if healthcare incident reports

---

Box 4.4 Understanding incident reports: lessons from aviation

(Adapted from Billings 1998 p 55–56)

Counting incident reports is a waste of time. Why? Because incident reporting is inherently voluntary. Because the population from which the sample is drawn is unknown, and therefore can not be characterized, and because you lose too much information and gain too little in the process of condensing and indexing these reports unless you do what we were fortunate enough to do blindly, and that is to keep all the narratives.

Incident reports are unique and not easily classified or pigeonholed. Generalizations might be possible in retrospect, given enough detailed data and enough understanding of the data. But this requires understanding the details of the task, the context, the environment and its constraints, which can be appreciated only by those with relevant expertise. This is why you have to have experts looking at the reports. Simply constructing taxonomies is grossly insufficient.

Too many people have thought that incident reporting was the core and primary component of what was needed. These people thought that simply from the act of collecting incidents, solutions and fixes would be generated *sui generis* and that this would enhance safety. Although much is unclear about incident reporting systems, this one fact is quite clear: incident reporting is only one component of what you need.

---

are to be of real value they need to be reviewed by clinicians and, ideally, also by people who can tease out the human factors and organizational issues.

Incident reports are therefore only the first step; few problems are solved solely from the review of incidents reports. Analytical studies and other research remain critical to a full understanding of the problem. Following that, interventions and means of prevention need to be tested and trialled. Incident reporting is useful but is only one component of the whole safety process.

REPORTING SYSTEMS IN HEALTHCARE

Many countries already operate reporting systems for adverse effects of drugs, problems with medical devices, the safety of blood products and other issues. In response to concerns about patient safety, new reporting systems have been initiated, which are intended to cover a much wider range of adverse outcomes, errors and near misses. These might operate at local level (risk management systems in hospitals) or at national level (the National Patient Safety Agency). Sophisticated systems have also been established to investigate and understand a variety of specific issues, such as transfusion problems or safety in intensive care. Some of the more sophisticated systems now include an assessment of factors that cause or contribute to errors. We will review some reporting systems to illustrate how the different kinds of systems operate and what their respective purposes are.

Local reporting systems

The development of risk management in the US, UK and elsewhere led to the establishment of local incident reporting systems in hospitals. Typically, there is a standard incident form, asking for basic clinical details and a brief narrative describing the incident. Sometimes, staff are asked to report any incident that concerns them or might endanger a patient; in practice serious incidents are followed by an urgent telephone call to a trusted risk manager. In more sophisticated systems where staff within a unit may be trying to routinely monitor and address specific problems, there might be a designated list of incidents, although staff are free to report other issues that do not fall into these categories (Table 4.2). Notice that the incidents to be reported are not necessarily errors and that harm to the patient might be unavoidable or have natural causes (e.g. very low birth weight). However, they are all 'flags' of possible problems in the delivery of care and vehicles for reflection on clinical practice.

Local systems are ideally used as part of an overall safety and quality improvement strategy but, in practice, might be dominated by managing claims and complaints. There is sometimes a conflict between the risk management function and the broader patient safety function, at least in terms of time and resources. The risk management function is nevertheless an important one. Early warning of specific incidents allows the healthcare organization to investigate the problem rapidly, collect witness statements while

Table 4.2 Examples of designated clinical incidents to be reported

Type of incident		
Obstetric	**Paediatric**	**Mental health**
Infant	Extravasation of i.v. fluid leading to tissue necrosis	Over-dose taken by inpatient on unit or while on leave
Neonatal deaths and stillbirths		
Apgar score <4 at 5 min	Drug prescription or administration error	Deliberate self-harm by patient
Subdural haematoma		
Unanticipated admission to Special Care Baby Unit	Failure to recognize the severity of an infant's condition or to recognize a serious diagnosis	Discovery of an object in patient's possession that could be used for self-harm
Major abnormality first detected at birth		
Fracture or paralysis	Child protection procedures not followed	Discharge against medical advice by a patient detoxing from alcohol or drugs
Shoulder dystocia		
Meconium aspiration	Problems during transportation to a tertiary referral centre	Absconding from unit
Fits in nursery within first 48 h		Fire-setting in unit
Mother	Major organization problems during resuscitation	Unexpected or sudden death of patient
Maternal death		
Transfer to ITU		Serious physical assault or aggression
Convulsions	Failure to act on a pathology or imaging result	
Major anaesthetic problems		Discovery of illicit drugs/alcohol on unit
Postpartum haemorrhage > 1 litre	Equipment failure impeding medical provision	Injury of unknown origin
30-min delay in caesarean section		Drug error
Soft tissue injury, 3rd-degree tear	Unexpected death	
Ruptured uterus, bladder injury		
Drug errors		

recollection is fresh and secure the relevant medical records. Risk managers, at least the more proactive ones, often play a key role in communicating with injured patients, attending to their needs and maintaining a relationship with them at a time when they might, understandably, be distressed and angry.

Early warning of potential claims through incident reporting can facilitate the opening and closing of claims and produce substantial savings in time and legal costs. Incident reports also allow the organization to manage any subsequent media coverage in a proactive manner instead of being caught on the back foot. Hospitals usually operate a Claims and Incidents Review Committee, ideally led by the medical director or other board level figure, which monitors litigation and should also have the authority to institute changes in clinical practice when necessary.

These basic reporting systems will hopefully evolve over time to have a stronger emphasis on patient safety, while still fulfilling a risk management function. Paper-based systems will give way to electronic or web-based systems. When a national system is being established, as in the UK, standardization of reporting forms and approaches should simplify systems, make the

Reporting and learning systems

process less haphazard and embed reporting more firmly in both organizations and healthcare culture.

SPECIALTY REPORTING SYSTEMS

Many different clinical specialities, particularly anaesthesia, have established reporting systems to assist them in improving clinical practice. These systems are designed to provide information on specific clinical issues, which can be shared within the professional group. As an example, we will look at Peter Pronovost and Albert Wu's Intensive Care Reporting System (ICU-SRS; Wu et al 2002), which is based in Johns Hopkins University in the US. ICU-SRS is based in part on the AIMS-ICU study (Beckmann et al 1996), which is in turn derived from the Australian Incident Monitoring System (AIMS) which is discussed below.

ICU-SRS is a web-based safety reporting system that examines clinical issues but also has a strong focus on contributory factors, incorporating a framework of factors developed for the analysis of clinical incidents (see Chapter 5). The explicit goal of ICU-SRS is to identify high-risk situations so that providers and risk managers can adjust the clinical processes and systems to reduce the risk of error. Reports are analysed and feedback given to the 30 participating units on a regular basis. Each ICU has a designated physician and nurse as leads on the project to ensure local ownership and clear lines of communication.

The web-based form elicits a narrative description of the incident, contextual information about the patient and staff, factors that contribute to incidents and measures that might be taken to prevent similar incidents in the future. The structure of the web-based form, with pull-down menus, means that staff have to complete only those sections that are strictly relevant to the incident in question. Staff use check boxes to describe information relating to the incident, such as patient demographics, location of the incident, degree of harm, and system factors that might have contributed to or prevented the incident, or mitigated the resulting harm. System factors include the availability of adequate equipment, factors in the physical environment, work practices, policies and protocols, communication and team issues. To evaluate types of harm, incidents are classified according to whether the patient died, suffered physiological changes, physical injury, psychological distress, discomfort, dissatisfaction, anticipated or actual increased length of stay. All incident reports are anonymous to patient and provider. It is voluntary whether the reporter identifies his or her ICU.

An initial analysis of 250 cases from 15 of the ICUs revealed that an average of about three incidents a month were reported from each ICU; most did not lead to harm but some involved the death of a patient or a prolonged stay. The system places great emphasis on identifying factors that contributed to the incidents reported; the two most frequently identified were excessive workload and inadequate communication. Whereas high workload might seem to be a natural response from busy nurses and doctors, the finding turned out to have serious implications for safety. In subsequent empirical studies, Pronovost and colleagues showed that workload was clearly related to quality of care and to patient morbidity (Pronovost et al 1999).

The other major problem was communication, specifically missing or mis-heard messages when staff were under pressure. The units are now experimenting with a 'check-back' system in which important messages are repeated back to ensure correct communication; this simple, resource-neutral solution is proving very effective. Wu et al (2002) emphasize that many of these safety initiatives emerged directly from a careful analysis of the reports from their system. They suggest that, in time, specialty systems such as their own must be integrated with other reporting systems, such as risk management, State or national systems, to minimize duplication of effort and reduce the burden on the staff.

NATIONAL AND OTHER LARGE SCALE SYSTEMS

National and other large-scale systems are expensive to run and tend to have the disadvantage of being entirely reliant on the written reports, perhaps supplemented by telephone checking. On the positive side their sheer scale gives a wealth of data, and their particular power is in picking up events that might be rare at a local level, with patterns of incident only appearing at national level. The British National Patient Safety Agency's 'National Reporting and Learning System' is as yet the only truly national system but the Veterans Affairs system in the US is very wide ranging, as is the Australian AIMS system. Many other countries are either in the process of setting up large-scale reporting systems or considering doing so. Here we will examine the AIMS system, the grandfather of all large-scale systems in healthcare.

Australian Incident Monitoring System (AIMS)

The pioneer of large-scale reporting systems in healthcare is undoubtedly Bill Runciman who, in addition to developing the Australian Incident Monitoring System (AIMS) and publishing widely, finds time to run the intensive care unit in Adelaide, which covers an area reaching from the Southern Australian coast up to Sumatra. AIMS provides a mechanism for reporting healthcare incidents of any kind using a single, standard form, either paper- or web-based. A classification has been established that allows information from various sources (such as coroners' recommendations, complaints, claims and incident reports) to be entered into the system. AIMS was introduced in 1996 but it derives from an incident-monitoring study in anaesthesia (AIMS-Anaesthesia) that began in 1988 (Beckmann et al 1996). AIMS has been implemented in several Australian states, as well as individual health units.

Incident information is collected on a form, which asks for specific information about the patient, a description of the incident and contributory factors; there are prompting questions on the type of incident and the possible contributory factors the reporter might consider. Management action taken on the incident is also recorded, although this is not a requirement of the report. The coding of the information provides the means for understanding the underlying causes of the incident and for analysing the contributing factors.

AIMS has led to an impressive number of publications, over 100 in peer-reviewed academic and medical journals. The majority are in anaesthetics, with additional studies carried out in family practice, psychiatry, intensive care and obstetrics. Results usually provide a description of clinical material, a classification of different types of error and a consideration of the causes of error. As an example, consider a review of 2000 anaesthesia incident reports involving circuit disconnection, oesophageal intubation, aspiration, regurgitation, severe hypotension, failure of oxygen delivery, hypoxic gas mixture and other problems all threatening to the patient's oxygen supply (Runciman et al 1993). About half of these incidents were first detected by staff, and about half by monitors. Careful review of these incidents suggested that a pulse oximeter was not in use during the majority of these incidents but would have detected over 80% of them and would have generally prevented any serious organ damage. The paper argues strongly for routine use of pulse oximetry (Runciman et al 1993).

The UK has recently seen the launch of the National Reporting and Learning system (Katikreddi 2004), which collects reports of patient safety incidents of all kinds from health professionals in England and Wales. To begin with, the system will mostly extract data from local risk management systems, gradually harmonizing the approach to incident reporting across the NHS. However, staff will also be able to report directly, if they prefer, through the web and other means. The aim is to steadily increase the number of reports and, in time, to see a reduction in incidents that lead to harm; the system has been piloted, with considerable success, but, at the time of writing, no results are available from the main system.

DO HEALTHCARE REPORTING SYSTEMS REFLECT THE UNDERLYING RATE OF INCIDENTS?

There is a great deal of confusion about the relationship between errors, adverse events and incidents that are reported. Risk managers, knowing that about 10% of patients admitted to hospital suffer adverse events, sometimes assess the success of their reporting systems on the basis of whether the number of reports they have equates to 10% of admissions. If it does, so the logic goes, they are capturing all the relevant incidents. This approach is seriously misguided. To begin with, all adverse events by definition involve patient harm or additional time in hospital; by contrast, most reported incidents do not involve harm but concern more general safety issues such as equipment problems. Some incidents will also be adverse events but most will not. To compound the problem, the extent and nature of what is reported varies widely according to the incident in question, the nature of the reporting system, the culture of the institution, how easy it is to report, the incentives or disincentives and other factors. Rates of reporting vary widely, as can be seen in Table 4.3, which illustrates the reporting of adverse drug event rates (Leape 1997). As the table shows, there can be a 50-fold difference between rates of reporting of adverse drug events depending on method and context. The table and rates are not definitive in any sense, and apply only to adverse drug

Table 4.3 Rates of detection of adverse drug events	
Method for detection	**Event rate (%)**
Self-reporting (voluntary)	0.2
Population record review	0.7
Computer screening	3.8
Chart review and stimulated report	6.5
Combination chart and computer	10.0
Adapted from Leape 1997	

reactions, although they do illustrate the general point that reported incidents usually provide only a very incomplete reflection of actual incidents. As was said earlier, reporting is not a good way of counting.

Can reporting be improved with sufficient dedicated staff and resources? After all most healthcare staff are under pressure and cannot spare time to report routine, and possibly frequently occurring, minor incidents. Nicola Stanhope and colleagues examined the reliability of adverse incident reporting systems in two obstetric units, each of which had dedicated risk managers who were also trained midwives. In addition to reporting systems, the risk managers would proactively check for incidents by visiting the wards and attending meetings, in an effort to produce complete data on a designated list of reportable incidents. A retrospective review of the obstetric notes, 500 deliveries in all, identified 196 incidents. Staff had reported 23% of these and the risk managers identified a further 22%. The remaining 55% of incidents were identified only by retrospective case note review and were not known to the risk manager. Staff were more likely to report serious incidents but the risk managers identified an additional 16% of serious incidents that staff did not report. Even with a dedicated person receiving reports and actively seeking out incidents, reporting does not reveal the full range of designated incidents (Stanhope et al 1999). Does this matter? Not necessarily. As long as the system receives sufficient reports to identify the main safety issues the absolute number of reports is not critical; however, to achieve this staff do have to be encouraged to report and to communicate their concerns.

Barriers to reporting

As we have seen errors, adverse events and incidents of all kinds are common, but reporting rates are low. Why is this? Admittedly it might not be necessary to report all incidents, or even the majority of them, but a higher flow of information on safety issues would undoubtedly assist the identification of potential problems. Nicola Stanhope and colleagues (1999) examined this question in a survey of 42 obstetricians and 142 midwives. On the two units concerned there were lists of specific incidents to report but a number of staff, particularly temporary nurses, did not know how to report. Even with a list of designated incidents, staff made their own assessments about whether to report, either because the event was not preventable (i.e. practice was of a good standard) or because there was no possibility of a complaint or claim.

Box 4.5 Obstetricians and midwives reasons for not reporting incidents

(adapted from Stanhope et al 1999)

- The circumstances or outcome of the case often make reporting unnecessary
- Increases workload
- Junior staff are often unfairly blamed for adverse incidents
- When the ward is busy I forget to make a report
- I am worried about litigation
- My colleagues might be unsupportive
- I do not know which incidents should be reported
- As long as staff learn from incidents it is unnecessary to discuss them further
- I am worried about disciplinary action
- I do not want the case discussed in meetings
- I do not know whose responsibility it is to make a report
- Incident reporting makes little contribution to the quality of care

Box 4.6 No action and no feedback, means no more reports

(adapted from Firth-Cozens et al 2004)

'These things go on for months and months before anything is done . . . This creates a feeling of apathy, that there is no point in filling in a needle-stick injury form or a blood splash form.'
'I've worked in three different ITUs and this [confusion of different dose infusion pumps] has happened in all three . . . I've suggested several times that they shouldn't be stored right next to each other but they're still stored together. And the error still happens.'
'They don't take action. They just listen to us, file it and tell me why the hospital cannot address the problem.'

This suggested in turn that there was considerable confusion about the purpose of incident reporting. Staff were also given a list of possible reasons for not reporting, which they ranked individually. Box 4.5 shows the reasons in order of importance and Box 4.6 some illustrative quotes from a later study (Firth-Cozens et al 2004). A lack of feedback, and a belief that nothing will be done in response to reporting, are major concerns.

Box 4.7 Encouraging incident reporting and learning

(adapted from Firth-Cozens 2002 and DoH 2000)

- Systems and mechanisms to make error-reporting easy and fast
- Clarifying the meaning of reportable error and incidents
- Time for multidisciplinary discussion of individual and accumulated error
- Feedback to individuals and the reporting community
- A working assumption that those who report should be thanked, rather than automatically blamed if something has gone wrong
- Providing support and understanding for those who have made errors
- Treating error and incidents consistently across organizations and professional groups
- Appropriate discretion in terms of nursing procedures and policy
- Providing training for clinicians on the management of risk and safety
- Having 'shop floor' staff on safety policy committees
- Ensuring reporting is followed by appropriate action

As Lucian Leape commented in an editorial accompanying these papers, many of the reasons for not reporting are grounded in fear and guilt: fear of embarrassment, punishment by oneself or others, and fear of litigation (Leape 1999). In a more recent survey, almost all American physicians reported that fear of litigation was a major barrier to reporting (Robinson et al 2002). Junior staff felt these problems particularly acutely and it is clear that if incident reporting is going to be effective, whether at local or national level, considerable effort must be expended in reassuring staff that the purpose is enhancing safety not blame or discipline. One of the key aims of an 'open and fair culture' is to increase reporting and open discussion of safety issues (Box 4.7).

REPORTING, SURVEILLANCE AND BEYOND

Reporting, whether voluntary or mandatory, is an attractive option because it is a relatively inexpensive method of detection. Nevertheless, as a data source it is unreliable, erratic and could never qualify as a measure of errors or adverse events, however defined. Reflecting on the enthusiasm for reporting, and the vast amounts of money poured into it (Vincent 2004), it is hard to see why such faith has been placed in establishing reporting systems and why anyone ever thought that reports could provide a good picture of the overall nature and scale of harm. In no other area of medicine could voluntary reporting ever be regarded as a substitute for systematic data collection. One reason perhaps, is that it seemed as if aviation and other industries were using reporting to establish rates of serious incidents. In fact, aviation had already established the epidemiology of harm, in the form of comprehensive accident databases; reporting was always a supplement to systematic data collection, a complementary activity providing warnings and additional safety information.

Reporting will always be important but has probably been overemphasized as a means of enhancing safety. In the future, we should see information on error and harm collected from a wider range of sources, and hopefully a move towards active surveillance of salient events, as discussed in Chapter 3. When the move to electronic medical records is achieved, records could be searched using data mining techniques to identify problems and detect patterns. These searches would not necessarily be able to detect specific kinds of errors or adverse events but could certainly identify records with a high probability of such an event. Much further work needs to be done on improving the performance and detection rates of such systems, in expanding them to a wider range of adverse outcomes and in testing their use in different settings. Nevertheless, if such routine monitoring could be developed, patient safety initiatives could be much more proactive in character, with adverse events and patient outcomes being monitored in near real time (Bates & Gawande 2003). If this could be done, we would be less reliant on reporting, although it would still have value for the unusual cases or those not monitored routinely.

In summary, reporting systems can provide warnings, point to important problems and provide some understanding of causes. They serve an important function in raising awareness and generating a culture of safety, as well

Reporting and learning systems

as in providing data. However, the results of reporting are often misunderstood in that they are mistakenly held to be a true reflection of the underlying rate of errors and adverse events. The reality is that rates of reporting vary widely; this does not necessarily affect the usefulness of the systems as long as it is clearly understood. Incident reports in themselves are primarily flags and warnings of a problem area, but then they must be analysed and understood which is the subject of the next two chapters.

REFERENCES

Barach P, Small SD 2000 Reporting and preventing medical mishaps: lessons from non-medical near miss reporting systems. British Medical Journal 320:759–763

Bates DW, Gawande AA 2003 Improving safety with information technology. New England Journal of Medicine 348:2526

Beckmann U, West LF, Groombridge GJ et al 1996 The Australian Incident Monitoring Study in Intensive Care: AIMS-ICU. The development and evaluation of an incident reporting system in intensive care. Anaesthesia and Intensive Care 24:314–319

Billings C 1998 Incident reporting systems in medicine and experience with the aviation reporting system. In: Cook RI, Woods DD, Miller CA (eds) A tale of two stories: contrasting views of patient safety. US National Patient Safety Foundation, North Adams, MA. Online. Available at: http://www.npsf.org/exec/front.html

Department of Health (DoH) 2000 An organization with a memory: learning from adverse events in the NHS. The Stationery Office, London

Firth-Cozens J 2002 Barriers to incident reporting. Quality and Safety in Health Care 11:7

Firth-Cozens J, Redfern N, Moss F 2004 Confronting errors in patient care: the experiences of doctors and nurses. Clinical Risk 10:184–190

Katikireddi V 2004 National reporting system for medical errors is launched. British Medical Journal 328:481

Kohn L, Corrigan J, Donaldson ME 1999 To err is human. National Academy Press, Washington, DC

Leape L 1997 A systems analysis approach to medical error. Journal of Evaluation in Clinical Practice 3:213–222

Leape LL 1999 Why should we report adverse incidents? Journal of Evaluation in Clinical Practice 5:1–4

Pronovost PJ, Jenckes MW, Dorman T et al 1999 Organizational characteristics of intensive care units related to outcomes of abdominal aortic surgery. Journal of the American Medical Association 281:1310–1307

Robinson AR, Hohmann KB, Rifkin JI et al 2002 Physician and public opinions on quality of health care and the problem of medical errors. Archives of Internal Medicine 162:2186–2190

Runciman WB, Webb RK, Barker L et al 1993 The Australian Incident Monitoring Study. The pulse oximeter: applications and limitations – an analysis of 2000 incident reports. Anaesthesia and Intensive Care 21:543–550

Stanhope N, Crowley-Murphy M, Vincent C et al 1999 An evaluation of adverse incident reporting. Journal of Evaluation in Clinical Practice 5:5–12

Vincent C 2004 Analysis of clinical incidents: a window on the system not a search for root causes. Quality & Safety in Health Care 13:242–243

Wu AW, Provonost P, Morlock L 2002 ICU incident reporting systems. Journal of Critical Care 17:86–94

Human error and systems thinking

I kept my tea in the right hand side of a tea caddy for some months and when that was finished kept it in the left, but I always for a week took off the cover of the right hand side, though my hand would sometimes vibrate. Seeing no tea brought back memory.
(Charles Darwin, from his *Notebooks*, quoted in Browne 2003 p 383)

Rather than being the instigators of an accident, operators tend to be the inheritors of system defects . . . their part is usually that of adding the final garnish to a lethal brew whose ingredients have already been long in the cooking.
(Reason 1990 p 173)

Human error is routinely blamed for accidents in the air, on the railways, in complex surgery and in healthcare generally. Immediately after an incident people make quick judgements and, all too often, blame the person most obviously associated with the disaster. The pilot of the plane, the doctor who gives the injection, the train driver who passes a red light are quickly singled out. However, these quick judgements and routine assignment of blame prevent us uncovering the second story (Cook et al 1998). This is the story in its full richness and complexity, which only emerges after thoughtful and careful inquiry. Whereas a particular action or omission might be the immediate cause of an incident, closer analysis usually reveals a series of events and departures from safe practice, each influenced by the working environment and the wider organizational context (Vincent et al 1998).

This chapter and the next explore the themes of human error, systems thinking and the analysis of accidents and disaster. This chapter is somewhat more conceptual; the next chapter more practical but, as with medicine itself, until you have the concepts the practice will elude you. We begin by examining the lessons of major accidents, which will bring out the themes to be covered in the two chapters. We then examine the difficult topic of human error, addressing the concept and definitions, the nature of medical error, the psychology of error and the different ways error can be managed.

THE LESSONS OF MAJOR ACCIDENTS

Our understanding of how the events preceding a disaster unfold has been greatly enhanced in the last 20 years by the careful examination of a number of high profile accidents (Boxes 5.1 and 5.2). The brief summaries of major accidents, and the account of the Columbia Space Shuttle accident, allow us to reflect on the many ways in which failure can occur and the complexity of the story that can unfold during a serious investigation. Human beings have the opportunity to contribute to an accident at many different points in the process of production and operation. Problems and failures might occur in the design, testing, implementation of a new system, its maintenance and operation. Technical failures, important though they can be, often play a relatively minor part. Looking at other industries, although they are often very different from healthcare, helps us understand the conceptual landscape and some of the practicalities of accident investigation.

The most obvious errors and failures are usually those that are the immediate causes of an accident, such as a train driver going through a red light or a doctor picking up the wrong syringe and injecting a fatal drug. These failures are mostly unintentional, although occasionally they are deliberate, but misguided, attempts to retrieve a dangerous situation. Some of the 'violations of procedure' at Chernobyl were in fact attempts to use unorthodox methods

---

Box 5.1 Major disasters involving human error

(adapted from Lucas 1997)

Chernobyl (April 1986)
Chernobyl's 1000 MW reactor no. 4 exploded, releasing radioactivity over much of Europe. Although much debated since the accident, a Soviet investigation team admitted 'deliberate, systematic and numerous violations' of safety procedures.

Piper Alpha (1988)
A major explosion on an oil rig, resulting in a fire and the deaths of 167 people. The Cullen enquiry (1990) found a host of technical and organizational causes rooted in the culture, structure and procedures of Occidental Petroleum. The maintenance error that led to the initial leak was the result of inexperience, poor maintenance procedures and deficient learning mechanisms.

Space Shuttle Challenger (January 1986)
An explosion shortly after lift-off killed all the astronauts on board. An 'O ring' seal on one of the solid rocket boosters split after take off, releasing a jet of ignited fuel. The causes of the defective O-ring involved a rigid organizational mindset, conflicts between safety and keeping on schedule, and the effects of fatigue on decision making.

Herald of Free Enterprise (March 1987)
The roll-on-roll-off ferry sank in shallow water off Zeebruge, Belgium, killing 189 passengers and crew. The inquiry highlighted the commercial pressures in the ferry business and the friction between ship and shore management that led to safety lessons not being heeded. The company was found to be 'infected with the disease of sloppiness'.

Paddington rail accident (October 1999)
31 people died when a train went through a red light onto the main 'up line' from Paddington, where it collided head-on with an express train that was approaching the station. The inquiry identified failures in training of drivers, a serious and persistent failure to examine reported poor signal visibility, a safety culture that was slack and less than adequate and significant failures of communication in the various organizations.

Box 5.2 The Loss of Space Shuttle Columbia

(adapted from the US National Aeronautics and Space Administration 2003)

The Columbia Accident Investigation Board's independent investigation into the loss of the Space Shuttle Columbia and its seven-member crew lasted nearly 7 months. A staff of more than 120, along with some 400 NASA engineers supported the Board's 13 members. Investigators examined more than 30,000 documents, conducted more than 200 formal interviews, heard testimony from dozens of expert witnesses, and reviewed more than 3000 inputs from the general public. In addition, more than 25,000 searchers combed vast stretches of the Western US to retrieve the spacecrafts debris. The Board recognized early on that the accident was probably not an anomalous, random event, but likely to be rooted to some degree in NASA's history and the culture of the human space flight programme. The Board's conviction regarding the importance of these factors strengthened as the investigation progressed, with the result that this report placed as much weight on these causal factors as on the more easily understood and corrected physical cause of the accident.

The physical cause of the loss of Columbia and its crew was a breach in the thermal protection system on the leading edge of the left wing, caused by a piece of insulating foam, which separated from the external tank 81.7 seconds after launch and struck the wing. During re-entry, this breach in the thermal protection system allowed superheated air to penetrate the leading edge insulation and progressively melt the aluminium structure of the left wing, resulting in a weakening of the structure until increasing aerodynamic forces caused loss of control, failure of the wing and break-up of the orbiter.

The organizational causes of this accident are rooted in the Space Shuttle programme's history and culture, including the original compromises that were required to gain approval for the Shuttle, subsequent years of resource constraints, fluctuating priorities, schedule pressures, mischaracterization of the Shuttle as operational rather than developmental, and lack of an agreed national vision for human space flight. Cultural traits and organizational practices detrimental to safety were allowed to develop, including: reliance on past success as a substitute for sound engineering practices; organizational barriers that prevented effective communication of critical safety information and stifled professional differences of opinion; lack of integrated management across programme elements; and the evolution of an informal chain of command and decision-making processes that operated outside the organization's rules.

Although the report does not provide a detailed organizational prescription, it discusses the attributes of an organization that could more safely and reliably operate the inherently risky Space Shuttle. Among those attributes are: a robust and independent programme technical authority that has complete control over specifications and requirements; an independent safety-assurance organization with line authority over all levels of safety oversight; and an organizational culture that reflects the best characteristics of a learning organization.

Human error and systems thinking

to prevent disaster. Attempts to control an escalating crisis can make matters worse, as when police officers believed they needed to contain rioting football fans who were in fact trying to escape from a fire. Problems can also occur in the management of escape and emergency procedures, as when train passengers were unable to escape from carriages after the Paddington crash.

The immediate causes described above are the result of actions, or omissions, by people at the scene. However, other factors further back in the causal chain can also play a part in the genesis of an accident. These 'latent conditions' as they are often termed, lay the foundations for accidents in the sense that they create the conditions in which errors and failures can occur (Reason 1997). The accidents described allude to poor training, problems with scheduling, conflicts between safety and profit, communication failures, failure to address known safety problems and to general sloppiness of management and procedures.

Some of these failures might have been known at the time, in that communication failures between management and supervisors may have been a long-standing and obvious problem. However, latent conditions can also be created by decisions that might have been perfectly reasonable at the time but are felt in retrospect to have contributed to an accident. For instance, the training budget for maintenance workers might have been cut to avoid staff redundancies. In any organization there are always pressures to reduce training, eliminate waste, act quickly to keep on schedule and so on. Safety margins are eroded bit by bit, sometimes without anyone noticing, eventually leading to an accident.

Another feature of these explanations for accidents, especially the more recent ones, are the references to safety culture and organizational culture. The safety culture of a train company, for instance, is described as 'slack and less than adequate'. The Columbia investigation refers to a number of 'cultural traits and organizational practices detrimental to safety', such as reliance on past success rather than formal testing, barriers to passing on safety information, stifling of dissenting voices and informal decisions that bypassed organizational rules and procedures. These are all, broadly speaking, cultural, in that they refer to or are embedded in the norms, attitudes and values of the organizations concerned.

Safety culture is hard to define precisely but can become more tangible when one reflects on one's own experience of organizations. In some hospital wards, for instance, the atmosphere might be friendly and cheerful but it is clear that there is little tolerance for poor practice and the staff are uniformly conscientious and careful. By contrast, others develop a kind of subculture in which sloppy practices are tolerated, risks are run and potentially dangerous practices are allowed to develop. These cultural patterns develop slowly but erode safety and morale. Sometimes these features of the ward or organization are ascribed to the personalities of the people working there, who are viewed as slapdash, careless and unprofessional. The use of the term 'culture', however, points to the powerful influence of social forces in moulding behaviour; we are all more malleable than we like to think and to some extent develop good or bad habits according to the prevailing ethos around us.

We should also note that major accidents in high-hazard industries are often the stimulus for wide-ranging safety improvements. For instance, the enquiry into the Piper Alpha oil disaster led to a host of recommendations and the implementation of a number of risk-reduction strategies, which covered the whole industry and addressed a wide range of issues. These included the setting-up of a single regulatory body for offshore safety, relocation of pipeline emergency shutdown valves, the provision of temporary safe refuges for oil workers, new evacuation procedures and requirements for emergency safety training (Vincent et al 1998). In healthcare, the process of systematic learning from accidents, as opposed to personal reflection by individual clinicians, is a relatively recent phenomenon but, fortunately, gaining ground. Safety needs to be addressed proactively as well of course. The investigation of minor incidents, 'free lessons' as they are sometimes called, and the direct assessment of safety culture and procedures are vital.

Finally, consider the resources that have been put into understanding these accidents. In the case of Columbia, hundreds of people were involved in intense investigation of all aspects of NASA's functioning. Certainly these accidents were all tragedies; many people died unnecessarily, there was a great deal at stake for the organizations concerned and enormous political and media pressures to contend with. Unnecessary deaths in healthcare, in comparison, receive relatively little attention and are only occasionally the subject of major enquiries. Large sums of money are spent on the roads and railways on safety measures, again relatively little in health. Patient safety is, thankfully for staff and patients alike, now firmly on the healthcare agenda in many countries. But the resources for keeping patients safe are still pretty minimal.

IS HEALTHCARE LIKE OTHER INDUSTRIES?

Aviation, nuclear power, chemical and petroleum industries are, like healthcare, hazardous activities carried out in large, complex organizations by, for the most part, dedicated and highly trained people. Commercial, political, social and humanitarian pressures have compelled these industries to raise their game and make sustained efforts to improve and maintain safety. Healthcare, by contrast, has relied on the intrinsic motivation and professionalism of clinical and managerial staff, which, while vital, is not sufficient to ensure safety. Studying other industries helps us realize that a range of other factors also need to be considered and might even allow us to discern the general properties of safe, or unsafe, organizations. We might also consider adapting specific industrial procedures and practices, whether for the analysis of error and harm or techniques for making processes safer. However, the most important lesson might be less the specific safety practices and more a matter of motivation and inspiration. Hearing other people working in dangerous environments talk about how they treat safety as something to be discussed, analysed, managed and resourced tells us that safety is not just a byproduct of people doing their best but a far more complex and elusive phenomenon.

We should, however, be cautious about drawing parallels between healthcare and other industries. The high technology monitoring and vigilance of anaesthetists and the work of pilots in commercial aviation are similar in some respects, but the work of surgeons and pilots is very different. Emergency medicine might find better models and parallels in the military or in fire fighting than in aviation. The easy equation of the work of doctors and pilots has certainly been over-stated, even though many useful ideas and practices have transferred from aviation to medicine. For instance, simulation and team training in anaesthesia and other specialties was strongly influenced by crew resource management in aviation. The idea that team training is crucial to the management of error and to safe operation transfers well. However, in developing training for surgical teams, our group has found that we have to take full account of the particular tasks and challenges faced by surgical teams. We cannot just import aviation team training wholesale. Aviation acts as a motivator and source of ideas but the actual training has to be developed and tested within the healthcare setting.

Differences between healthcare and other industries

What differences can be identified between healthcare and other industries? First, healthcare encompasses an extraordinarily diverse set of activities: it encompasses the mostly routine, but sometimes highly unpredictable and hazardous world of surgery; primary care, where patients can have relationships with their doctors over many years; the treatment of acute psychosis, requiring rapid response and considerable tolerance of bizarre behaviour; some highly organized and ultra-safe processes, such as the management of blood products, and the inherently unpredictable, constantly changing environment of emergency medicine. To this list we can add hospital medicine, care in the community, patients who monitor and treat their own condition and, by far the most important in poorer cultures, care given in people's homes. Even with the most cursory glance at the diversity of healthcare, the easy parallels with the comparatively predictable high-hazard industries, which usually have a limited set of activities, begin to break down.

Work in many hazardous industries, such as nuclear power is, ideally, routine. Emergencies and departures from usual practice are unusual and to be avoided. Many aspects of healthcare are also largely routine and would, for the most part, be much better organized on a production-line basis. Much of the care of chronic conditions, such as asthma and diabetes, is routine and predictable, which is not to say that the people suffering from these conditions should be treated in a routine and standardized manner. However, in some areas, healthcare staff face very high levels of uncertainty. In hospital medicine, for example, the patient's disease might be masked, difficult to diagnose, the results of investigations not clear cut, the treatment complicated by multiple co-morbidities and so on. Here, a tolerance for uncertainty on the part of the staff, and indeed the patient, is vital. The nature of the work is very different from most industrial settings.

A related issue is that pilots and nuclear power plant operators spend most of their time performing routine control and monitoring activities, rather than actually doing things. For the most part, the plane or the plant runs itself, and the pilot or operator is simply checking and watching. Pilots do, of course, take over manual control and need to be highly skilled but actual 'hands on' work is a relatively small part of their activities (Reason 1997). By contrast, much of healthcare work is very 'hands on' and, in consequence, much more liable to error. The most routine tasks – putting up drips, putting in lines to deliver drugs – all require skill and carry an element of risk. Finally, and most obviously, passengers in trains and planes are generally in reasonable health. Many patients are very young, very old, very sick or very disturbed, and in different ways vulnerable to even small problems in their care.

The organization of safety in healthcare and other industries

As well as comparing specific work activities, we can also consider more general organizational similarities and differences. David Gaba (2000) has argued that these contrasts are illuminating and have implications for safety. Gaba points out that most high-risk industries are very centralized, with a clear control structure; healthcare, even national systems such as in the UK, is fragmented and decentralized in comparison. (In countries with more mixed systems, such as the US, making changes across the entire system is monumentally difficult.) Gaba is not suggesting that safety is achieved simply by top-down command and control but forcefully points to the necessity for some standardization of process and approach to common problems. Standardizing the design of infusion pumps, for instance, is highly desirable but very difficult to achieve in practice. Other industries also put much more emphasis on standardizing both the training and the work process. Rene Amalberti (2001) has pointed out that it is a mark of the success and safety of commercial aviation that we do not worry about who the pilot is on a particular flight; we assume they, in his phrase, are 'equivalent actors' who are interchangeable. This is not an insult but a compliment to their training and professionalism. Gaba points out that in healthcare the autonomy of the individual physician, although necessary at a clinical level, does permit a variability in practice that can be detrimental to safety. If nurses, for instance, are constantly responding to different practices of senior physicians in intensive care, unnecessary variability and potential for error is introduced.

Safe organizations devote a great deal of attention and resources to ensuring that workers have the necessary preparation and skills for the job; medical school is a long and intensive training but a young doctor will still arrive on a new ward and be expected to pick up local procedures informally, sometimes with catastrophic consequences, as we will see in Chapter 6. Finally, Gaba points out that healthcare is comparatively unregulated compared to other industries. In the UK, there is in fact a plethora of regulatory bodies, each with responsibility for some aspect of education, training or clinical practice. There are undoubtedly too many organizations, consuming too much clinical and management time. However, regulation still has very little effect on day-to-day clinical practice. All of these issues are complex and we will return to many of them later in the book. For now, however, it is sufficient to note there are many differences, as well as some similarities, between healthcare and other industries in both activity and organization.

WHAT IS ERROR?

Patient safety is beset by difficulties with terminology and the most intractable problems occur when the term error is used. For instance, you might think that it would be relatively easy to define the term 'prescribing error'. Surely, a drug is either prescribed correctly or not? Yet achieving a consensus on this term required a full study and several iterations of definitions among a group of clinicians, and there was still room for disagreement (Dean et al 2000). Such definitional and classification problems are long standing and certainly not confined to healthcare. Regrettably, we are not going to resolve the problems here. However, we can at least draw some distinctions and show the different ways that error is defined and discussed. Hopefully this will clear some of the fog that envelops the term and allow us to discern the various uses and misuses in the patient safety literature.

Defining error

In everyday life, recognizing error seems quite straightforward, although admitting it might be harder. My own daily life is accompanied by a plethora of slips, lapses of memory and other 'senior moments', in the charming American phrase, that are often the subject of critical comment from those around me. (How can you have forgotten already?). Immediate slips, such as making tea instead of coffee, are quickly recognized. Other errors might not be recognized until long after they occur. You might only realize you took a wrong turning some time later when it becomes clear that you are irretrievably lost. Some errors, such as marrying the wrong person, become apparent only years later. An important common theme running through all these examples is that an action is only recognized as an error after the event. Human error is a judgement made in hindsight (Woods & Cook 2002). There is no special class of things we do or do not do that we can designate as errors; it is just that some of the things we do turn out to have undesirable or unwanted consequences. This does not mean that we cannot study error or examine how our otherwise efficient brains lead us astray in some circumstances, but it does suggest that there will not be specific cognitive mechanisms to explain error that are different from those that explain other human thinking and behaviour.

Eric Hollnagel (1998) points out that the term 'error' has historically been used in three different senses: as a cause of something, as the event itself (the action) and as the outcome of an action. These three senses all appear in the media and the medical literature (Box 5.3). The distinctions are not absolute in that many uses of the term involve both cause and consequence to different degrees, but they do have a very different emphasis. For instance, the UK National Patient Safety Agency has found that patients equate 'medical error' with a preventable adverse outcome for the patient. Terms like 'adverse event', although technically much clearer, just seem like an evasion or a way of masking the fact that someone was responsible. The term 'medical error' cannot, however, be used simply to refer to adverse outcomes for patients, if only because numerous errors occur that never lead to harm.

The most precise definition of error, and the one most in accord with everyday usage, ties it to observable behaviours and actions. As a working

---

Box 5.3 Different senses of the word error

As a cause
- Plane crash due to 'human error'
- Errors by doctor cause death of child

As an event or action
- I forgot to check the water level
- I picked up the wrong syringe

As a consequence or outcome
- Salt in my coffee
- 98,000 medical errors each year in US

definition, John Senders and Neville Moray (1991) proposed that an error means that something has been done which:

- was not desired by a set of rules or an external observer
- led the task or system outside acceptable limits
- was not intended by the actor.

This definition of error, and other similar ones (Hollnagel 1998), implies a set of criteria for defining an error. First, there must be a set of rules or standards, either explicitly defined or at least implied and accepted in that environment; second, there must be some kind of failure or 'performance shortfall'; third, the person involved did not intend this and must, at least potentially, have been able to act in a different way. All three of these criteria can be challenged, or at least prove difficult to pin down in practice. Much clinical medicine for instance is inherently uncertain and there are frequently no guidelines or protocols to guide treatment. In addition, the failure is not necessarily easy to identify; it is certainly not always clear, at least at the time, when a diagnosis is wrong or at what point blood levels of a drug become dangerously high. Finally, the notion of intention, and in theory at least being able to act differently, is challenged by the fact that people's behaviour is often influenced by factors, such as fatigue or peer pressure, of which they might not be aware and have little control over. So, although the working definition is reasonable, we should be aware of its limitations and the difficulties of applying it in practice.

Classifying errors

Classifications of error can be approached from several different perspectives. An error can be described in terms of the behaviour involved, the underlying psychological processes and in terms of the factors that contributed to it. Giving the wrong drug, for instance, can be classified in terms of the behaviour (the act of giving the drug), in psychological terms as a slip (discussed below) and be due, at least in part, to fatigue. To have any hope of a coherent classification system these distinctions have to be kept firmly in mind, as some schemes developed in healthcare mix these perspectives together indiscriminately.

Human factors experts working in high-risk industries often have to estimate the likelihood of accidents occurring when preparing a 'safety case' to persuade the regulator that all reasonable safety precautions have been taken. The preparation of a safety case usually involves considering what errors might occur, how often and in what combinations. To facilitate this, a number of classification schemes have been proposed. One of the most detailed, incorporating useful features of many previous schemes is the one used in the Predictive Human Error Analysis (PHEA) technique (Embrey 1992, Hollnagel 1998) (Box 5.4).

PHEA has been developed for industries where the actions of a particular person controlling operations can be fairly closely specified (operations here meaning the operation of the system, not the surgical type). The scheme is deliberately generic, a high-level classification scheme that can be applied in different environments. It covers errors of omission (failure to carry out an

Box 5.4 PHEA classification of errors

(adapted from Hollnagel 1998)

Planning errors
- Incorrect plan executed
- Correct but inappropriate plan executed
- Correct plan, but too soon or too late
- Correct plan, but in the wrong order

Operation errors
- Operation too long/too short
- Operation incorrectly timed
- Operation in wrong direction
- Operation too little/too much
- Right operation, wrong object
- Wrong operation, right object
- Operation omitted
- Operation incomplete

Checking errors
- Check omitted
- Check incomplete
- Right check on wrong object
- Wrong check on right object
- Check incorrectly timed

Retrieval errors
- Information not obtained
- Wrong information obtained
- Information retrieval incomplete

Communication errors
- Information not communicated
- Wrong information communicated
- Information communication incomplete

Selection errors
- Selection omitted
- Wrong selection made

operation), errors of commission (doing the wrong thing) and extraneous error (doing something unnecessary). Generally, there is quite high agreement when independent judges are asked to classify errors with schemes of this kind, which at least gives a starting point in describing the phenomena of interest. Looking at such schemes gives one new respect for human beings; the wonder is not how many errors occur but, given the numerous opportunities for messing things up, how often things go well.

These generic schemes can seem very remote from healthcare: too abstract, too conceptual and only of interest to researchers such as myself, and other impractical boffins. However, many healthcare classification schemes would be considerably more coherent if a scheme such as PHEA had been used as a starting point. Consider the checking of anaesthetic equipment before an operation; there are several different types of check to be made but all the ways of failing to check probably fall into one of the six types listed in PHEA. In operating the anaesthetic equipment, anaesthetic drugs can be given for too long, at the wrong time, the dials can be turned in the wrong direction, the wrong dial can be turned and so on. Communication between the surgeon and anaesthetist about, say, blood loss, might not occur, might be incomplete or might be misleading.

Describing and classifying error in medicine

Conceptual confusion about error is not just an obsession of academics; it has real practical consequences. Classifications of medical errors often leave a lot to be desired, frequently grouping and muddling very different types of concept. Reporting systems, for instance, might ask the person reporting to define the error made, or select the type of error from a list. In one system I reviewed, the causes of error included 'wrong drug given', 'a mistake' and 'fatigue', and the clinician was meant to choose between them. In reality, any or all of these might be applicable. If the clinician is not presented with a sensible set of choices, there is no hope of learning anything useful from the incident. Realizing the extent and implications of these conceptual problems, some researchers have sought to clarify the definitions in use and build classification schemes that everyone can agree on. We will briefly examine work on prescribing error and diagnostic error.

Prescribing error

Studies suggest that prescribing errors occur in 0.4–1.9% of all medication orders written and cause harm in about 1% of inpatients. A major problem with interpreting and comparing these studies is that many of the definitions of prescribing error used are either ambiguous or not given at all. To bring some rigour and clarity to the area, Bryony Dean and colleagues (Dean et al 2000) carried out a study to determine a practitioner-based definition of prescribing error, using successive iterations of definitions until broad agreement was obtained. The final agreed list is shown in Box 5.5 and we can see that this definition of prescribing error covers a wide range of specific failures. A strength of working 'from the ground up' and basing such decisions on the views of pharmacists, doctors and nurses is that the final definition is clinically meaningful and the descriptions of acts and omissions that results are also clearly defined. The descriptions are, as the box shows, sensibly couched in terms of behaviour as far as possible, although like PHEA and other schemes, terms such as 'intention' creep in; these are not strictly observable. Writing such definitions without any reference to what the doctor intended, however, would be more or less impossible because there would often be any other point of reference. Many of the specific types of prescribing error do fall into more general categories in the PHEA scheme. There are, for instance, failures of planning (not prescribing what was intended), failures of operation (writing illegibly, using abbreviations), failures of communication of various kinds (transcription errors) and so on. There might not be a complete mapping of one scheme to another but comparing the two schemes does show the relationship between generic and specific schemes and that the same errors can, even in behavioural terms, be classified in more than one scheme.

Box 5.5 Varieties of prescribing error

(adapted from Dean et al 2000)

Prescriptions inappropriate for patient
- Drug that is contraindicated
- Patient has allergy to drug
- Ignoring potentially significant drug
- Inadequate dose
- Drug dose will give serum levels above/below therapeutic range
- Not altering drug in response to serum levels outside therapeutic range
- Continuing drug in presence of adverse reaction
- Prescribing two drugs where one will do
- Prescribing a drug for which there is no indication

Pharmaceutical issues
- Intravenous infusion with wrong dilution
- Excessive concentration of drug to be given by peripheral line

Failure to communicate essential information
- Prescribing a drug, dose or route that is not that intended
- Writing illegibly
- Writing a drug's name using abbreviations
- Writing an ambiguous medication order
- Prescribing 'one tablet' of a drug that is available in more than one strength
- Omission of route of administration for drug that can be given by more than one route
- Prescribing an intermittent infusion without specifying duration
- Omission of signature

Transcription errors
- Not prescribing drug in hospital that patient was taking prior to admission
- Continuing a GP's prescribing error when patient is admitted to hospital
- Transcribing incorrectly when rewriting patient's chart
- Writing 'milligrams' when 'micrograms' was intended
- Writing a prescription for discharge that unintentionally deviates from in hospital prescription
- On admission to hospital writing a prescription that unintentionally deviates from pre-admission prescription

---

Diagnostic errors

Prescribing errors are a relatively clearly defined type of error in that they do at least refer to a particular act – writing or otherwise recording a drug, a dose and route of administration. Diagnosis, by contrast, is not so much an act as a thought process; whereas prescribing happens at a particular time and place, diagnosis is often more an unfolding story. Diagnostic errors are much harder to specify and the category 'diagnostic error' wider and less defined. The list of examples of diagnostic error in Box 5.6 shows how the label 'diagnostic error' can indicate either a relatively discrete event (missing a fracture when looking at an X-ray) or something that happens over months or even years (missed lung cancer because of failures in the coordination of outpatient care). These examples show that the term error can be an oversimplification of very complex phenomena and sometimes a long story of undiagnosed illness.

Diagnostic errors have not yet received the attention they deserve considering their probable importance in leading to harm or substandard treatment for

> **Box 5.6 Examples of diagnostic errors**
>
> (adapted from Graber et al 2002)
>
> **Errors of uncertainty (no-fault errors)**
> - Missed diagnosis of appendicitis in elderly patient with no abdominal pain
>   *Comment*: unusual presentation of disease
> - Missed diagnosis of Lyme disease in an era when this was unknown
>   *Comment*: limitations of medical knowledge
> - Wrong diagnosis of common cold in patient found to have mononucleosis
>   *Comment*: diagnosis reasonable but incorrect
> - Missed diagnosis of colon cancer in patient who refused screening
>   *Comment*: lack of patient co-operation
>
> **Errors precipitated by system factors (system errors)**
> - Missed colon cancer because flexible sigmoidoscopy performed instead of colonoscopy
>   *Comment*: lack of appropriate equipment or results
> - Fracture missed by emergency department
>   *Comment*: radiologist not available
> - Delay in diagnosis of pulmonary embolus
>   *Comment*: policy failure; nuclear medicine section not open at weekends
> - Delay in diagnosis due to ward team not informed of patient's admission
>   *Comment*: failure to coordinate care
>
> **Errors of thinking and reasoning (cognitive errors)**
> - Wrong diagnosis of ventricular tachycardia on ECG with electrical artefact simulating dysrhythmia
>   *Comment*: inadequate knowledge
> - Missed diagnosis of breast cancer because of failure to perform breast examination
>   *Comment*: faulty history taking and inadequate assessment
> - Failing to perceive lung nodule on patient's chest X-ray
>   *Comment*: faulty information processing
> - Wrong diagnosis of degenerative arthritis (no further test ordered) in a patient with septic arthritis
>   *Comment*: premature decision made before other possibilities considered

patients. Graber et al (2002), among others, have argued for a sustained attack on diagnostic errors, dividing them into three broad types that require different kinds of intervention to reduce them (Box 5.6). They distinguish 'no-fault errors', which primarily arise because of the difficulty of diagnosing the particular condition, 'system errors' primarily due to organizational and technical problems and 'cognitive errors', which are due to faulty thinking and reasoning.

We should be cautious about accepting a sharp division between no-fault, system and cognitive errors, because this distinction, although broadly useful, is potentially misleading. First, separating out some errors as 'cognitive' is slightly curious; in a sense all error is 'cognitive' in that all our thinking and action involves cognition. The implication of the term 'cognitive error' is really to locate the cause of the diagnostic error in failures of judgement and decision making. Second, the term 'system error', although widely used, is to my mind a rather ghastly and nonsensical use of language. Systems might fail, break down or fail to function but only people make errors. System error as a term is usually a rather unsatisfactory shorthand for factors that contributed to the failure to make an accurate diagnosis, such as a radiologist not being available or poor coordination of care. In reality, diagnosis is always an interaction between the patient and the doctor or other professional, who are both influenced by the system in which they work. This theme, of the interaction of person and system, will emerge again in Chapter 6 and later in the book.

THE PSYCHOLOGY OF ERROR

In the preceding two sections, error has mainly been examined in terms of behaviour and outcome. However, errors can also be examined from a psychological perspective. The psychological analyses to be described are mainly concerned with failures at a particular time and probe the underlying mechanisms of error. (There is therefore not necessarily a simple correspondence with medical errors, which, as discussed, can refer to events happening over a period of time.) In his analysis of different types of error, James Reason (1990) divides them into two broad types: slips and lapses (which are errors of action) and mistakes (which are, broadly speaking, errors of knowledge or planning). Reason also discusses violations, which, as distinct from error, are intentional acts that, for one reason or another, deviate from the usual or expected course of action.

Slips and lapses

Slips and lapses occur when a person knows what he or she wants to do but the action does not turn out as intended. They are failures of execution, rather than failures of knowledge or planning. Slips relate to observable actions and are associated with attentional failures, whereas lapses are internal events and associated with failures of memory. When Charles Darwin went to the wrong tea caddy, he had a lapse of memory. If, on the other hand, he had remembered where the tea was but had been momentarily distracted and knocked the caddy over rather than opening it, he would have made a slip.

Slips and lapses occur during the largely automatic performance of some routine task, usually in familiar surroundings. They are often associated with some form of distraction, either from the surroundings or from the person's own preoccupation with something in his or her mind. They are also provoked by change, either in the current plan of action or in the immediate surroundings.

Mistakes

Slips and lapses are errors of action: you intend to do something but it does not go according to plan. With mistakes, the actions might go entirely as planned but the plan itself deviates from some adequate path towards its intended goal. Here the failure lies at a higher level: with the mental processes involved in planning, formulating intentions, judging and problem solving (Reason 2001). If a doctor treats someone with chest pain as if the cause was a myocardial infarction, when in fact it is not, then this is a mistake. The intention is clear, the action corresponds with the intention, but the plan was wrong.

Mistakes can occur for various different reasons. One important division is between rule-based mistakes that occur through not following the right rule or procedure and knowledge-based mistakes that occur because the person does not know what rule or procedure to follow in the first place. Rule-based mistakes occur when the person already knows some rule or procedure, acquired as the result of training or experience. Rule-based mistakes might occur through applying the wrong rule, such as treating someone for asthma when you should follow the guidelines for pneumonia. Alternatively, the mistake might occur because the procedure itself is faulty; deficient clinical guidelines for instance.

Knowledge-based mistakes occur in novel situations when the solution to a problem has to be worked out on the spot. These situations are probably more common in medicine than in more proceduralized industries. For instance, a doctor might simply be unfamiliar with the clinical presentation of a particular disease, or there might be multiple diagnostic possibilities and no clear way at the time of choosing between them; a surgeon might have to guess at the source of the bleeding and make an understandable mistake in his or her assessment in the face of considerable stress and uncertainty. In none of these cases do the clinicians have a good 'mental model' of what is happening to base their decisions on, still less a specific rule or procedure to follow.

Violations

Errors are, by definition, unintended in the sense that we do not want to make them. Violations, by contrast, are deliberate deviations from safe operating practices, procedures, standards or rules. This is not to say that people intend that there should be a bad outcome, as when someone deliberately sabotages a piece of equipment; more usually, people hope that the violation of procedures won't matter 'on this occasion' or will actually help get the job done. Deliberate violations differ from errors in several important ways. Whereas errors are primarily due to our human limitations in thinking and remembering, violations are more closely linked with our attitudes, motivation or the work environment. The social context of violations is very important and understanding them, and if necessary curbing them, requires attention to the culture of the wider organization as well as the attitudes of the people concerned.

Reason (2001) distinguishes three types of violation:

- A routine violation is basically cutting corners for one reason or another, perhaps to save time or simply to get on to another more urgent task.
- Necessary violations occur when a person flouts a rule because it seems the only way to get the job done. Suppose a nurse gives a drug that should be double-checked by another nurse but there is no one around and the patient needs the medication? The nurse will probably give the drug, knowingly violating procedure but in the patient's interest. This can, of course, have disastrous consequences as we will see in the next chapter.

- Optimizing violations are for personal gain, sometimes just to get off work early or, more sinister, to alleviate boredom 'for kicks'. Think of a young surgeon carrying out a difficult operation in the middle of the night, without supervision, when the case could easily wait until morning. The motivation is partly to gain experience, to test oneself out, but there might be a strong element of the excitement of sailing close to the wind in defiance of the senior surgeon's instructions.

The psychological perspective on error has been very influential in medicine, forming a central plank of one of the most important papers in the patient safety literature (Leape 1994). Errors and violations are also a component of the organizational accident model, discussed in Chapter 6. However, attempts to use these concepts in practice in healthcare, in reporting systems for instance, have often foundered. Why is this? One important reason is that in practice the distinction between slips, mistakes and violations is not always clear, either to an observer or the person concerned. The relationship between the observed behaviour, which can be easily described, and the psychological mechanism is not one to one. Giving the wrong drug might be a slip (attention wandered and picked up the wrong syringe), a mistake (misunderstanding about the drug to be given) or even a violation (deliberate over-sedation of a difficult patient). The concepts are not easy to put into practice, except in circumstances where the action, context and personal characteristics of those involved can be quite carefully explored.

PERSPECTIVES ON ERROR AND ERROR REDUCTION

As must now be clear, error has many different facets and the subject of error, and how to reduce error, can be approached in different ways. Although there is a multitude of different taxonomies and error reduction systems, some broad general perspectives, or 'error paradigms' as they are sometimes called, can be

---

Box 5.7 Perspectives on error

(after Lucas 1997 and Reason 2001)

Engineering perspective
Focuses on the technical aspects of the system. Human beings tend to be viewed as unreliable components to be eliminated as far as possible.

Individual perspective: the 'person model'
Focuses on characteristics of people that lead to error, such as motivation, personality and cognitive characteristics. In its crude form it focuses on blame.

Psychological perspective
Focuses on the psychological processes underlying error.

Organizational perspective: the 'system model'
Highlights the role that wider system and organizational factors play in precipitating errors. Might see the major causes of accidents and harm in organizational factors rather than in the actions of those 'at the sharp end'.

discerned. Following Deborah Lucas (1997) and James Reason (1997), four perspectives can be distinguished (Box 5.7). The psychological perspective has been discussed above and we will not consider it further here. The various perspectives are seldom explicitly discussed in medicine but, once you have read about them, you will certainly have seen them in action in discussions of safety in healthcare. Each perspective leads to different kinds of solution to the problem of error. Some people just blame doctors for errors and think discipline and retraining is the answer; some want to automate everything; others put everything down to 'the system'. Each perspective has useful features, but unthinking adherence to any particular one is unlikely to be productive.

Engineering perspective

The central characteristic of the engineering perspective is that human beings are viewed as potentially unreliable components of the system. In its extreme form, this perspective implies that humans should be engineered out of a system by increasing automation, so avoiding the problem of human error. In its less extreme form, the engineering approach regards human beings as important parts of complex systems but places a great deal of emphasis on the ways people and technology interact. For instance, the design of anaesthetic monitors needs to be carefully considered if the wealth of information displayed is not to lead to misinterpretation and errors at times of crisis.

In the manufacture of computers and cars on assembly lines, less human involvement in repetitive tasks has undoubtedly led to higher reliability. However, automation does not always lead to improvements in safety and might actually introduce new problems – the 'ironies of automation' as Lisanne Bainbridge expressed it (Bainbridge 1987). In particular, the operators of equipment become much less 'hands on' and spend more time monitoring and checking. This is well expressed in the apocryphal story of the pilot of a commercial airliner, who turned to his co-pilot and said, of the onboard computer controlling the plane, 'I wonder what it's doing now?' There have, however, been some real life tragedies in which automation led human beings astray with tragic consequences (Box 5.8).

Errors are sometimes portrayed as a kind of virus that must be stamped out if we are ever to achieve safe healthcare. It is certainly true that some kinds of error need to be reduced but the ambition to eliminate all error, as opposed to eliminating harm, does not capture the real aims of patient safety

---

Box 5.8 The Vincennes incident

(adapted from Lucas 1997)

In 1988 the USS *Vincennes* erroneously shot down a civilian Airbus carrying 290 passengers. The *Vincennes* had been fitted with a very sophisticated tactical information co-ordinator (TIC), which warned of a hostile aircraft close to the ship. The captain also received a warning that the aircraft might be commercial but, under great time pressure, and considering the safety of ship and crew, he accepted the TIC warning and shot down the airliner. In another US warship with, paradoxically, a less sophisticated warning system, the crew relied less on the automated system and had decided the aircraft was civilian.

and might, in fact, not be the most effective way of improving safety. Errors can be useful, as in trial and error learning. For instance, surgeons learning to remove gall bladders in laparoscopic cholecystectomy (keyhole surgery) have to avoid severing the common bile duct; if the duct is severed bile is released into the abdomen, which carries serious risks for the patient. However, while they are learning surgeons inevitably make many minor errors, such as going too close to the duct, which help in calibrating their movements as they gradually build the hand–eye coordination needed for the subtleties of laparoscopic surgery. This suggests that we should be aiming not so much to eliminate error as to work within safe boundaries. This insight, most powerfully expressed by Jens Rasmussen, is discussed further below.

Individual perspective: the person model

In daily life errors are frequently attributed to stupidity, carelessness, forgetfulness, recklessness and other personal defects. The implication is that the person who makes an error has certain characteristics that produce the error and, furthermore, that these characteristics are under the person's control and that he or she is therefore to blame for the errors they make. This is error seen from the individual perspective; when applied to understanding accidents, Reason refers to this as the 'person model' (Reason 2000).

Efforts to reduce error are, from this perspective, targeted at individuals and involve exhortations to 'do better', retraining or adding new rules and procedures. For errors with more serious consequences, more severe sanctions come into play, such as naming and shaming, disciplinary action, suspension, media condemnation and so on. Legal perspectives on error, and the whole notion of medical negligence, are built on the concepts of personal responsibility, fault, blame and redress. This view is strongly entrenched in healthcare, as seen by the immediate suspension of nurses who make serious errors, with reflection on the incident and investigation coming later, if at all. It is also reflected in the deep shame many professionals experience if they make a serious error: 'How could I, as a responsible professional, do such a thing?'

Blame, when thoughtless and automatic, penalizes individuals sometimes to the point of destroying careers. However, it is also a major barrier to improving safety, hence the enormous importance given to creating an 'open and fair culture', discussed later in the book. Learning from error, discussing error, reporting safety issues and incidents in which patients are harmed require that the people involved are supported and even praised for coming forward. If there is no free flow of information about error and safety, the organization cannot learn, cannot address safety issues and is destined to remain forever unsafe.

The folly of the crude person model is apparent. However, it is important not to swing to the other extreme and attribute everything to 'the system'. Rather, one needs to preserve individual accountability but understand the interplay between the person, the technology and the organization. Individual characteristics might well play a part in the occurrence of an error or in a poor clinical outcome. For instance, motivation and attitude are important determinants of how people behave and whether they work conscientiously. A strong sense of personal responsibility is fundamental to being a good clinician. Patient safety is not a never-never land in which everyone is always motivated and principled. People who deliberately behave recklessly and without regard to their patients' welfare deserve to be blamed, whether or not they make errors.

There are other individual characteristics that we might need to understand to improve safety and which have been given relatively little attention as yet. People's beliefs and attitudes to safety, and to their work generally, will determine how safe they are as practitioners. Being completely rule-and-procedure-bound might, for instance, be as unsafe as being overly reckless, because it leaves one unable to adapt and respond to changing circumstances. Similarly, although accident-proneness as a concept is now discredited (in the sense of a life-long predisposition), people might have cognitive dispositions to respond in a certain way, which make them more liable to certain types of error (Croskerry 2002). More obviously relevant to healthcare, and closely tied to wider organizational and societal considerations, stress, fatigue, alcohol and drug addiction and other personal crises can have major safety implications. Blame might not be appropriate but action might need to be taken to protect patients and help a doctor or nurse whose work is affected by illness or personal crisis.

Organizational perspective: the system model

The quote from James Reason at the beginning of this chapter perfectly expresses the essence of the organizational view of accidents, often referred to in healthcare as the 'system' model. The essential idea underlying this approach is that errors and human behaviour cannot be understood in isolation, but only in relation to the context in which people are working. Clinical staff are influenced by the nature of the task they are carrying out, the team they work in, their working environment and the wider organizational context; these are the system factors. From this perspective, errors are seen not so much as the product of personal fallibility but as consequences of more general problems in the working environment.

In considering how people contribute to accidents, therefore, we have to distinguish between 'active failures' and 'latent conditions' (Reason 2001). The active failures are unsafe acts of various kinds (errors and violations) that have already been described. These are committed by people at the 'sharp end' of the system who are actually operating it or working with a patient. The active failures are wrongly opening the bow door of a ferry, shutting down the wrong engine on an airliner or misreading the anaesthetic monitor. These unsafe acts can, and often do, have immediate consequences. However, these unsafe acts all occur in a particular context and they can be precipitated by what Reason terms 'latent conditions'. Perhaps the ferry company has become progressively more lax, and the procedures for opening the bow doors are ill defined or ambiguous; the cockpit design and warning signals are misleading; syringe labels do not sufficiently distinguish dangerous drugs; anaesthetists are working excessive hours, become tired and less vigilant. These are the latent conditions that stem from decisions made by designers, people who write procedures and guidelines, senior management and others. Note that, whereas errors can be made by anyone, it is not easy to foresee the long-term effects of design or management decisions, which are themselves made in the face of many competing demands. For instance, there might be pressure on surgical teams to clear the waiting lists of patients waiting for operations. These are, in some respects, well-intentioned decisions and yet, pushed too far, make the delivery of healthcare unsafe. Decisions made years before, such as in the design of instruments, can have consequences later when a particular combination of circumstances puts the people and the system under stress. The system model, and its application in healthcare, will be discussed further in Chapter 6 when we examine the causes of harm to patients in more detail.

MYTHS ABOUT ERROR

The picture of error and its causes that is emerging is rather different from our everyday understanding of error, accidents and the behaviour of skilled professionals. We tend to think that experts are trained to perfection, that errors are caused by recklessness or carelessness and we all too easily blame people who appear to be the cause of accidents. This is in many ways a comforting picture of a world in which we are in safe hands, cared for by infallible professionals who, while of course compassionate, are able to perform with machine like regularity and perfection. James Reason (2004) has pointedly tackled our naïve understanding by setting out seven widespread myths about human error, which nicely highlight some of the ways that our common understanding is adrift (Box 5.9). It should be clear by now why most of them are myths, but we will consider two of them in more detail.

The myth of the rarity of error

We have seen in earlier chapters that errors in medicine are all too common. However, this is slightly different from the sense intended here, which is the myth that people who are highly trained make few errors. Reason points out that even in successful, and extremely safe, enterprises minor errors occur all the time. For instance, studies by both Robert Helmreich's team in the US and Rene Amalberti and colleagues in France have shown that minor errors are very frequent, even in commercial aviation (Amalberti & Wioland 1997, Helmreich & Merrit 1998). Amalberti & Wioland estimated from their observations that

---

Box 5.9 Seven myths about human error and its management

(adapted from Reason 2004)

- Errors are intrinsically bad
- Bad errors are made by bad people
- Errors are random and highly variable
- Practice makes perfect
- The errors of highly trained professionals are very rare
- The errors of highly trained professionals are usually sufficient to cause bad outcomes
- It is easier to change people than situations

each year 100 million errors are made by flight crews but that, as official statistics show, these contribute to around 100 major incidents and 25–30 actual crashes. Errors are very frequent but usually have no consequences either because they do not impact on the activity in question or because they are recognized and corrected.

In our own observations of surgical teams (Healey et al 2004) we have observed a multitude of ways in which basic procedures are not fully carried out, and yet the outcome of the operation is successful. In 50 laparoscopic cholecystectomies we observed that equipment checks, although broadly adhered too, were frequently not completed. The surgeon often did not inform the anaesthetist, as he or she is meant to, that the operation was about to start. The scrub nurses uncovered the surgical equipment before they should have done, thus increasing the risk of contamination. This level of omission is worrying and hardly ideal. Yet, in all these operations, the patients' outcome was good and the team was composed of committed, serious individuals who would have been horrified if a patient had been harmed in what is, nowadays, a routine operation. This points, among other things, to the fact that teams are adjusting constantly, correcting errors that actually threaten the patient and anticipating what is going to happen next. The anaesthetist is aware, because he or she is watching, that the surgeon is about to start. Even so, if the surgeon does explicitly state that the operation is starting, this is an additional safety measure that, on rare occasions, will prevent disaster.

In more challenging settings a similar picture is seen. In a study carried out by Marc de Leval, a paediatric cardiac surgeon, and colleagues (de Leval et al 2000), 165 arterial switch operations were observed. This is a complex operation, with a significant mortality, performed on very young children in whom the great arteries are transposed. de Leval and colleagues classed the errors and other threatening events they observed into two kinds: major events, which threatened the patient, and minor events, which were not directly threatening but interrupted the surgical flow. On average there were seven major events per procedure and six minor ones. Teams who were able to compensate for the major events, that is recognize and recover from them, had better outcomes. Minor events usually went unchecked but cumulatively appeared to degrade the performance of the surgical team and affect outcome. The recovery from error seen here points to another important feature of expertise. Experts are not so much people who never make mistakes (although they might make fewer than novices) but people who are always aware that they do make mistakes and might make one at any moment. They are therefore on the alert and able to recover from dangerous situations.

The myth of bad people

The next myth is that bad errors are made by bad people. This is the extreme version of the 'person model' in which people are blamed and castigated for their errors.

Most general talks, papers and books on patient safety give tremendous prominence to the need to get away from blaming people and to create a fair culture. Without doubt, healthcare has a culture of blame, people are fearful of reporting and changing this culture is an essential step in enhancing safety. Yet I have chosen not to discuss the issue of blame until near the end of a chapter on error, which might seem eccentric. The reason is straightforward. The issue of error and blame is often presented without any background understanding of the nature of error and can, at worst, seem to be little more than a plea to be nice to people. More usually it is a very reasonable plea for a fairer and more thoughtful approach to people involved in serious accidents or bad outcomes for patients. However, with more understanding of error, the arguments for a just and fair culture become much more powerful. Error is frequent; errors are committed by even the best people; error is often precipitated by circumstances beyond our control, indeed is often outside our conscious control; major accidents are seldom due to one person alone and so on. When all these considerations are taken into account, blame becomes not so much morally wrong as largely irrelevant to the quest for safety. With understanding comes a very different perspective of both the causes of harm to patients and of what an appropriate response might be.

THE CONCEPT OF ERROR: IS IT USEFUL FOR THE DESIGN OF SAFE HEALTHCARE SYSTEMS?

After raising the issue of blame so late on, it might seem still more curious, even perverse, to ask whether the concept of error is useful for patient safety. The heading comes from the title of a chapter written by Jens Rasmussen (1997) whose work has influenced every field of safety and has been a major influence on many of the leading figures in patient safety. We cannot do more than hint at some of his ideas here but they will set the scene for a later chapter on creating safety.

Rasmussen was very influenced in his thinking by his studies of the operators of nuclear power plants (Rasmussen 1990). Even here in, what one would imagine to be the most highly proceduralized environment, he found enormous flexibility and adaptability to circumstances and departure from guidelines and procedures. This was not because nuclear power workers were especially reckless or wished to endanger others; quite the contrary. The point is that although they were trained in standard procedures and knew about them, they often did not follow them in the practice; rather they tried to get the job done in the way that seemed best at the time. Rasmussen's view of human work is that of our own everyday experience; we are constantly adapting to new circumstances, doing the best we can and coping with a variety of organizational pressures. He further argues, in a wide-ranging critique, that error is often an oversimplification, that the accident investigator can never really capture the choices and conflicts facing those involved in the accident, that error often plays a crucial role in learning and that recovery from error is as worthy of study as error. Studying errors and accidents, although certainly illuminating, will never be sufficient. We need to understand how people work and how they adapt to pressures and circumstances.

Furthermore, because of the shifting and changing nature of systems, safety measures themselves affect the system in unanticipated ways. When radar was introduced to improve safety at sea, captains of ships (and their owners) were more able to anticipate bad weather. They were therefore more able to travel in bad weather, could travel more efficiently and thus increase the number of journeys made. A measure to improve safety therefore simultaneously increased danger by exposing ships to worse weather. Similarly, anaesthetics, being generally extremely safe, are vulnerable to pressure from patients and management to achieve more and so put safety at risk (Healzer et al 1998). Paradoxically, as a system becomes safer, there is more pressure for increased performance, cutting corners and the eventual degrading of safety–until the next accident occurs.

Reading and reflecting on this helps one to understand that safety in a system is a much more fluid and dynamic concept than is often thought. Many charged with improving safety regard increasing standardization, more automation, better training and a general tightening up of procedures as the way forward. Although we should not underestimate the importance of these approaches, particularly in disorganized healthcare systems, Rasmussen helps us understand that this can never be a complete solution. Safety is, both at the individual and organizational level, very much a question of steering a course in a shifting and changing landscape, rather than setting standards and expecting people to stick to them for all time. The people who work in the system will always be adapting to circumstances, sometimes degrading safety in the process, but more often enhancing safety by their anticipation and improvization in a complex, changing environment.

REFERENCES

Amalberti R 2001 The paradoxes of almost totally safe transportation systems. Safety Science 37:109–126

Amalberti R, Wioland L 1997 Human error in aviation. In: Soekkha H (ed) Aviation safety: human factors, system engineering, flight operations, economics, strategies, management. VSP, Utrecht

Bainbridge L 1987 Ironies of automation. In: Rasmussen J, Duncan K, Leplat J (eds) New technology and human error. Wiley, Chichester

Browne J 2003 Charles Darwin. Voyaging. Pimlico Books, London

Cook RI, Woods DD, Miller CA 1998 A tale of two stories: contrasting views of patient safety. US National Patient Safety Foundation, North Adams, MA. Online. Available at: http://www.npsf.org/exec/front.html

Croskerry P 2002 Achieving quality in clinical decision making: cognitive strategies and detection of bias. Academic Emergency Medicine 9:1184–1204

Dean B, Barber N, Schachter M 2000 What is a prescribing error? Quality in Health Care 9:232–237

de Leval M, Carthey J, Wright DJ et al 2000 Human factors and cardiac surgery: a multi-center study. Journal of Thoracic and Cardiovascular Surgery 119:661–672

Embrey DE 1992. Quantitative and qualitative prediction of human error in safety assessments. Institute of Chemical Engineering, Rugby

Gaba DM 2000 Anaesthesiology as a model for patient safety in health care. British Medical Journal 320:785–788

Graber M, Gordon R, Franklin N 2002 Reducing diagnostic errors in medicine: what's the goal? Academic Medicine 77:981–992

Healey AN, Undre S, Vincent CA 2004 Developing observational measures of performance in surgical teams. Quality and Safety in Health Care 13:i33–i40

Healzer JM, Howard SK, Gaba DM 1998 Attitudes toward production pressure and patient safety: a survey of anesthesia residents. Journal of Clinical Monitoring and Computing 14:145–146

Helmreich RL, Merrit AC 1998 Culture at work in aviation and medicine: national, organisational and professional influences. Ashgate, Aldershot

Hollnagel E 1998 Cognitive reliability and error analysis method. Elsevier, Oxford

Leape LL 1994 Error in medicine. Journal of the American Medical Association 272:1851–1857

Lucas D 1997 The causes of human error. In: Redmill F, Rajan J (eds) Human factors in safety critical systems. Butterworth Heinemann, Oxford

Rasmussen J 1990 The role of error in organizing behaviour, Ergonomics 33:1185–1199.

Rasmussen J 1997 The concept of human error: is it useful for the design of safe systems? In: Vincent C, de Mol B (eds) Safety in medicine. Elsevier Science, Oxford

Reason JT 1990 Human error. Cambridge University Press, New York

Reason JT 1997 Managing the risks of organisational accidents. Ashgate, Aldershot

Reason JT 2000 Human error: models and management. British Medical Journal 320:768–770

Reason JT 2001 Understanding adverse events: the human factor. In: Vincent C (ed) Clinical risk management: enhancing patient safety, 2 edn. BMJ Publications, London

Reason JT 2004. Beyond the organisational accident: the need for 'error wisdom' on the front line. Quality and Safety in Health Care 13: ii28–ii33

Senders JW, Moray N 1991 Human error: course, prediction and reduction. Lawrence Erlbaum Associates, Hillsdale, NJ

US National Aeronautics and Space Administration 2003 Report of the Columbia Accident Investigation Board. Online. Available at: http://www.naa.gov

Vincent C, Taylor-Adams S, Stanhope N 1998 Framework for analysing risk and safety in clinical medicine. British Medical Journal 316:1154–1157

Woods DD, Cook RI 2002 Nine steps to move forward from error. Cognition, Technology & Work 4:137–144

Understanding how things go wrong

At approximately 17.00 hours on Thursday 4th January 2001, Mr Wayne Jowett, a day case patient on Ward E17 at the Queen's Medical Centre Nottingham (QMC), was prepared for an intrathecal (spinal) administration of chemotherapy as part of his medical maintenance programme following successful treatment of leukaemia.

After carrying out a lumbar puncture and administering the correct cytotoxic therapy (cytosine) under the supervision of the Specialist Registrar Dr Mulhem, Dr Morton, a Senior House Officer, was passed a second drug by Dr Mulhem to administer to Mr Jowett, which he subsequently did. However, the second drug, vincristine, should never be administered by the intrathecal route because it is almost always fatal.

Unfortunately, whilst emergency treatment was provided very quickly in an effort to rectify the error, Mr Jowett died at 8.10 a.m. on the 2nd February 2001.
(Toft 2001 p 9)

Following an internal inquiry at QMC, Professor Brian Toft was commissioned by the Chief Medical Officer of England to conduct an inquiry into Mr Jowett's death and to advise on the areas of vulnerability in the process of intrathecal injection of these drugs and ways in which fail-safes might be built in (Toft 2001). The orientation of the inquiry was therefore, from the outset, one of learning and change. We will use this sad story, and Brian Toft's thoughtful report, to introduce the subject of analysing cases. This case illustrates many general principles and acts as an excellent, although tragic, illustration of models of organizational accidents and systems thinking.

The systems view of medical error was not, however, the approach taken by the courts. Dr Mulhem was charged with manslaughter, pleaded guilty and was sentenced to 8 months imprisonment. Wayne Jowett's parents considered the sentence ridiculous, pointing out that he would have probably served a longer sentence for theft of hospital equipment (Balen 2004). The anger and desire for justice is more than understandable and some would argue that no one, in whatever profession, should be exempt from charges of manslaughter. Conversely, criminalizing fatal medical mistakes and destroying careers and people might not actually help us improve patient safety. As Dr Mulhem said, when interviewed by police, 'I know it's a lame excuse, but

I am a human being' (Holbrook 2003). The proper role of the law in healthcare is too complex an issue to be discussed properly here, and in any event heavily dependent on culture and wider societal attitudes and values. However, we should note the contrast between, on the one hand, the judicial view of error and the concept of manslaughter and, on the other, the view that emerges from Brian Toft's enquiry. After considering the full circumstances of the case and the way the odds stacked up against the unfortunate patient and doctors involved in this tragedy, the reader can reappraise the verdicts.

BACKGROUND TO THE INCIDENT

Provided vincristine is administered intravenously (i.v.), it is a powerful and useful drug in the fight against leukaemia. The dangers of inadvertent intrathecal administration of vincristine are well known: there are product warnings to that effect, a literature that stresses the dangers and well-publicized previous cases. Medical staff at QMC had put a number of measures in place to prevent inadvertent intrathecal use and it was clear that these precautions were taken seriously. There was a standard written protocol, which, at the request of hospital staff, had been changed so that cytosine and vincristine would be administered on different days to avoid any potentially fatal confusion. Drugs for intravenous and for intrathecal use were also supplied separately to the wards, again to reduce the chances of mixing up the different types of drug. Nevertheless, because of a combination of circumstances, all these defences were breached and Mr Jowett died (Box 6.1).

Defences, discussed further below, are the means by which systems ensure safety. Sometimes the term is used to encompass almost any safety measure but it more usually refers to particular administrative, physical or other barriers that protect or warn against deviations from normal practice. Usually these defences and barriers will 'capture' an error and block the trajectory of an accident. In this example, many defences and barriers existed, in the form of procedures and protocols, custom and practice. Administering cytosine and vincristine on separate days, for instance, is clearly intended to be a defence against incorrect administration. The separation of the two drugs in pharmacy and the separate delivery to the ward are other examples of defences against error. Having two doctors present checking labels and doses is another check, another barrier against potential disaster. If one or other of these checks fails, the outcome is usually still good. For instance, as long as the correct drug has been delivered, no harm will result if the doctor does not check conscientiously or is distracted while checking. It is nevertheless, good practice to always check 'just in case'. Sometimes, however, as in this case, a series of defences and barriers are all by breached at once. This is brilliantly captured in James Reason's Swiss cheese metaphor of the trajectory of an accident, which gives us the sense of hazard being ever present and occasionally breaking through when all the holes in the Swiss cheese line up (Fig. 6.1).

From the chronology, one can see the classic 'chain of events' leading toward the tragedy. Dr Mulhem was quite new to the ward, unfamiliar with the chemotherapy regime and did not know the patient. The pharmacy, some-

Box 6.1 Chronology of events

(adapted from Toft 2001)

Mr Jowett arrived on the ward at about 4.00 p.m. He was late for his chemotherapy but staff tried to accommodate him. The pharmacist for the ward had made an earlier request that the cytosine should be sent up and that the vincristine should be 'sent separately' the following day. The pharmacy made up the drugs correctly and they were put on separate shelves in the pharmacy refrigerator. During the afternoon, the ward day-case coordinator went to the pharmacy and was given a clear bag containing two smaller bags each containing a syringe – one vincristine and one cytosine. She did not know they should not be in the same bag.

Dr Mulhem was informed and approached by Dr Morton to supervise the procedure, as demanded by the protocol. When it had been established that Mr Jowett's blood count was satisfactory, Dr Mulhem told Dr Morton that they would go ahead with Mr Jowett's chemotherapy. The staff nurse went to the ward refrigerator and removed the transparent plastic bag, placed there by the day-case coordinator, within which were two separate transparent packets, each one containing a syringe. She noted that the name 'Wayne Jowett' was printed on each of the syringe labels, delivered it and went to carry on her work.

Dr Mulhem looked at the prescription chart noting that the patient's name, drugs and dosages corresponded with the information on the labels attached to the syringes. He did not, however, notice that the administration of vincristine was planned for the following day or that its route of administration was intravenous. Dr Mulhem, anticipating a cytotoxic drugs system similar to the one at his previous place of work, had presumed that, as both drugs had come up to the ward together, both were planned for intrathecal use. He had previously administered two types of chemotherapy intrathecally and it did not therefore seem unusual.

A lumbar puncture was carried out successfully and samples of cerebrospinal fluid taken for analysis. Dr Mulhem then read out aloud the name of the patient, the drug and the dose from the label on the first syringe and then handed it to Dr Morton. Dr Mulhem did not, however, read out the route of administration. Dr Morton, having received the syringe, now asked if the drug was 'cytosine', which Dr Mulhem confirmed. Dr Morton then removed the cap at the bottom of the syringe and screwed it onto the spinal needle, after which he injected the contents of the syringe.

Having put down the first syringe, Dr Mulhem handed the second syringe containing vincristine to Dr Morton, again reading out aloud the name of the patient, the drug and dosage. Once again, he did not read out the route of administration. However, Dr Mulhem could not later recall if he:

> . . . actually said the word 'vincristine' but once again I had clearly fixed in my mind that the drug was methotrexate and not a drug for administration other than intrathecally. If I had consciously appreciated that the drug was vincristine I would have stopped the procedure immediately and would never allowed Dr Morton to administer it.

Dr Mulhem could not explain the fact that he mentally substituted the word 'methotrexate' for 'vincristine', except for the fact that his mindset was that drugs for administration by a route other than intrathecal would simply not be available at the same time.

Dr Morton was surprised when he was passed a second syringe, because on the only other occasion that he had performed a supervised intrathecal injection only one syringe had been used. However, he assumed that on this occasion that '. . . the patient was either at a different stage in his treatment or was on a different treatment regime than the other patient.' Dr Morton, with the second syringe in his hand, said to Dr Mulhem 'Vincristine?' Dr Mulhem replied in the affirmative. Dr Morton then said 'Intrathecal vincristine?' Dr Mulhem again replied in the affirmative. After which Dr Morton removed the cap at the bottom of the syringe and screwed it onto the spinal needle. He then administered the contents of the syringe to Mr Jowett, with ultimately fatal results.

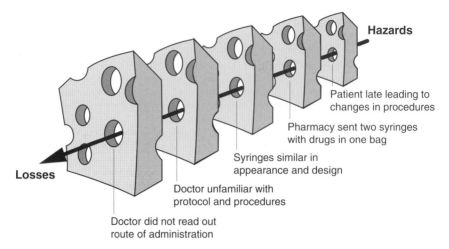

Hazards

Patient late leading to
changes in procedures

Pharmacy sent two syringes
with drugs in one bag

Syringes similar in
appearance and design

Losses

Doctor unfamiliar with
protocol and procedures

Doctor did not read out
route of administration

Fig. 6.1 Swiss cheese model of failed defences (adapted from Reason 1997 British Medical Journal 320:768–770, amended and reproduced with permission from the BMJ Publishing Group).

how, although separating the two drugs, placed them in a single bag. Although the doctors involved can be held responsible for their specific actions and omissions, one can also see that circumstances conspired against them. However, the case also illustrates some much more general themes, issues that pervade healthcare and indeed other organizations, and which are right now, as you read this, putting patients at risk.

DEATH FROM SPINAL INJECTION: A WINDOW ON THE SYSTEM

Recognizing hazards in the workplace

The unit where Wayne Jowett died had used these drugs for many years without a major incident. After an event of this kind, and a subsequent analysis, we can see that the systems, although reasonably robust, were nevertheless far from fault free. Huge reliance was placed on custom and practice and on people simply knowing what they were doing. With experienced staff who know the unit's procedures, this works reasonably well, but when new staff join a unit without clear induction and training the system inevitably becomes unsafe. People are assumed to be competent when in fact they are necessarily 'winging it', doing the best they can in the circumstances. In healthcare this happens all the time as junior staff battle with situations that are unfamiliar to them, or when more senior staff new to a unit feel that they must display more competence than they actually feel.

In fact, the unit where Wayne Jowett died seems to have been a well-run unit, where professionals respected each other's work and things went well on a day-to-day basis. Paradoxically, safety creates its own dangers in that an uneventful routine lulls one into a false sense of security. The safer one becomes, the more necessary it is to remind oneself that the environment is inherently unsafe. This is what James Reason means when he says that the price of safety is chronic unease (Reason 2001). In fact, the very assumption that all is well can itself be dangerous.

Assumptions about people and organizations

Brian Toft introduces his examination of the tacit assumptions of those involved in this case with an apposite quote:

> A newcomer assumes that he knows what the organisation is about, assumes that others in the setting have the same idea, and practically never bothers to check out these assumptions.
> **(Toft 2001 p 31)**

Dr Mulhem, the newest member of staff involved, assumed for instance that chemotherapy for different routes of administration could never be on the ward at the same time. He also assumed that he was competent to supervise Dr Morton, and that Dr Morton was allowed to give these drugs under supervision. More rashly still, he assumed that Dr Morton was familiar with Mr Jowett's case and so they did not need to consult his records. Dr Morton, in his turn, assumed that Dr Mulhem knew what he was doing and was authorized to supervise him. He also assumed that, although he should not have administered the drugs, it was permissible when authorized by Dr Mulhem. These assumptions, made by each doctor, were unfortunately perfectly matched, each tacitly reassuring the other of their mutual competence and the essential normality of the situation.

Senior doctors on the ward, although not directly involved, made their own assumptions. They assumed that Dr Mulhem knew about the dangers of vincristine, that there was no need for a formal induction for junior staff, that Dr Mulhem understood that 'shadowing' meant that he should not administer cytotoxic drugs.

None of the assumptions made by anyone was completely unreasonable. We all make such assumptions, in fact we need to just to get through the day. We cannot check everything all the time. However, one can at least realize that many of one's assumptions are likely to be wrong and begin to look, before disaster strikes, for the holes in the Swiss cheese that permeate one's own organization. We will return to this theme of vigilance and the anticipation of error and hazard later in the book.

The influence of hierarchy on communication

When asked why he did not challenge Dr Mulhem, Dr Morton said:

> First of all, I was not in a position to challenge on the basis of my limited experience of this type of treatment. Second, I was an SHO [junior doctor] and did what I was told to do by the registrar. He was supervising me and I assumed he had the knowledge to know what was being done. Dr Mulhem was employed as a registrar by QMC, which is a centre for excellence, and I did not intend to challenge him.
> **(Toft 2001 p 29)**

Dr Morton was in a very difficult position. He assumed Dr Mulhem, as a registrar, knew what he was doing and reasonably points out that he himself had limited experience of the treatment. However, he did have sufficient knowledge to query the intrathecal vincristine but did not feel able to speak up more forcefully and challenge a senior colleague. Criticism might be made here of both Dr Morton, for not having the courage to request further checks, and of Dr Mulhem for not taking the junior doctor's query more seriously and at least halting the procedure while checks were made.

The interaction can also be seen as reflecting the more general problem of authority gradients in clinical teams. In a survey asking whether junior members of a team should be able to question decisions made by senior team members, pilots were almost unanimous in saying that they should (Helmreich 2000). The willingness of junior pilots to question decisions is not seen as a threat to authority but as an additional defence against possible error. By contrast, in the same survey, almost a quarter of consultant surgeons stated that junior members of staff should not question seniors.

Physical appearance of syringes containing cytotoxic drugs

Syringes containing vincristine were labelled 'for intravenous injection' and syringes containing cytosine 'for intrathecal use'. You might think this is fairly clear cut, but on a busy ward with numerous injections being given every day, the design and packaging of drugs is an important determinant of the likelihood of error. In the final few minutes leading up to the fatal injection, the doctors involved were not helped by the similarity in appearance and packaging of the drugs. First, the labels were similar and, although the bold type of the drug and dose stood out there were no other strong visual cues to draw a reader's eye to the significance of the route of administration. Second, the syringes used to administer the two drugs were of similar size; the size of the syringe did not give any clues as to the route of administration to be used. Third, both drugs were clear liquids administered in similar volumes; neither colour nor volume gave any indication of the proper route of administration. Finally, the most dangerous physical aspect of all, in Toft's opinion, is:

> . . . that a syringe containing vincristine can also be connected to the spinal needle that delivers intrathecal drugs to patients. Clearly, once such a connection has been made the patient's life is in danger as there are no other safeguards in place to prevent the vincristine from being administered.
> (Toft 2001 p 14)

We can see, therefore, first that the syringes and labelling are unnecessarily similar and second that there are potential design solutions that would reduce, or even eliminate, this type of incident. Most obviously, syringes of drugs for intrathecal use could have their own specific, unique fitting, colour and design. Although this might not eliminate the possibility of injecting the correct drug, it does add a powerful check to wrong administration. In the same way, fatalities in anaesthesia that resulted from switching oxygen and nitrous oxide supplies were eliminated by the simple expedient of making it impossible to connect the nitrous oxide line to the oxygen input. In daily life there are thousands of such checks and guides to behaviour. When you fill your car with unleaded petrol you use a small nozzle; larger nozzles for leaded or diesel will simply not fit into the filling pipe. Manufacturers of syringes appear to be less safety conscious than car manufacturers.

Unnecessary differences in practice between hospitals

The Joint Council for Clinical Oncology had published guidelines for the administration of cytotoxic chemotherapy. However, these were only advisory, and indeed the Council probably did not have the power to make them mandatory. Thus, what any particular doctor knew about the practice of administering cytotoxic drugs depended, to some extent at least, on local custom and practice. When moving from post to post, therefore, new practices are encountered and there is every possibility of confusion, particularly in the first few weeks.

This in turn might make us wonder why healthcare is so casual about widespread variations in practice and their potential dangers. Doctors rightly regard clinical autonomy as an important aspect of professional practice and a necessary accompaniment to professional responsibility and accountability. In healthcare, much less can be standardized or mandated than in other industries. But the administration of cytotoxic drugs cries out for the adoption of national standards, aided by good design and training. Simply having the same procedures in place throughout the country would, if they were well designed, in itself be a safety measure. As an example of a much overdue standardization, the British National Patient Safety Agency (NPSA) has done the NHS a great service by the simple expedient of standardizing the hospital crash call number across the country; previously several different numbers were in use.

Much more could, and has, been said about the death of Wayne Jowett. Our purpose here, however, is not to resurrect this particular tragedy or to criticize the people involved, but to use the story to show the complexity of events that lead to harm and illuminate the many facets of patient safety. We can see that a combination of individual errors, assumptions about the workplace, poor design, communication problems, problems in team working and other contributory factors brought about this death. In fact, as we saw in the last chapter, this same blend of personal, design and organizational factors underlies many accidents and disasters. We will now look at this more formally by examining James Reason's model of organizational accidents and its application in healthcare (Reason 2001).

AETIOLOGY OF 'ORGANIZATIONAL' ACCIDENTS

Many of the accidents in both healthcare and other industries need to be viewed from a broad systems perspective if they are to be fully understood. The actions and failures of individual people usually play a central role but their thinking and behaviour is strongly influenced and constrained by their immediate working environment and by wider organizational processes.

James Reason has captured the essentials of this understanding in his model of an organizational accident (Reason 1997). We should emphasize though, before describing the model, that not every slip, lapse or fall needs to be understood in terms of the full organizational framework; some errors are confined to the local context and can be largely explained by individual factors and the characteristics of the particular task at hand. However, major incidents almost always evolve over time, involve a number of people and a considerable number of contributory factors; in these circumstances the organizational model (Fig. 6.2) proves very illuminating.

The accident sequence begins (from the left) with the negative consequences of organizational processes, such as planning, scheduling, forecasting, design, maintenance, strategy and policy. The latent failures so created are transmitted along various organizational and departmental pathways to the workplace (the operating theatre, ward, etc.) where they create the local conditions that promote the commission of errors and violations (for example, high workload or poor human equipment interfaces). Many unsafe acts are likely to be committed, but very few of them will penetrate the defences to produce damaging outcomes. The fact that engineered safety features, such as alarms or standard procedures, can be deficient due to latent failures as well as active failures is shown in the figure by the arrow connecting organizational processes directly to defences.

The model presents the people at the sharp end as the inheritors rather than as the instigators of an accident sequence. Reason points out that this might simply seem as if the 'blame' for accidents has been shifted from the sharp end to the system managers. However, managers too are operating in a complex environment and the effects of their actions are not always apparent; they are no more, and no less, to blame than those at the sharp end of the clinical environment (Reason 2001). Also, any high-level decision, whether within a healthcare organization or made outside it by government or regulatory bodies, is a balance of risks and benefits. Sometimes, such decisions are obviously flawed but even prima facie reasonable decisions might later have unfortunate consequences.

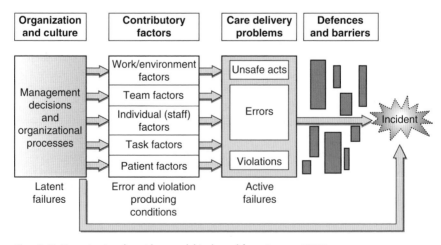

Fig. 6.2 Organizational accident model (adapted from Reason 2001).

One might argue, for instance, that the increasing regulation of healthcare should make patients safer, as it will promote good practice, standardization of essential procedures, better design of equipment and so on. The downside to this is the unwitting creation of a plethora of regulatory bodies, a great increase in paperwork and the fact that people within healthcare organizations have to devote considerable time to being seen to meet standards and targets, time that might be better spent making direct improvements to the quality and safety of care. Thus regulation, as so much else, can impact both positively and negatively on patient care.

As well as highlighting the difficulty of assessing the wisdom of strategic decisions, this analysis also extends the analysis of accidents beyond the boundaries of the organization itself to include the regulatory environment. In healthcare, many external organizations (such as manufacturers, government agencies, professional and patient organizations) also impact on the safety of the patient. The model shown in Fig. 6.2 relates primarily to a given institution but the reality is considerably more complex, with the behaviour of other organizations impinging on the accident sequence at many different points.

Seven levels of safety

We have extended Reason's model and adapted it for use in a healthcare setting, classifying the error producing conditions and organizational factors in a single broad framework of factors affecting clinical practice (Vincent et al 1998) (Table 6.1).

At the top of the framework are patient factors. In any clinical situation the patient's condition will have the most direct influence on practice and outcome. Other patient factors, such as personality, language and psychological problems, can also be important because they influence communication with staff. The design of the task, the availability and utility of protocols and test results can influence the care process and affect the quality of care. Individual factors include the knowledge, skills and experience of each member of staff, which will obviously affect their clinical practice. Each staff member is part of a team within the inpatient or community unit, and part of the wider organization of the hospital, primary care or mental health service. The way an individual practises, and his or her impact on the patient, is constrained and influenced by other members of the team, and the way they communicate, support and supervise each other. The team is influenced in turn by management actions and by decisions made at a higher level in the organization. These include policies for the use of locum or agency staff, continuing education, training and supervision and the availability of equipment and supplies. The organization itself is affected by the institutional context, including financial constraints, external regulatory bodies and the broader economic and political climate.

The framework provides the conceptual basis for analysing clinical incidents, in that it includes both the clinical factors and the higher-level, organizational factors that can contribute to the final outcome. In doing so, it allows the whole range of possible influences to be considered and can therefore be used to guide the investigation and analysis of an incident. However, it has

Table 6.1 Framework of contributory factors influencing clinical practice (from Vincent et al 1998)

Factor types	Contributory influencing factors
Patient factors	Condition (complexity and seriousness)
	Language and communication
	Personality and social factors
Task and technology factors	Task design and clarity of structure
	Availability and use of protocols
	Availability and accuracy of test results
	Decision-making aids
Individual (staff) factors	Knowledge and skills
	Competence
	Physical and mental health
Team factors	Verbal communication
	Written communication
	Supervision and seeking help
	Team leadership
Work environmental factors	Staffing levels and skills mix
	Workload and shift patterns
	Design, availability and maintenance of equipment
	Administrative and managerial support
	Physical environment
Organizational and management factors	Financial resources and constraints
	Organizational structure
	Policy, standards and goals
	Safety culture and priorities
Institutional context factors	Economic and regulatory context
	National health service executive
	Links with external organizations

also been used in the analysis of a series of 88 potentially serious prescribing errors (Dean et al 2002). Interviews with prescribers who made 44 of these errors provided a rich account of the factors contributing to these errors, which were analysed and classified using the seven levels framework, although in practice the influence of higher level factors could not be identified directly (Box 6.2). The importance of an analysis of this kind is that it begins to identify cross-cutting system issues and, more importantly still, to rank and prioritize them according to their frequency of occurrence. Staff identified staffing and workload issues as fundamental, followed by lack of skills and knowledge and physical health as being the most important contributory factors.

THE INVESTIGATION AND ANALYSIS OF CLINICAL INCIDENTS

A clinical scenario can be examined from a number of different perspectives, each of which will illuminate facets of the case. Cases have, from time immemorial, been used to educate and reflect on the nature of disease. They can also

> **Box 6.2 Classification (and number) of factors contributing to 88 potentially serious prescribing errors**
>
> (from Dean et al 2002)
>
> **Work environment**
> - Physical environment (13)
> - Staffing (37)
> - Heavy workload (31)
>
> **Team**
> - Communication (8)
> - Supervision (4)
> - Responsibility (11)
>
> **Individual**
> - Physical health: tired, hungry or unwell (18)
> - Mental health: low morale (8)
> - Skills and knowledge (24)
>
> **Task**
> - Protocols (8)
> - Not routine (9)
>
> **Patient**
> - Unhelpful (2)
> - Complex clinical disease (7)
> - Language and communication (2)

be used to illustrate the process of clinical decision making, the weighing of treatment options and sometimes, particularly when errors are discussed, the personal impact of incidents and mishaps. Incident analysis, for the purposes of improving the safety of healthcare, can encompass all of these perspectives but, critically, also includes reflection on the broader healthcare system.

Methods of investigation

A number of methods of investigation and analysis are available in healthcare, although these tend to be comparatively under-developed in comparison with methods available in industry. In the US, the most familiar is the root cause analysis approach of the Joint Commission, an intensive process with its origins in total quality management approaches to healthcare improvement (Spath 1999). The Veterans Hospital Administration has developed a highly structured system of triage questions, which is being disseminated throughout its system (National Center for Patient Safety (NCPS) 2003). A sample of the questions posed in the Veterans system is shown in Box 6.3. In our unit we have developed a method based on Reason's model and our framework of contributory factors. The method of root cause analysis developed by the NPSA in the UK is an amalgam of elements of all these approaches. We do not have space to examine all potential methods, which vary in their orientation, theoretical basis and basic approach. All, however, to a greater or lesser extent, uncover factors contributing to the final incident. We will summarize the approach developed by the Clinical Safety Research Unit

---

Box 6.3 Veterans Administration approach to root cause analysis

(adapted from NCPS 2003)

Examples of triage questions

Was communication a factor in this event?

• If Yes, go to Communications questions

Were appropriate rules/policies/procedures – or lack thereof – a factor in this event?

• If Yes, go to Rules/Policies/Procedures questions

Were issues related to staff training or staff competency a factor in this event?

• If Yes, go to Training questions

Examples of training questions

Was there a program to identify what is actually needed for training of staff?

• If No, this could be a root cause/contributing factor

Was training provided prior to the start of the work process?

• If No, this could be a root cause/contributing factor

Was training adequate? If not, consider the following factors:

• supervisory responsibility

• procedure omission

• flawed training rules, policy or procedure

Had procedures and equipment been reviewed to ensure a good match between people and the task they did?

• If procedures were not followed as intended go to Rules/Policies/Procedures questions

---

over the years with many London-based colleagues known, imaginatively, as the London protocol (Adams & Vincent 2004).

Systems analysis or root cause analysis?

For reasons that are now lost in history, most approaches to analysing incidents in healthcare are called 'root cause analysis'; by contrast we have described our own approach to the analysis of incidents as a systems analysis because we believe that it is a more accurate and more fruitful description. The term 'root cause analysis', although widespread, is misleading in a number of respects. To begin with it implies that there is a single root cause, or at least a small number. Typically, however, the picture that emerges is much more fluid and the notion of a root cause a gross over-simplification. There is usually a chain of events and a wide variety of contributory factors leading up to the eventual incident. However, a more important and fundamental objection to the term 'root cause analysis' relates to the very purpose of the investigation. Surely the purpose is obvious? To find out what happened and what caused it. Certainly it is necessary to find out what happened and why in order to explain to the patient, their family and others involved. However, if the purpose is to achieve a safer healthcare system then it is necessary to go further and reflect on what the incident reveals about the gaps and inadequacies in the healthcare system in which it occurred. The incident acts as a 'window' on the system, hence systems analysis.

Incident analysis, properly understood, is not a retrospective search for root causes but an attempt to look to the future. In a sense, the particular causes of the incident in question do not matter because they are now in the past.

However, the system weaknesses revealed are still present and could lead to the next incident (Vincent 2004); the London protocol aims to guide reflection on incidents in order to reveal these weaknesses.

Systems analysis of clinical incidents: the London protocol

During an investigation, information is gleaned from a variety of sources. Case records, statements and any other relevant documentation are reviewed. Structured interviews with key members of staff are then undertaken to establish the chronology of events, the main care delivery problems and their respective contributory factors, as perceived by each member of staff. The key questions are 'What happened? (the outcome and chronology); How did it happen? (the care delivery problems) and Why did it happen? (the contributory factors). Examples of care delivery problems and a summary of the process are shown in Boxes 6.4 and 6.5.

Once the chronology of events is clear there are three main considerations: the care delivery problems identified within the chronology, the clinical context for each of them and the factors contributing to the occurrence of the care delivery problems. Any combination of contributory factors might contribute to the occurrence of a single care delivery problem. The investigator needs to differentiate between those contributory factors that are relevant only to that particular occasion and those that are longstanding or permanent features of the unit. For instance, there might be a failure of communication between two midwives contributing to a care delivery problem. If this is unusual, and seldom occurs otherwise, then it is unlikely to have any wider implications and might not need to be considered further. If, however, this problem is more general then the incident is clearly reflecting a wider systemic problem, which needs to be addressed. Ideally, the patient, or a member of the patient's family, should also be interviewed, although as yet this does not often happen.

Although a considerable amount of information can be gleaned from written records, interviews with those involved are the most important method

---

Box 6.4 Examples of care delivery problems

(from Adams & Vincent 2004)

- Failure to monitor, observe or act
- Delay in diagnosis
- Inadequate risk assessment (for instance of suicide risk)
- Inadequate handover
- Failure to note faulty equipment
- Failure to carry out preoperative checks
- Not following an agreed protocol (without clinical justification)
- Not seeking help when necessary
- Incorrect protocol applied
- Treatment given to incorrect body site
- Wrong treatment given

Box 6.5 A summary of the process of investigation and analysis

(from Adams & Vincent 2004)

Care delivery problems (CDPs)

The first step in any analysis is to identify the care delivery problems. These are actions or omissions, or other deviations in the process of care, which had a direct or indirect effect on the eventual outcome for the patient.

Clinical context and patient factors

For each care delivery problem identified, the investigator records the salient clinical events or condition of the patient at that time (e.g. bleeding heavily, blood pressure falling) and other patient factors affecting the process of care (e.g. patient very distressed, patient unable to understand instructions).

Contributory factors

Having identified the CDP, the investigator then considers the conditions in which errors occur and the wider organizational context. These are the contributory factors. For each CDP the investigator uses the framework both during interviews and afterwards, to identify the factors that led to that particular care delivery problem. For example:

- Individual factors may include lack of knowledge or experience of particular staff
- Task factors might include the non-availability of test results or protocols
- Team factors might include inadequate supervision or poor communication between staff
- Work environment might include high workload, inadequate staffing or limited access to vital equipment

---

of identifying the contributory factors. This is especially so if the interview systematically explores these factors and so allows the member of staff to collaborate in the investigation. In the interview, the story and 'the facts' are just the first stage. The member of staff is also encouraged to identify both the care delivery problems and the contributory factors, which greatly enriches both the interview and investigation.

Analyses using this method have been conducted in hospitals, primary care settings and mental health units. The protocol can be used in a variety of formats, by individual clinicians, researchers, risk managers and by clinical teams. A clinical team might use the method to guide and structure reflection on an incident, to ensure that the analysis is full and comprehensive. For serious incidents, a team of individuals with different skills and backgrounds would be assembled, although often only a risk manager or an individual clinician will be needed. The protocol could also be used for teaching as a vehicle for introducing systems thinking. Whereas reading about systems thinking is helpful, actually analysing an incident brings systems thinking alive.

The contributory factors that reflect more general problems in a unit are the targets for change and systems improvement. When obvious problems are identified, action might be taken after a single incident, but when more substantial changes are being considered other incident analyses and sources of data (routine audits and outcome data) should also be taken into account. Recommendations might be made in a formal report but it is essential to follow these up with monitoring of action and outcome and to specify who is responsible for implementation.

AN ILLUSTRATIVE CASE EXAMPLE

Stephen Rogers (2002) adapted this method for use in primary care and family medicine settings, also producing a very clear format for presenting the findings of both the analysis and recommendations for action. He describes the following case:

Case example

(adapted from Rogers 2002 p 31)

Mrs G was a 70-year-old widow who was living alone in a ground floor Housing Association flat. Her first language was Portuguese and her English was poor. The patient had some genuine health problems but was excitable and tended to over-state the severity of her symptoms. The patient had suffered from osteoarthritis of the knees for years. She was prescribed regular analgesia and had been treated by a physiotherapist, but without perceiving any benefit. She had been referred for an orthopaedic opinion but was still waiting for an appointment.

After a fall at home, an ambulance was called and the patient was taken to an accident and emergency department. She was admitted for assessment and during her hospital stay she was seen by an orthopaedic surgeon, who included her in his operating list for a knee replacement the following week. The patient developed pyrexia after the operation but no cause was found and she was discharged, with instructions to complete a course of antibiotics. A week after discharge, a neighbour called the district nurses' office because 'no-one had been'. A nurse visited and noted that the patient's wound was moist. On a second visit the nurse told the patient to telephone for a doctor's visit, which she did later that day.

On the following day her doctor visited. He was concerned to find that the patient's knee was hot and painful, and admitted her to hospital with a provisional diagnosis of septic arthritis. A methicillin-resistant *Staphylococcus aureus* infection of the knee joint was confirmed and the patient required arthroscopic washout and long-term antibiotics. The patient's hospital discharge letter arrived on the day of her re-admission. The doctor reviewed the case, because he felt that the patient's diagnosis had been unnecessarily delayed.

The analysis and action plan are summarized in Tables 6.2 and 6.3. In this case, the analysis centres around the delay in diagnosis and summarizes the contributory factors from several points in the process of care. Rogers focuses on one particular problem in the process care – the delay in diagnosis of infection following discharge from hospital. In this instance, this spans a period of several days and involves quite a number of clinical staff. The initial problem in fact stemmed from the patient being discharged from hospital without the cause of the infection being ascertained, which could have been separately examined as a care delivery problem. However, once discharged, a combination of misunderstanding of the purpose of the antibiotics, inadequate communication from the hospital, slow communication between members of the primary care team and other factors led to a week during which

Table 6.2 Care delivery problem: there was delay in recognizing the seriousness of the patient's complaint (adapted from Rogers 2002)

Factor	Contributory influencing factors
Patient factors	The patient was not able to make her worries and concerns clear to her doctor The patient had an anxious temperament and had tended to over-state the severity of her symptoms in the past
Individual factors	The visiting nurse assumed that the antibiotics prescribed by the hospital were for the patients 'wound infection' The doctor interpreted the patient's call as a request for a 'routine review' at the request of the visiting district nurse
Task factors	District nurses typically communicated with the doctors in the practice by passing messages via reception The patient's discharge letter arrived 9 days after the patient was sent home
Team factors	There was no call from the orthopaedic ward to indicate a need for district nurse input The visiting nurse did not discuss the case in detail with nursing colleagues, nor with the doctors
Work environment factors	There was no strong culture of communication between the district nursing team and the practice doctors The visiting nurse was temporarily seconded to the team on account of staffing shortages. She was not familiar with the local doctors The district nursing sister was on holiday and the deputy did not have any explicit system for staff supervision in the sister's absence
Organizational management and institutional factors	Measures designed principally to optimize bed management can compromise other aspects of the hospital admission and discharge process Recruitment problems in district nursing lead to teams being understaffed and to frequent relocations of individuals

the infection went unrecognized. This delay certainly had consequences for the patient, although the eventual outcome was good. The importance of the example lies in the fact that even a relatively ordinary incident can be used to examine weaknesses in the process of care and to suggest points where improvements might be made. The suggested action plan in Table 6.3 clearly shows how the basic framework of contributory factors also forms the basis for the action plan and how the contributory factors themselves are the targets for change.

HUMAN RELIABILITY ANALYSIS

Analyses of specific incidents, especially when systematic and thorough, can illuminate systemic weaknesses and help us understand how things go wrong. We have seen how there is frequently a chain of events leading to an incident and a variety of contributing factors. Having understood these principles, we are now able to approach the examination of system weaknesses

Table 6.3 Suggested action plan (adapted from Rogers 2002)

Changes for consideration	What	Who	How
Individuals	Appraise possible learning needs of visiting community nurse	District nursing sister	Informal discussion Include needs identified in appraisal cycle
Tasks	Review clinical issues around management and discharge of patients with post-operative pyrexia of unknown origin	Hospitals consultant(s) and/or infection control officer	Review of case series Establish consensus and develop protocol Implement protocol and review
	Review practice policy on home visits	General practice partners	Review of case series Establish consensus and develop guidance Implement and review
Teams	Avoid delay in communicating discharge details to primary care staff	Senior hospital clinicians and management	Consider faxing discharge details to practice doctors Reinforce hospital policy of telephoning community teams on discharge of elderly patients
Work environment	Ensure that overall levels of staffing and supervisory arrangements are not compromised by absences for leave, sickness, etc	District nursing sister and trust nurse managers	Review and monitor arrangements for cross-cover
	Ensure mechanisms are in place for effective communication between district nursing staff and GPs	District nursing sister, general practice doctors	Group discussion Explore mechanisms for meeting Implement and review
Organizational and institutional management	Improve incentives and support for recruitment to district nursing	Hospital nurse managers, strategic health authority	Review manpower planning and recruitment activities

from a different perspective. Rather than take a case, analyse it and see where it leads us, an alternative approach is to begin with a process of care and systematically examine it for possible failure points. This is the province of human reliability analysis.

Human reliability analysis or assessment (HRA) has been defined as the application of relevant information about human characteristics and behaviour to the design of objects, facilities, and environments that people use (Kirwan 1994). HRA techniques can be used in the analysis of incidents but are more usually used to examine a process or system. HRA techniques of various kinds have been in use in high-risk industries and military settings for over 50 years. For instance, failure modes and effects analysis (FMEA) was developed in 1949 by the US military to determine the effects of system and equipment failures, and was used by NASA in the 1960s to predict failures, plan preventative measures and back-up systems in the Apollo Space Programme (Kirwan 1994). Since then, HRA has been applied in many 'high-risk' industries, including aviation and aerospace, rail, shipping, air traffic control, automobile, offshore oil and gas, chemical, and all parts of the military. In more mundane settings, HRA has been applied to the installation of telecommunications equipment, design of computer software and hardware and to manual tasks such as lathe operation. HRA has been applied at all stages of the 'life-cycle' of a process from design of a system, normal functioning of the process, maintenance and decommissioning (Lyons et al 2005).

Techniques that purport to assess reliability of systems in advance of their operations have been particularly closely associated with the development of the nuclear industry; to gain public acceptance and an operating licence, designers and builders of nuclear power plants have to demonstrate *in advance* that the designs and proposed methods of operation are safe. This requires a minutely detailed specification of the actual processes, a quantitative assessment of the likelihood of different kinds of failure, a quantitative assessment of the likelihood of different kinds of human error and, finally, modelling the combined effects of all possible combinations of error and breakdown to give an overall assessment of safety.

Techniques of human reliability analysis

There are a vast number of these analytic techniques, derived by different people in different industries for different purposes. Most are commercial in origin, often not published in the academic literature and not subject to formal evaluation or validation. To add to the confusion, the reader is faced with a wealth of opaque acronyms, such as FMEA, HRA, PSA, PRA, SLIM, HEART, THERP, HAZOP (Lyons et al 2005).

Some techniques are primarily aimed at providing a close description of a task or to map out the work sequence. For instance, in hierarchical task analysis, the task description is broken down into subtasks or operations; this approach has been applied with much success to error analysis in endoscopic surgery (Joice et al 1998). Human error identification and analysis techniques build on a basic task analysis to provide a detailed description of the kinds of error that can occur and the points in the sequence where they are likely to occur: some involve highly structured taxonomies that assist the analyst in defining ways in which a task can fail; some of the methodologies also take situational, contextual or environmental factors into account that might impact on an individual or system and make errors more or less likely to occur.

The goal of human error quantification is to produce error probabilities, building on task analysis and error identification techniques to provide a probabilistic risk assessment. This provides numerical estimates of error likelihood and of the probability of overall likelihood of system breakdown. Quantification of error is the most difficult aspect of HRA. Assigning numbers to necessarily uncertain events, that is, the expected probability of an unknown individual making an error, is an enormous challenge. Often the quantification is heavily reliant on expert judgement, rather than the more rigorous approach of actual observation and recording of error frequencies. Such techniques are little used in healthcare but have been successfully applied to anaesthesia (Paté-Cornell 1999). Nevertheless, some hospital tasks, such as blood transfusion, are highly structured and the quantification of errors probabilities would seem to be eminently feasible (Lyons et al 2005).

Box 6.6 summarizes some of the best-known approaches to give a general sense of the range of methods. Some of the approaches focus on mapping a process and identifying points of weakness or hazard. These include event tree analysis, fault tree analysis and failure modes and effects analysis; these are all general approaches used in a variety of ways. HAZOP (hazard and operability study), which is used particularly in the chemical industry, offers a specific methodology and approach to this basic question. Probabilistic reliability analysis (PRA) goes one step further, taking a basic fault tree and adding specific probabilities to the various branches so that an overall assessment of risk can be derived. Finally, there are approaches that address the conditions in which people work rather than the process itself emphasizing, as Reason's accident model does, the importance of assessing latent factors and organizational processes. These include Tripod Delta, developed by Reason and colleagues for use in the oil industry, and HEART, developed by Jeremy Williams, an ergonomist, to assess the influence of error producing conditions in various contexts (Reason 1997, Williams 1985).

Human reliability techniques are, ideally, used at the design stage of a process and subsequently during actual operation. In healthcare, such analyses could certainly be used in this way when, for instance, designing a new infusion pump or setting up a new outpatient cancer centre. However, these techniques are just

---

Box 6.6 Techniques of human reliability analysis

(from Redmill & Rajan 1997 and Reason 1997)

- *Fault tree analysis* starts with a potential, or actual, undesirable event and works backwards seeking the immediate cause, preceding causes and combinations of causes.
- *Event tree analysis* works forward from events (such as equipment failure) and assesses their possible consequences in different unfolding scenarios.
- *Failure modes and effects analysis (FMEA)* analyses potential failures of systems, components or functions and their effects. Each component is considered in turn, its possible modes of failure defined and the potential effects delineated.
- *Hazard analysis and critical control points (HACCP)* is a systematic methodology for the identification, assessment and control of hazards, mostly used in food production.
- *Hazard and operability study (HAZOP)* is a team-based, systematic, qualitative method to identify hazards (or deviations in design intent) in process industries.
- *Probabilistic risk assessment (PRA)* builds on such techniques as FMEA and HAZOP by adding modelling of fault and event trees and assignment of probabilities to events and outcomes.
- *Tripod delta* is an integrated system of safety management that assesses general failure types, such as maintenance and design problems, and their potential impact on safety.
- *Human error assessment and reduction technique (HEART)* examines particular task types and their associated error probabilities using tables of task types and factors which impact on the performance of the task.

beginning to be explored systematically in healthcare and are mainly being applied to existing systems. Examples of successful application are few and far between as yet, but are very likely to increase in both number and importance in the next few years. We will examine the most common technique used in healthcare so far and provide examples of its application.

FAILURE MODES AND EFFECTS ANALYSIS (FMEA)

The Joint Commission in the US, the NPSA in the UK and the US Veterans Administration (VA) all encourage the use of failure modes and effects analysis (FMEA). The Joint Commission now requires organizations to carry out at least one FMEA each year as part of their accreditation programme. Guidelines are provided on the respective websites and the VA in particular has taken steps to review available methods and customize them for use in healthcare, using elements of classical FMEA, their own root cause analysis framework and the HACPP approach (see Box 6.6). Their guidance provides a very clearly delineated process, specific terminology, decision trees, severity scoring matrix and worksheets. The main steps of the VA process are summarized in Box 6.7 (DeRosier et al 2002). Immediately, we can see that this is a

---

Box 6.7 Healthcare failure modes and effects analysis: a summary of the Veterans Administration process

(adapted from DeRosier et al 2002)

Step 1: define the HFMEA topic
This will usually be a high-volume or high-risk area that warrants a sustained safety programme.

Step 2: assemble a multidisciplinary team
It is helpful to have different disciplines represented. Including people who are not familiar with the process under review encourages critical and innovative thinking.

Step 3: map out the process using flowcharts and diagrams
- Develop and check the flow diagram.
- If the process is complex, identify the area to focus on.
- Identify all subprocesses (e.g. the analysis phase of PSA testing).
- Create a flow diagram for subprocesses.

Step 4: conduct a hazard analysis
- List all potential failures modes for each process and subprocess, using the expertise of the whole team.
- Assess the severity of failure at any particular point.
- Decide whether the failure mode warrants further action.
- Repeat for all phases of the process.

Step 5: actions and outcome measures
- Determine whether you want to eliminate, control or accept each potential cause of failure.
- Identify possible courses of action to eliminate or control failure modes.
- Identify outcome measures that will be used to test the redesigned process.
- Identify a single responsible individual to act and monitor the outcomes.
- Indicate whether top management has backed the recommended action.
- Test to make sure that new vulnerabilities have not been introduced in the system as a result of the changes.

---

substantial undertaking, but clearly necessary when dealing with a complex, sophisticated and hazardous process. A great strength of the VA approach is the insistence on the involvement and backing of senior management.

To give a sense of how FMEA works in practice, we will review an analysis carried out in the Good Samaritan Hospital, Ohio (Burgmeier 2002). The hospital's Safety Board, aware of healthcare's vulnerability to error, decided to proactively assess high-risk processes. Blood transfusion was the first process to be studied because it affected a large number of patients, because haemolytic reactions to blood could be fatal and because the procedure had become very complicated – numerous steps and double checks had been added to safeguard patients and meet regulatory requirements; well-intentioned efforts to increase safety, by adding checks, had introduced a new hazard, that of complexity. The team assembled followed the JCAHO approach but the essential process is similar to that outlined above.

The team assembled was quite large and appropriately senior and multidisciplinary. There were representatives from risk management, blood transfusion services, administration, surgery, intensive care and high-use patient areas. Roles were defined and a total of 4 days set aside for the initial mapping and analysis. The difficulties in simply producing the flow chart were extremely illuminating. There were two organizational policies, five nursing procedures and a multitude of special considerations, for example, certain kinds of filtered tubing are inappropriate for some blood products. We can speculate that probably no one person in this organization fully understood this process until they sat down and mapped it out. The final process had multiple steps and, as a consequence, multiple potential sources of failure. Looking at these processes, one marvels not so much at the level of error as at people's ability to navigate these complex, imperfect systems.

For each step in the process the team considered what could go wrong (the failure mode), why the failure might occur (cause) and what could happen if it did occur (effects). An example of the analysis of a failure mode is shown in Box 6.8. A total of 40 failure modes were identified, each of which was then rated on a 10-point scale for occurrence (how easily it could happen), severity and detectability (if it did occur how likely it is that the failure would go undetected). These three scores are then multiplied together to give a rough index of hazard. The most highly rated potential failure modes are shown in Box 6.9.

The FMEA process produced a series of recommendations for immediate change and for longer-term moves to computerized physician order entry and bar coding. The immediate changes included the introduction of a standardized form for blood products that allowed physicians to check boxes for ordering while documenting the reasons for the transfusion; a blood barrier system that restricted access to the blood until a patient code was dialled in and a video to provide the required training. Most importantly, the multitude of policies and procedures relating to blood transfusion were combined into a single comprehensive policy that incorporated a flow chart of the new process

Looking at these changes in a more generic way, we can see a strong element of simplification and standardization at the core. Simplify the policies and procedures, make the flow chart explicit, develop a standard form used by everyone and provide training to get the new systems started. In addition,

---

Box 6.8 A failure mode in the blood transfusion process

(adapted from Burgmeier 2002)

Failure mode

Two people do not always check order entry for blood products.

Causes
- Immediate patient care elsewhere is often more important.
- Nurses do not fully understand the consequences of a decision not to enter an order when they give priority to a patient elsewhere.
- Nurses do not fully use each other as resources.
- Nurse entering order prefers to 'get things done' rather than follow process carefully and correctly.
- Current policy is not explicit that two people must check the order.

Potential effects of failure
- Waste of personnel and resources.
- Delay in treatment to appropriate patient.
- Ties up scarce blood resources.
- Increases patient's level of risk.
- Increases length of stay.
- Demoralizes people involved ('I could have harmed someone!').

Design action (solutions)
- Blood-specific order form used by all departments and on computer screen that is completed by physician.
- Order form faxed through to Blood Transfusion Service and double-checked against computer entry.
- Training on use of form will be given to everyone participating in blood transfusion process.
- In the longer term, physician will enter order directly into computer.

Validation and monitoring
- Incidents of documented variance are recorded and analysed.
- Manager will discuss variances with staff as necessary.

---

an additional 'defence' was put in place in the form of the blood barrier system. Monitoring of the changes showed a steady reduction in variances and problems as the system bedded down and no instances of serious error or harm to patients in the initial months.

Box 6.9 Most serious failure modes in blood transfusion process

(adapted from Burgmeier 2002)

- Failure to accurately match the right blood to the right patient.
- Nurse might not remain with patient for full 15 minutes after start of transfusion.
- The patient's stated name and ID band might not be compared when the type and cross-match specimen is drawn.
- The person applying the label to the type and cross-match specimen might not verify the patient's ID band.
- The person applying the label to the type and cross-match specimen might accept verbal instructions instead of requiring a printed requisition.
- Two people might not check the order entry.
- The order might be interpreted differently from the physician's intent.

Although a formal evaluation of the FMEA and changes made was not attempted (there were no before-and-after measures) this appears to have been a very worthwhile exercise resulting in a much clearer and safer system. Nevertheless, it is important to realize that safety improvements of this kind require significant time and resources. The final judgement of the team was that although FMEA had many advantages as an approach, it was not to be employed lightly. Tackling FMEA had involved substantial investment of time, money and energy and they planned to reserve its use for high-priority processes only (Burgmeier 2002).

INTEGRATION AND EVALUATION OF ANALYTIC TECHNIQUES

Incident analysis is usually seen as retrospective, whereas techniques such as FMEA, which examine a process of care, are seen as prospective and, therefore, potentially superior. The idea is that by using prospective analysis we can prevent the next incident, rather than using case analysis to look back at something that has already gone wrong. We might think that, as healthcare becomes safer, these prospective analyses will eventually supplant incident analysis. Leaving aside the fact that healthcare has rather a long way to go before the supply of incidents dries up, there are a number of reasons for continuing to explore individual incidents as well as examining systems prospectively.

To begin with, there is no sharp division between retrospective and prospective techniques; as argued above, the true purpose of incident analysis is to use the incident as a window onto the system, in essence looking at current weakness and future potential problems. Conversely, so-called prospective analysis relies extensively on the past experience of those involved. Probabilities and hazards assessed in failure modes and effects analysis are derived almost exclusively from groups of clinicians on the basis of their past experience. Techniques such as FMEA are, in addition, very expensive in terms of time and resources. The analysis of single incidents, whether or not they have a bad outcome, can be scaled to the time and resource available, be it 10 minutes or 10 days. A single incident, a story, almost always engages a clinical group and can be analysed by an individual risk manager or a whole clinical team.

The future probably lies in a judicious application of both forms of techniques, using systems analyses of incidents to generate both enthusiasm and hypotheses as a basis for more resource intensive analyses of whole processes and systems. A major concern with all the techniques discussed is the lack of formal testing and evaluation. Most of these methods are in what might be termed a 'development' phase, analogous to the initial testing of a drug in clinical populations. In one of the few reviews of these techniques, Jeremy Williams began by saying 'It must seem quite extraordinary to most scientists engaged in research into other areas of the physical and technological world that there has been little attempt by human reliability experts to validate the human reliability assessment techniques which they so freely propagate, modify and disseminate' (Williams 1985). By 1997 little had changed, and Redmill & Rajan (1997) could write that human reliability techniques were developed independently, without an intention to standardize, or even to define, the boundaries between them and suggest that there was a considerable need for standardization, evaluation, consistency in terminology and exploration of the strengths and limitations of the various methods. Healthcare, although coming late to these approaches, might in fact have much to offer because of the much stronger tradition of use of evidence, comparative clinical trials, evaluation and quantitative research. As patient safety becomes a more professional and better-founded enterprise, we should hope that the various approaches will be more rigorously evaluated to assess their strengths, limitations and individual contributions.

REFERENCES

Adams S, Vincent C 2004 Systems analysis of clinical incidents: the London protocol. Online. Available at: http://www.csru.org.uk

Balen P 2004 Gross negligence manslaughter: Wayne Jowett. Clinical Risk 10:25–27

Burgmeier J 2002 Failure mode and effect analysis: an application in reducing risk in blood transfusion. Joint Commission Journal on Quality Improvement 28:331–339

Dean B, Schachter M, Vincent CA et al 2002 Causes of prescribing errors in hospital inpatients: a prospective study. Lancet 359:1373–1378

DeRosier J, Stalhandske E, Bagian JP et al 2002 Using health care failure mode and effect analysis: the VA National Center for Patient Safety's prospective risk analysis system. Joint Commission Journal on Quality & Safety 28:248–267

Helmreich RL 2000 On error management: lessons from aviation. British Medical Journal 320:781–785

Holbrook J 2003 The criminalisation of fatal medical mistakes. British Medical Journal 327:1118–1119

Joice P, Hanna GB, Cuschieri A 1998 Errors enacted in endoscopic surgery. Surgery 29:409–414

Kirwan B 1994 A guide to practical human reliability assessment. Taylor and Francis, London

Lyons M, Adams S, Woloshnowych M et al 2004 Human reliability techniques in healthcare. International Journal of Risk and Safety in Medicine 16:223–227

National Centre for Patient Safety (NCPS) 2003 NCPS home page. Online. Available at: http://www.patientsafety.gov

Paté-Cornell ME 1999 Medical application of engineering risk analysis and anesthesia patient risk illustration. American Journal of Therapeutics 6:245–255

Reason JT 1997 Managing the risks of organisational accidents. Ashgate, Aldershot

Reason JT 2001 Understanding adverse events: the human factor. In: Vincent C (ed) Clinical risk management: enhancing patient safety, 2 edn, BMJ Publications, London

Reason JT 1990 Human error. Cambridge University Press, New York

Redmill R, Rajan J 1997 Human factors in safety critical systems. Butterworth Heinemann, Oxford

Rogers S 2002 A structured approach for the investigation of clinical incidents in health care: application in a general practice setting. British Journal of General Practice 52:S30–S32

Spath P (ed) 1999 Error reduction in health care: a systems approach to improving patient safety. AHA Press, Washington

Toft B 2001 External inquiry into the adverse incident that occurred at Queen's Medical Centre, Nottingham. Department of Health, London

Vincent C 2004 Analysis of clinical incidents: a window on the system not a search for root causes. Quality & Safety in Health Care 13:242–243

Vincent C, Taylor-Adams S, Stanhope N 1998 Framework for analysing risk and safety in clinical medicine. British Medical Journal 316:1154–1157

Williams JC 1985 Validation of human reliability assessment technique. Reliability Engineering 11:149–162

The aftermath: caring for patients harmed by treatment

If only I had been told honestly, I could have faced it so much better.
(Vincent, personal communication from a patient.)

Previous chapters have shown that many patients experience errors during their treatment, whether they realize it or not, and some are inadvertently harmed by healthcare. The harm might be minor, involving only inconvenience or discomfort, but can involve serious disability or death. Almost all bad outcomes will have some psychological consequences, ranging from worry and distress through to depression and even despair. Most of this book has been devoted to understanding how adverse events occur and how they can be prevented. However, what happens after such events can be just as important as what happens before. Thankfully, there are now initiatives in several countries for policies of open disclosure about errors, an important first step to the more humane and thoughtful treatment of patients and families. As yet, however, much less attention has been paid to the long-term consequences for injured patients and very few healthcare organizations have shouldered the full responsibility of looking after people they have harmed. The experiences of these people tend not to be fully appreciated, and yet understanding the impact of such injuries is a prerequisite of providing useful and effective help. The aim of this chapter is to convey something of the experience of injured patients and their families and to give some guidance on how they can be helped.

PSYCHOLOGICAL RESPONSES TO MEDICAL INJURY

Patients are often in a vulnerable psychological state, even when diagnosis is clear and treatment goes according to plan. Even routine procedures and normal childbirth can produce post-traumatic symptoms (Clark et al 1997, Czarnocka & Slade 2000). When they experience harm or misadventure therefore, patients' reactions are likely to be particularly severe.

Traumatic and life-threatening events produce a variety of symptoms, over and above any physical injury. Sudden, intense, dangerous or uncontrollable events are particularly likely to lead to psychological problems, especially if accompanied by illness, fatigue or mood disturbances (Brewin et al 1996). Awareness under anaesthesia is an example of such an event. When people experience such a terrifying, if short lived, event they often later suffer from anxiety, intrusive and disturbing memories, emotional numbing and flash-backs. Almost everyone experiences such memories after stressful events, such as a divorce or bereavement and, although unpleasant, they gradually die down. However, they can be intense, prolonged and cause considerable suffering. In severe cases the person might suffer from the full syndrome of post-traumatic stress disorder, discussed below.

The full impact of some incidents only becomes apparent in the longer-term. A perforated bowel, for example, might require a series of further oper-ations and time in hospital. The long-term consequences can include chronic pain, disability and depression, with a deleterious effect on family relation-ships and ability to work (Vincent et al 1993). Depression appears to be a more common long-term response to medical injury than post-traumatic stress dis-order (Vincent & Coulter 2002), although there is little research in this area. Whether people actually become depressed and to what degree will depend on the severity of their injury, the support they have from family, friends and health professionals and a variety of other factors (Kessler 1997).

When a patient dies, the trauma is obviously more severe still and can be particularly severe after a potentially avoidable death (Lundin 1984). For instance, many people who have lost a spouse or child in a road accident con-tinue to ruminate about the accident and what could have been done to pre-vent it for years afterwards. They are often unable to accept, resolve or find any meaning in the loss (Lehman et al 1987). Relatives of patients whose death was sudden or unexpected might therefore find the loss particularly difficult to bear. If the loss was avoidable in the sense that poor treatment played a part in the death, the patient's relatives can face an unusually trau-matic and prolonged bereavement. They might ruminate endlessly on the death and find it hard to deal with the loss.

INJURY FROM MEDICAL TREATMENT IS DIFFERENT FROM OTHER INJURIES

The impact of a medical injury differs from most other accidents in some impor-tant respects. First, patients have been harmed – unintentionally – by people in whom they placed considerable trust and so their reactions might be especially powerful and hard to cope with. Second, patients are often cared for by the same professions, and perhaps the same people, as those involved in the origi-nal injury. As they might have been very frightened by what has happened to them, and have a range of conflicting feelings about those involved, this too can be very difficult, even when staff are sympathetic and supportive.

Patients and relatives can also suffer in two distinct ways from the injury itself. First from the injury itself and second from the way the incident is han-dled afterwards. Many people harmed by their treatment suffer further trau-ma through the incident being insensitively and inadequately handled. Conversely, when staff come forward, acknowledge the damage and take the necessary action, the support offered can ameliorate the impact both in the short and long term. Injured patients need an explanation, an apology, to know that changes have been made to prevent future incidents and often also practical and financial help (Vincent et al 1994). This is not to say that they necessarily need unusual treatment or that staff should be wary of talking to them. The problems tend to arise when ordinary impulses to help are blunted by anxiety, shame or just not knowing what to say.

THE EXPERIENCES OF INJURED PATIENTS AND THEIR RELATIVES

Reports of studies help us understand the main effects of injury to patients but it is still difficult to grasp the full extent of the trauma that people sometimes face. Appreciating and understanding their experiences is essential if one is going to provide individually appropriate and practical help. The two true stories retold here illustrate some of the principal forms of trauma that result from serious adverse events: chronic pain and depression, anxiety and other post-traumatic reactions. The focus of each case description is on the effects on the people involved, rather than the clinical events that preceded them. The quotations are the patient's or relative's own words taken from the interviews. Names and other details have been changed to protect the identity of those involved.

Perforation of the colon leading to chronic pain and depression

Mrs Long suffered a series of avoidable surgical complications over a period of several months, which left her in considerable pain (Box 7.1). Traumatic experiences, chronic pain and physical weakness combined to produce a serious depression that lasted several years. The depression was marked by classic symptoms of low mood, tiredness, fatigue, low self-esteem and sleep disturbance (Box 7.2) but nevertheless went unnoticed by any of the health professionals involved in her care. Clearly there were many problems with her surgical treatment and care on the wards. However, her problems were compounded by the lack of explanation or apology, a lack of interest or response from the hospital where all the problems occurred and the complete failure of anyone involved in her care to realize how deeply she had been affected (Vincent 2001).

Neonatal death: bereavement and post-traumatic stress disorder

Many of the symptoms and experiences reported by Mr Carter (Box 7.3) are common in any bereavement. Depression, distressing memories, feelings of anger and dreams of the person who has died are not unusual. However, the intensity, character and duration of Mr Carter's reaction indicates that this was far from an ordinary bereavement. Anger of this intensity and violent daydreams are not usual, and show that he was suffering from post-traumatic stress disorder (Box 7.4). The staff of the paediatric unit clearly tried to help Mr and Mrs Carter, although they did not seem to appreciate what he was

---

Box 7.1 Perforation of the colon leading to chronic pain and depression

(adapted from Vincent 2001)

A woman underwent a ventrosuspension – the fixation of a displaced uterus to the abdominal wall. After the operation she awoke with a terrible pain in her lower abdomen, which became steadily worse over the next 4 days. She was very frightened and repeatedly told both doctors and nurses but they dismissed it as 'wind'.

On the fifth day the pain reached a crescendo and she felt a 'ripping sensation' inside her abdomen. That evening the wound opened and the contents of her bowel began to seep through the dressings. Even then, no one seemed concerned. Finally, the surgeon realized that the bowel had been perforated and a temporary colostomy was carried out.

The next operation, to reverse the colostomy, was 'another fiasco'. After a few days there was a discharge of faecal matter from the scar, the wound became infected and the pain was excruciating, especially after eating. She persistently asked if she could be fed with a drip but the nursing staff insisted she should keep eating. For 2 weeks she was 'crying with the pain, really panicking – I just couldn't take it any more'. She was finally transferred to another hospital where she was immediately put on a liquid diet.

A final operation to repair the bowel was successful but left her exhausted and depressed. She began to recover her strength only after a year of convalescence. Three years later she was still constantly tired, irritable, low in spirits and 'I don't enjoy anything any more'. She no longer welcomes affection or comfort and feels that she is going downhill, becoming more gloomy and preoccupied.

Her scars are still uncomfortable and painful at the time of her periods. Her stomach is 'deformed' and she feels much less confident and attractive as a result. As her depression has deepened, she has become less interested in sex and more self-conscious about the scar. Three years later the trauma of her time in hospital is still very much alive. She still has nightmares about her time in hospital and is unable to talk about it without breaking into tears. She feels very angry and bitter that no one has ever apologized to her or admitted that a mistake has been made.

---

suffering and did not ask about traumatic reactions. Given the strength of Mr Carter's emotional reaction, it would probably still have been very difficult for him to accept an explanation early on even if the death had been unavoidable. The necessary explanation would have to have been given gradually, over several meetings, and combined with some attempts to support him and ease the intensity of his reaction (Vincent 2001).

Post-traumatic stress disorder is a term that is bandied about fairly indiscriminately, and a word of caution is needed about its use. Properly conceived,

---

Box 7.2 Principal symptoms of depression

(adapted from American Psychiatric Association (APA) 1994)

- Continual depressed mood
- Loss of interest or pleasure in daily activities
- Significant weight loss (when not dieting), or loss of appetite
- Insomnia or excessive sleeping
- Fatigue and loss of energy nearly every day
- Strong and frequent feelings of worthlessness or guilt
- Diminished ability to think, concentrate or make decisions
- Recurrent thoughts of death, suicidal ideas or suicide attempts

---

Box 7.3 Neonatal death: bereavement and post-traumatic stress disorder

(adapted from Vincent 2001)

Mr Carter's son, Jamie, sustained injuries at birth, due to inadequate obstetric care, causing irreparable spinal cord injury. He died when he was 2 months old without regaining consciousness.

Three days after the birth a paediatrician confirmed that their son was, as they suspected, severely handicapped. He suffered from fits and was partially sighted. He never cried or made any sounds because his vocal cords had been damaged. In spite of these injuries he continued to grow and put on weight. Two weeks after Jamie's birth they were told that he would not live. They then spent two terrible months, mostly at the hospital, waiting for him to die.

Mr and Mrs Carter had a number of meetings with hospital staff but Mr Carter never felt he had received a full explanation. He remembers being told that 'it was just one of those things – that really sent me sky-rocketing. No one said it was a mistake, that's what wound me up. Till this day I've got many questions. No one acted quickly enough. No doctor came at all until the paediatrician arrived'.

Mr Carter's reaction to Jamie's death was intense, violent and prolonged. For a year he suffered from disturbing memories and horrific dreams. He became quiet, withdrawn and remote even from his wife, feeling 'empty and hopeless'. He was tormented by disturbing images and memories of Jamie, of the birth, his slow death and particularly of his small, shrunken skull toward the end. Images of Jamie's birth still 'popped into my head at the most unexpected times. Very vivid, just like looking in on it. It just grabs you round the throat'. He suffered from a persistent stress-related stomach disorder. His sleep was interrupted by violent nightmares of a kind he had never previously experienced. 'There was all this blood and gore, fantasy-like stuff.' During the day violent images, sometimes of killing people, would come into his head, which absolutely horrified him.

Before Jamie's death, Mr Carter had always been a relaxed and easy-going person. Now he was easily irritated and there were many arguments between him and his wife. At work his irritability would often turn to anger, leading to confrontations and sometimes to fights. 'I was really angry all the time, so aggressive – I wanted to hurt people, and I'm not like that at all. I felt I had to blame someone all the time for everything.'

About a year later Mrs Carter became pregnant again. Mr Carter was very anxious during the pregnancy but his symptoms began to subside after their daughter was born. Two years on he still breaks down and cries occasionally, and is generally a sadder and quieter person. When he passes the cemetery where his son is buried he still becomes angry but now the feelings subside.

The aftermath: caring for patients harmed by treatment

it is a formal psychiatric diagnosis with strict, specific criteria. We have no idea how many people suffer from the full syndrome after medical treatment, like Mr Carter, but the number is probably small. However, the incidence of some of the symptoms is probably very much greater. Many injured patients I have spoken to, for instance, suffered from nightmares about their treatment and time in hospital, from persistent and intrusive recollections of their care and other problems. They were not, however, suffering the full constellation of symptoms that makes up post-traumatic stress disorder. Many of these reactions to trauma are ordinary, if very unpleasant, responses to traumatic events. Anyone working with patients who have been harmed needs to know about them though, because many of the patients will be experiencing such reactions. Just talking about them and finding out that they are common responses can be a considerable relief for the people concerned.

> **Box 7.4 Principal symptoms of post-traumatic stress disorder**
>
> (adapted from APA 1994)
>
> - The person has been exposed to a traumatic event in which there was actual or threatened death or serious injury, to themselves or someone close to them.
> - The person's response involves intense fear, helplessness or horror.
> - The traumatic event is persistently re-experienced in one or more of the following ways:
>   - recurrent and intrusive distressing recollections of the event
>   - recurrent distressing dreams
>   - acting or feeling as if the event was re-occurring
>   - intense distress at thoughts and or reminders of the event.
> - Persistent avoidance of reminders of the event:
>   - avoiding thoughts and feelings associated with the event
>   - avoiding activities and places associated with the event
>   - inability to recall important aspects of the trauma
>   - feelings of detachment from others
>   - restricted range of feelings.
> - Persistent symptoms of increased arousal:
>   - difficulty falling or staying asleep
>   - irritability or outbursts of anger
>   - difficulty concentrating
>   - hypervigilance
>   - exaggerated startle response.

In earlier chapters we covered dozens of studies of errors and adverse events. 'Adverse event' is a useful but deliberately neutral technical term. It does not, and is not intended to, capture the often awful human stories that lie behind this innocuous term. These two stories, and many, many more are available, give some indication of what happens to people when things go wrong. This is really the heart of patient safety and its justification. We can also see, particularly in the first story, that the impact of the original incident was made very much worse by the way it was handled afterwards – the second trauma. So, how can we best help injured patients? The remainder of this chapter provides some ideas and guidance, but be warned that this aspect of patient safety is very little developed.

PRINCIPLES FOR HELPING PATIENTS AND THEIR FAMILIES

Every injured patient has his or her own particular problems and needs. Some will require a great deal of professional help whereas others will prefer to rely on family and friends. Some will primarily require remedial medical treatment whereas in others the psychological effects will be to the fore. Hospitals and other healthcare organizations are just beginning to take their responsibilities seriously and risk managers and clinicians are beginning to follow-up injured patients and consider their longer-term needs. Although the task of dealing with adverse outcomes falls mainly on individual clinicians, they need to be backed by those senior to them and by the organization as a whole. Successful handling of adverse outcomes relies on the sensitivity and courage of individual clinicians and risk managers, but also requires a commitment to certain basic principles at the highest level of the organization. It is quite unrealistic, indeed quite unfair, to expect openness and honesty from individuals without the backing of a policy of honesty and openness approved by the governing body of the organization concerned.

A number of basic considerations will help in dealing with anyone who has been injured or seriously distressed by their treatment, whether or not negligence or litigation are involved. In the short term, the two most important principles are to believe the patient and to be as honest and open as possible.

Believe the patient

When a clinician is first faced with a patient who seems not to be doing as well as he or she should, in fact might even be getting worse, the immediate reaction might be that the patient is exaggerating the pain, or is even a neurotic complainer. In fact, patients who consider that they have been harmed by their treatment should in the first instance be believed. In many cases it might turn out that they had unrealistic expectations of their treatment, or had not fully understood the risks involved. In a few cases they might be malingering or hypochondriacal. However, given the frequency of adverse events, a report of such an injury should at least be seen as credible. It should certainly not be automatically seen as evidence of personality problems or of being 'difficult'. Being believed is extremely important for injured patients and, conversely, not being believed is always frustrating and can be intensely disturbing.

Honesty and openness

A patient harmed by treatment poses acute and painful dilemmas for the staff involved. It is natural to avoid that pain by avoiding the patient, yet the staff's response is crucial to the patient's recovery. When patients think that information is being concealed from them, or that they are being dismissed as trouble-makers, it is much more difficult for them to cope with the injury. A poor explanation fuels their anger, might affect the course of their recovery and can lead patients to distrust the staff caring for them. They might then avoid having further treatment – which in most cases they very much need. By contrast, an honest explanation and a promise to continue treatment can enhance the patient's trust and strengthen the relationship.

OPEN DISCLOSURE

Patients, whether or not they have suffered an adverse event, would generally like to be fully informed about any significant error. Both qualitative and quantitative studies have found that doctors generally underestimate the information that patients would like about errors and adverse outcomes.

In one focus group study, patients were strongly of the view that they wanted to be told about all harmful errors, and to know what happened, how it happened, how it would be mitigated and what would be done to prevent recurrence (Gallagher et al 2003). The physicians who took part agreed that harmful errors should be disclosed but were generally more circumspect in the language they used. Often, this simply meant speaking truthfully and very factually about what had occurred, without using the word error. 'You were given too much insulin. Your blood sugar was lowered and that's how you arrived in the intensive care unit . . .' (Gallagher et al 2003 p 1004). If the patient wanted to know more, they would go on to explain how the problem had arisen.

Opinions in both groups were more varied when near misses were considered, some patients and many physicians thinking disclosure would make patients unduly fearful and lead to unnecessary loss of trust. There is another, practical issue here, seldom discussed, which is simply the time it would take to disclose all errors fully. As yet we have yet to work out styles of disclosure appropriate to what has occurred. At one end of the scale, openness and honesty might require only a 10-second acknowledgment of a minor problem and a simple apology. At the other, it could involve a series of meetings over several months; in serious cases disclosure and ongoing support might literally have life-long implications for some patients.

Advocates of openness and proactive approaches to distressed or injured patients are frequently questioned by more cautious colleagues about the problems that could arise. Generally, clinicians want to be more open but are anxious about the disapproval of colleagues, complaints and litigation, the mindless assaults of the media or the anger and bitterness of patients and relatives. Problems certainly do occur, but rather less than those that arise from defensiveness and covering up. Being defensive and failing to explain after adverse outcomes is a major cause of litigation and a source of bitterness and anger from patients. Conversely, being open with patients can dramatically alter their reaction and promote a climate of trust. Bolsin and colleagues (2003) provide a vivid illustration of openness about a complication that even included discussion of the trainee's professional monitoring (Box 7.5). A family who initially wanted to sue the hospital ended up praising the systems and practices in place.

Box 7.5 A positive response to open disclosure

(adapted from Bolsin et al 2003)

An 81-year-old patient presented for coronary artery surgery and the following week underwent coronary artery bypass grafting. The patient experienced a very rare but recognized complication of internal jugular venous cannulation. This information was provided to the family during a discussion after the surgery.

The family's initial response was an angry denunciation of the standards of clinical practice within the hospital and a criticism of the Division of Perioperative Medicine for allowing a trainee to jeopardize the life of a patient. The clinicians involved in the case examined the trainee's record of performance of central venous line insertion. The implications of this disclosure of the performance record were discussed with the trainee and the specialist managing the case.

After the disclosure of the trainee's record, including the performance chart, there was an immediate and dramatic change in the family's opinions. The senior members of the family understood that the decision to allow the trainee to undertake the procedure had been made on the basis of valid performance data and was entirely justified. They were so impressed by the quality and clarity of the data they made formal compliments about the clinical service and to the anaesthetic service.

In some hospitals and other healthcare organizations, open disclosure is now moving from a rarely practised ideal towards being an organizational policy. These moves have been given considerable impetus by national bodies setting standards for open disclosure. One of the most impressive approaches has been that of the Australian Safety and Quality Council, which has produced a standard, information for patients (Box 7.6) and now educational and training materials for staff.

Box 7.6 Patient information sheet on open disclosure

(adapted from Australian Safety and Quality Council 2004)

When we need to visit a healthcare professional we can expect to receive the safest health care available. But sometimes things may not work out as expected. For example, a patient may be given the wrong dose of medicine. Or there may be complications after surgery that means the result is not as good as expected. Most adverse events are minor and do not result in harm. When a patient is harmed they have a right to know what has happened and why.

If an adverse event occurs the hospital needs to follow a process of open disclosure. This means that the patients and their family or carers are told, as soon as possible after the event, what has happened and what will be done about it. An important part of the process is finding out exactly what went wrong, why it went wrong and actively looking for ways to stop it happening again.

What can I expect if something goes wrong?

If something goes wrong during your hospital visit, a member of the hospital staff will talk to you and your family and carers about what happened. You can also discuss any changes to your ongoing care plan because of the adverse event.

In this situation you have the right:

- To have a support person of your choice present at the discussion
- To ask for a second opinion from another health care professional
- To pursue a complaints process
- To nominate specific people (family or carers) who you'd like to be involved
- To make the process easier we'll ask you to nominate someone (a member of your family, close friend or hospital patient advocate) to support you during your stay in hospital.

Who at the hospital will speak to me?

The person who talks to you about what happened is likely to be one of the healthcare team that is looking after you. However, if you have difficulty talking to this person you can nominate someone else. Ideally this will be someone who:

- You are comfortable with and can talk to easily
- Has been involved in your care and knows the facts
- Has enough authority to begin action to stop the problem happening again.

Who else will be present?

The person who be discussing what happened is also able to have someone there to assist and support them. When something goes wrong it is distressing for the patient and their carers, but is also traumatic for the healthcare team involved. Sometimes discussion after the event can become quite emotional or heated. Having someone there who is not as closely involved can help you to make the discussion more constructive. This is likely to assist you as well as the health team member.

What will happen afterwards?

As part of the open disclosure process, if something does go wrong, steps are taken to prevent it from happening again. The hospital will investigate what went wrong. You will be informed of the results and the changes that will be made to prevent the same thing from happening to someone else. If the investigation takes a long time, you will be kept up to date with its progress. If you wish, a meeting will be arranged for you to discuss the results of the investigation when it is finished.

The aftermath: caring for patients harmed by treatment

The open disclosure standard set out by the Safety and Quality Council is thoughtful and wide ranging. Many key themes have been built in: a commitment to openness, support over time, letting patients know the results of investigations, telling them what will be done to prevent future incidents and so on. Notice especially that open disclosure is spoken of as a process, not a one-off event. From the case histories at the beginning of the chapter, we can see that serious incidents can have a long time course to resolution. Even less serious incidents can require more than one meeting and some ongoing contact; in the first meeting patients might be too shocked to take much in, coming back later, having thought things over, to ask more questions.

Notice too that the Safety and Quality Council specifically says that the patient has a right to complain and, presumably, to seek compensation. Open disclosure is, occasionally, seen as a way of reducing complaints and litigation. Say sorry, and they won't sue. It is certainly true that a failure to receive explanations and apologies is a powerful motivator to legal action (Vincent et al 1994). However, finding out what happened is simply the patient's right. Whereas open disclosure might indeed reduce claims and complaints, that is not its purpose or rationale. People might still wish to seek compensation, and that is also their right in most healthcare systems. More importantly, they might *need* compensation, to care for an injured child for instance. At the moment, the legal process generally needs to be invoked for a patient to receive compensation. However, there is absolutely no need for a protracted legal process in less serious cases. Healthcare organizations could easily be much more proactive in stepping in with offers of help and, if necessary, financial assistance.

Finally, the patient information leaflet very sensibly draws attention to the impact on staff, discussed in Chapter 8. Patients might not, quite understandably, be thinking much about the staff when they have been injured but everyone involved is likely to be affected in a serious incident. However, it is perhaps unfortunate that, according to the leaflet, the patient and their carers are distressed but it is traumatic for the healthcare team. Much as we want to acknowledge the impact on staff, the outcome is more usually distress for the staff and trauma for the patient.

The challenge now for the open disclosure policy is in implementation. It is difficult for anyone to know at the moment how this document, which expresses an ideal open disclosure process, will work in practice and what resources will be needed, mainly staff time, to make it work effectively.

Open disclosure policies have not yet been widely adopted and it is not at all clear yet what the impact has been in practice. In the US, JCAHO mandated open disclosure as part of its accreditation policies but, 1 year later, only a third of its hospitals had a policy in place and there was still considerable reluctance to disclose preventable, as opposed to unpreventable, harm (Lamb et al 2003). From the little information available it does seem clear that those organizations that have followed the path of open disclosure have not been overwhelmed by lawsuits. To the contrary, the experience has been positive and they have argued strongly for others to follow. One hospital in the US initiated a policy of open disclosure in 1987, deciding to both take a more proactive approach to managing defensible claims and also to come forward and acknowledge when a serious error had been made. This commendable ethical position has led to five major settlements over the years of cases where the patient was unaware that an error had been made. Overall, however, the financial cost of claims since the policy was initiated has been moderate and comparable to other similar institutions (Kraman & Hamm 2002).

The initiatives of individual clinicians and risk managers must be strongly supported by board-level policy and directives. It is quite unreasonable to expect any clinician to be honest and open about problems that have occurred if that person will later face sanctions from senior management. All healthcare organizations need a strong proactive policy of active intervention and monitoring of those patients whose treatment has caused harm. Clearly there is an ethical imperative to inform patients of adverse outcomes, but the fear of legal action and media attention can act as a major disincentive.

BREAKING THE NEWS ABOUT ERROR AND HARM

A young doctor or nurse will not (and should not) be expected to shoulder the burden of breaking the news of a serious adverse outcome or to deal with the longer-term consequences. A senior doctor would usually discuss the incident with the family, although often accompanied by more junior staff. Nevertheless, it is important for clinicians to understand the principles at any stage in their career for two reasons. The first is that they will need to put these principles into practice at some point, and this could be sooner than they think. More importantly, though, even very junior staff will already be dealing with adverse outcomes, although they might be not seeing them as such. A painful injection, a prolonged infection, a frightening procedure are all, in a sense, adverse outcomes for the patient, especially if unexpected. The principles of accepting the patient's response, explaining patiently and being open about what has occurred still apply and are a useful basis for later coping with more serious incidents.

When something has gone wrong, doctors should take the initiative to seek out the patient and/or family and face the situation openly and honestly; avoiding or delaying such a meeting unnecessarily will only suggest there is something to hide. A senior member of staff needs to give a thorough and clear account of what exactly happened. At the first interview, junior staff involved with the patient might also be present. The patient and their relatives need to have time to reflect on what was said and to be able to return and ask further questions. Remember that people might be numb with shock after an incident and be unable to cope with very much information. Several meetings could be needed, over the course of weeks or months. Similar considerations apply when doctors are breaking bad news of any kind (Finlay & Dallimore 1991).

Telling patients or their families about disappointing results and dealing with their reactions is not easy. Nevertheless, if done with care and compassion, such communication maintains trust between the people involved and can greatly help the patient's adjustment to what has happened. Conversely, failing to explain, apologize, answer questions and explain the actions taken degrade trust and increase the chance of complaints and litigation. To help clinical staff faced with these difficult meetings, James Pichert and Gerald

Hickson have developed some guidelines (Box 7.7) (Pichert & Hickson 2001). Although they are aimed at fairly serious adverse outcomes, the general principles apply to explaining any unforeseen problem that has arisen in a patient's care and which has caused distress.

IN THE LONGER TERM

When serious harm has been done, acknowledging and discussing the incident is just the first stage. The longer-term needs of patients, families and staff need to be considered. We cannot possibly cover all the eventualities here and the different reactions to harm to a child as compared to an adult, the different reactions to sudden disaster compared with slow, gradual onset harm and the many other factors that affect response to harm. However, there are a few basic, useful things in bear in mind.

Ask specific questions about emotional trauma

A common theme in interviews with injured patients is that none of the professionals involved in their care appreciated the depth of their distress. I can recall several patients left in severe pain who were deeply depressed and at times suicidal; although great efforts were being made to deal with their physical problems, no one had thought to ask about their mental state. Risk managers, clinicians and others involved with these patients can ask basic questions without fear of 'making things worse'. The case histories illustrate some of the most common reactions and experiences of people suffering from depression and post-traumatic stress disorder. Other crucial areas of enquiry

---

Box 7.7 Communication after an error or adverse outcome

(adapted from Pichert & Hickson 2001)

- Give bad news in a private place where the patient and/or family may react and you can respond appropriately.
- Deliver the message clearly. The adverse outcome must be understood. 'I'm sorry to report that the procedure resulted in . . .'
- Wait silently for a reaction. Give the patient/family time to consider what has happened and formulate their questions.
- Acknowledge and accept the initial reaction. The usual reaction to bad news is a mixture of denial, anger, resignation, shock, etc. Listen.
- Resist the urge to blame or appear to blame other health professionals for the outcome.
- Discuss transition support. Tell the patient/family what steps will be taken to provide medical, social, or other forms of support.
- Finish by reassuring them about your continued willingness to answer any questions they might have. Discuss next steps.
- Consider scheduling a follow-up meeting. Some patients will want to talk only after the crisis has subsided.
- Afterwards, document a summary of the discussion. Ideally, share this with the patient and family.

are feelings of anger, humiliation, betrayal and loss of trust – all frequently experienced by injured patients.

When something truly awful has happened, staff are naturally also affected. In most clinical situations the need to think clearly and act decisively mean that emotions must be kept under control. Similarly, it is of no help whatever to patients, and might be quite damaging, if staff are obviously unable to cope with the tragedy that has occurred. However, this does not mean that staff need to be remote or uninvolved. Many patients have derived comfort from the empathy and sadness of staff involved in tragic incidents describing, for instance, the warmth and support they found in the staff's own sadness at the event.

A proportion of patients are likely to be sufficiently anxious or depressed to warrant formal psychological or psychiatric treatment. Although it is important that a senior doctor is involved in giving explanations and monitoring remedial treatment, it is unrealistic to expect the staff of say, a surgical unit, to shoulder the burden of formal counselling. They have neither the time nor the necessary training to deal with the more serious reactions. When a referral to a psychologist or psychiatrist is indicated it must be handled carefully. Injured patients are understandably very wary of their problems being seen as 'psychological' or 'all in the mind'.

Continuing care and support

Injured patients can receive support, comfort and practical help from many sources. It might come from their spouse, family, friends, colleagues, doctors or community organizations. An especially important source of support will be the doctors and other health professionals who are involved in their treatment. It is vital that staff continue to provide the same care and do not withdraw from the patient through guilt or embarrassment. After an initial mistake it is extremely reassuring for a patient to be overseen by a single senior doctor who undertakes to monitor all aspects of treatment, even if it involves a number of different specialties. When care has been substandard, the patient must be offered a referral elsewhere if that is what they wish but if the incident is dealt with openly and honestly then trust might even be strengthened.

Inform patients of changes

Patients and relatives wish to prevent future incidents, and this can be seen both as a genuine desire to safeguard others and as an attempt to find some way of coping with their own pain or loss. The pain might be ameliorated if they feel that, because changes were made, then at least some good came of their experiences. Relatives of patients who have died might express their motives for litigation in terms of an obligation to the dead person to make sure that a similar accident never happens again, so that some good comes of their death. The implication of this is that if changes have been made as a result of the adverse outcome, it is very important to inform the patients concerned. Although some will regret that the changes were made too late for them, most will appreciate the fact that their experience was understood and acted upon.

Financial assistance and practical help

Injured patients often need immediately practical help. They need medical treatment, counselling and explanations, but they might need money too. They might need to support their family while they are recovering, pay for specialist treatment, facilities to cope with disability and so on. In less serious cases, relatively small sums of money to provide therapy, alterations to the home or additional nursing can make an enormous difference to the patient, both practically and in his or her attitude to the hospital. Protracted and adversarial medicolegal negotiations can be very damaging, frustrating and above all incomprehensible to patients and their family. One only has to imagine oneself in a similar position to appreciate this. If you were injured in a rail or aviation accident you would hope and expect the organization concerned to help you. What would your reaction be if, as is still the case for many patients, the message you received was that 'you will be hearing from our lawyers in due course'?

SOME GOOD PRACTICE AND POSITIVE OUTCOMES

To close this chapter, and to mitigate the sense of gloom and despondency it might have induced, we will consider some examples of the benefits of a positive and proactive approach (Vincent 2001). Neither of these incidents had long-term consequences but both were very frightening to the patients concerned and, if handled badly, might well have affected their recovery and willingness to have future treatment. The examples show that even potentially disastrous events, like awareness under anaesthesia, can be handled in a sensitive and innovative way with great benefits to staff and patients alike.

Explanations and apology after iatrogenic cardiac arrhythmia

> Mrs A was admitted for minor day case surgery, expecting to return home later that day. A surgeon requested a weak solution of adrenaline to induce a blood free field, but was given a stronger solution than requested. As soon as the liquid was applied the patient developed a serious cardiac arrhythmia, the operation was terminated and she was transferred to the Intensive Therapy Unit, where she gradually recovered. **(Vincent 2001 p 474)**

The clinical risk manager was alerted immediately and assessed the likely consequences for the patient and her family. The first task was clearly to apologize and provide a full explanation. However, with both the patient and family in a state of shock, this had to be carried out in stages. The consultant and risk manager had a series of short meetings over a few days, to explain what had happened and keep the family informed about ongoing remedial treatment. Each time the family was given the opportunity to reflect on what they had been told and come back with further questions. A small package of compensation was also arranged, primarily aimed providing the necessary clinical and psychological support. The whole incident was resolved within 6 months and the patient expressed her thanks for the hospital for the way in which the incident had been handled, particularly the openness about the causes of the incident.

Anaesthetic awareness: reducing the fear of future operations

> A woman was admitted for an elbow replacement. During the operation she awoke, paralysed and able to hear the discussions amongst the surgical team. She was terrified, in great pain and absolutely helpless. The lack of anaesthetic was fortunately noticed, and she was next aware of waking in recovery screaming.
> **(Vincent 2001 p 475)**

The risk manager visited the patient at home as soon as practicable, maintained contact, offered psychological treatment for trauma and advised her on procedures for compensation, including an offer to pay for an independent legal assessment of the eventual offer of compensation. As in the first example, emotional trauma was the principal long-term concern, particularly anxiety about future operations. As this woman suffered chronic conditions requiring further surgery, this problem required some additional, imaginative measures.

Some months later, when the patient felt ready, she was given a tour of the operating theatre and the anaesthetic failure was explained in great detail, as were the procedural changes that had been made subsequent to the incident. This was immensely important in reducing her understandable fear of future operations and minimizing the long-term impact of the incident.

REFERENCES

American Psychiatric Association (APA) 1994 Diagnostic and Statistical Manual of Mental Disorders, 4th edn (DSM IV). American Psychiatric Association, Washington DC

Australian Safety and Quality Council 2004 What is open disclosure? Online. Available at: http://www.safetyandquality.org

Bolsin S, Solly R, Patrick A 2003 The value of personal professional monitoring performance data and open dislosure policies in anaesthetic practice: a case report. Quality and Safety in Healthcare 12:295–297

Brewin CR, Dalgleish T, Joseph S 1996 A dual representation theory of post-traumatic stress disorder. Psychological Review 103 670–686

Clarke DM, Russell PA, Polglase AL et al 1997 Psychiatric disturbance and acute stress response in surgical patients. Australia and New Zealand Journal of Surgery 67:115–118

Czarnocka J, Slade P 2000 Prevalence and predictors of post-traumatic stress symptoms following childbirth. British Journal of Clinical Psychology 39:35–52

Finlay I, Dallimore D 1991 Your child is dead. British Medical Journal 302:1524–1525

Gallagher TH, Waterman AD, Ebers AG et al 2003 Patients' and physicians' attitudes regarding the disclosure of medical errors. Journal of the American Medical Association 289:1001–1007

Kessler RC 1997 The effects of stressful life events on depression. Annual Review of Psychology 48:191–214

Kraman SS, Hamm G 2002 Risk management: extreme honesty may be the best policy. Annals of Internal Medicine 131:963–967

Lamb RM, Studdert DM, Bohmer RM et al 2003 Hospital disclosure practices: results of a national survey. Health Affairs 22:73–83

Lehman DR, Wortman CB, Williams AF 1987 Long-term effects of losing a spouse or child in a motor vehicle crash. Journal of Personality and Social Psychology 52:218–231

Lundin T 1984 Morbidity following sudden and unexpected bereavement. British Journal of Psychiatry 144:84–88

Pichert J, Hickson G 2001 Communicating risk to patients and families. In: Vincent C (ed) Clinical risk management: enhancing patient safety, 2nd edn. BMJ Publications, London

Vincent C 2001 Caring for patients harmed by treatment. In: Vincent C (ed) Clinical risk management: enhancing patient safety, 2nd edn. BMJ Publications, London

Vincent C, Coulter A 2002 Patient safety. What about the patient? Quality and Safety in Healthcare 11:76–80

Vincent C, Pincus T, Scurr JH 1993 Patients' experience of surgical accidents. Quality in Health Care 2:77–82

Vincent C, Young M, Phillips A 1994 Why do people sue doctors? A study of patients and relatives taking legal action. Lancet 343:1609–1613

Supporting staff after serious incidents

8

> Virtually every clinician knows the sickening feeling of making a bad mistake. You feel singled out and exposed – seized by the instinct to see if anyone has noticed. You agonize about what to do, whether to tell anyone, what to say. Later, the event replays itself in your mind. You question your competence but fear being discovered. You know you should confess, but dread the prospect of potential punishment and of the patient's anger.
> **(Wu 2000 p 726)**

Human beings make frequent errors and misjudgements in every sphere of activity, but some environments are less forgiving of error than others. Errors in academia, law or architecture, for instance, can mostly be remedied with an apology or a cheque. Those in medicine, in the air, or on an oil rig can have severe or even catastrophic consequences. This is not to say that the errors of doctors or pilots are more reprehensible, only that they bear a greater burden because their errors have greater consequences. Making an error, particularly if a patient is harmed because of it, might therefore have profound consequences for the staff involved, particularly if they are seen, rightly or wrongly, as primarily responsible for the outcome. The typical reaction has been well expressed by Albert Wu in the opening quotation for this chapter, which is taken from his aptly titled paper 'the second victim'.

For a proportion of junior doctors, mistakes are the most memorable events of their training and, at whatever stage of one's career, mistakes can be a devastating experience (Mizrahi 1984). All these observations apply to some degree to other health professionals, although the little research in this area is almost entirely restricted to doctors. In the last few years there has been a little more openness about the topic of error, with a realization of its importance for learning and its impact on staff.

The preventable death of a child under one's care is one of the worst clinical experiences for a doctor or nurse (Box 8.1). The brave and thoughtful account in the box foreshadows many of the themes of this chapter. The doctor concerned acknowledges his personal contribution and responsibility, yet it is clear that he was failed by others and that organizational problems contributed to the delays and difficulties and possibly to the final outcome. Although the impact on the doctor is not directly discussed it was probably profound, as the case is still vivid 8 years later. Although a child died, and he

Box 8.1 Death of a child

(adapted from Sutcliffe 2002)

When I was an inexperienced registrar some 8 years ago, a child died under my care. Her death was largely preventable but caused by a series of errors. I had been a registrar for 24 months and I had on duty with me a senior house officer who was new to paediatrics. It was an exceptionally busy day covering the wards and accident and emergency department, with cases including a child with tubercular meningitis and another with acute subdural haemorrhage from non-accidental injury. After 5 p.m. I was also responsible for the neonatal intensive care unit, which had 15 intensive care cots.

The child who died was admitted in the morning with a seizure. I had seen her before in the outpatient clinic and during a previous admission with an 'atypical febrile convulsion', when she had been noted to be hypoglycaemic and had had further tests. We initially checked her electrolytes, gave her rectal then intravenous diazepam, and did an infection screen in view of a low-grade fever. She was hypoglycaemic on admission, which we corrected.

After admission she appeared to stabilize but later started having another seizure. I ordered a clonazepam infusion and saw her several times during the day. The professor rang mid-afternoon and asked how things were. I expressed concern about the child but he suggested no new management. Later that evening, while I was busy on the neonatal unit, the nursing staff notified me that the child was having yet another seizure. I rang the sub-specialist. We discussed the case but he sounded uninterested. He suggested I perform a lumbar puncture. I thought this was too risky and my decision was fortunate in the end. She died 4 hours later from coning secondary to status epilepticus, and might have died during the lumbar puncture if I had done what was suggested. In retrospect I had confused the masking effect of clonazepam (half-life 72 hours) with cessation of her seizure. At her arrest call, resuscitation went reasonably smoothly but the child did not respond. I asked for flumazenil (an antidote drug to diazepam). It was not in the emergency drug cupboard. We called an anaesthetist who went to another ward by mistake. It took several hours for an intensive care bed to be found and she subsequently died.

Things could have gone better if there had been protocols for the management of status epilepticus (there were none on the ward). Double cover of busy neonatal and general paediatric units still goes on and should cease entirely. Intensive care availability has improved but needs to continue to do so. In retrospect there were various things I should have done, such as recognizing that the child was still having a seizure, arranging transfer to intensive care earlier and getting a neurological opinion.

I was never given an opportunity to discuss this case in a non-critical forum. If a more junior colleague rings a senior colleague at home the onus is on that colleague to offer to come in and review the case; I didn't feel able to ask. Rather than look ourselves in the mirror we tend to blame others when things go wrong. In a spirit of openness this needs to change.

was the clinician with immediate responsibility, he was never able to discuss the case in way that would have helped him personally or foster any clinical learning. The phrase 'a spirit of openness' exemplifies the cultural shift that he believes is needed.

THE WORSE THE OUTCOME, THE GREATER THE BLAME?

Reactions to error and adverse outcomes in medicine are greatly magnified because so much can be at stake. Few other professions face the possibility of causing the death of another person with such regularity, although the likelihood of this varies hugely in different areas of healthcare. Social, legal and personal imperatives drive us to condemn people who make serious mistakes and harm others. Our gut feeling, however much systems thinking we have absorbed, is that this is just appalling and the person concerned must be brought to book. Atul Gawande, an American surgeon, explores this theme, after a description of his own involvement in a near disaster:

> Consider some other surgical mishaps. In one, a general surgeon left a large metal instrument in a patient's abdomen, where it tore through the bowel and the wall of the bladder. In another a cancer surgeon biopsied the wrong part of a woman's breast and thereby delayed her diagnosis of cancer for months. A cardiac surgeon skipped a small but key step during a heart valve operation, thereby killing the patient . . .

> How could anyone who makes a mistake of that magnitude be allowed to practice medicine? We call such doctors 'incompetent', 'unethical' and 'negligent'. We want to see them punished. And so we've wound up with the public system we have for dealing with error: malpractice lawsuits, media scandal, suspensions, firings.

> There is, however, a central truth in medicine that complicates this tidy vision of misdeeds and misdoers: all doctors make terrible mistakes. Consider the cases I've just described. I gathered them simply by asking respected surgeons I know – surgeons at top medical schools – to tell me about mistakes they had made in the last year.
> **(Gawande 2002 p 55–56)**

When a patient is harmed, those involved are more likely to blame themselves than if an error occurred and no harm resulted. However, as discussed earlier in the book, the causes of adverse events are complex. Many could not have been prevented: some are the result of genuine uncertainty in diagnosis and decision-making. Even where errors have occurred, they are often only part of a chain of events inseparable from a web of organizational background causes. Seldom, after close analysis, is it possible to lay the blame for an adverse outcome solely at the door of one individual, however tempting this might be. Junior doctors, for instance, might find themselves forced to deal with events that are well beyond their competence. From this perspective, the junior doctor in the front line might be the inheritor of problems elsewhere in the organization; for them to then take responsibility and shoulder all the blame is both unwarranted and personally damaging.

ATTITUDES TO ERROR AND THE CULTURE OF MEDICINE

In his landmark paper on error in medicine, Lucian Leape (1994) speculated as to why high error rates in medicine have not stimulated more concern and efforts at error prevention. Leape argued that one of the most important reasons that clinicians have difficulty dealing with error is because of the culture of medical practice:

Physicians are socialized in medical school and residency to strive for error-free practice. There is a powerful emphasis on perfection, both in diagnosis and treatment. In everyday hospital practice, the message is equally clear: mistakes are unacceptable. Physicians are expected to function without error, an expectation that physicians translate into the need to be infallible. One result is that physicians, not unlike test pilots, come to view an error as a failure of character – you weren't careful, you didn't try hard enough. This kind of thinking lies behind a common reaction by clinicians: 'How can there be an error without negligence?' **(Leape 1994 p 1852)**

All clinicians recognize the inevitability (although perhaps not the frequency) of error. However, this seldom carries over into open recognition and discussion, still less into research on error. There is therefore a curious, and in some ways paradoxical, clash of beliefs. On the one hand we have an enterprise fraught with uncertainty, where knowledge is inadequate and errors are bound to occur. On the other hand, those working in this environment foster a culture of perfection, in which errors are not tolerated, in which a strong sense of personal responsibility both for errors and outcome is expected. The strong sense of responsibility is in many ways appropriate and necessary. However, there is a clash between reality and culture, and between reality and the expectations of both patients and clinicians. With this background it is not surprising that mistakes are hard to deal with, particularly when so much else is at stake in terms of human suffering.

THE IMPACT OF ERRORS AND MISTAKES

Although error is common, and the impact of error on clinicians undoubted, there is no sustained body of research on the subject and little public discussion. Those who have tried to bring the subject into the open have not always fared well at the hands of their colleagues. For instance, Hilfiker argued that 'We see the horror of our own mistakes, yet we are given no permission to deal with their enormous emotional impact . . . The medical profession simply has no place for its mistakes' (Hilfiker 1984 p 118). This paper drew some supportive correspondence but also comments such as 'This neurotic piece has no place in the *New England Journal of Medicine*' (Anderson 1984 p 1676). Hilfiker hoped that others would follow his example and write about their own errors but was apparently disappointed that progress was slow thereafter (Ely 1996). Since then, however, a few studies have emerged that have shed some light on the experience of errors and other traumatic events.

When Mizrahi (1984) asked young interns 'What were your most memorable experiences during training?', 21% of the replies concerned actual or potential mistakes; half of the young doctors he interviewed had made serious and even fatal mistakes in the first 2 months of their jobs. In Britain Jenny Firth-Cozens found that British junior doctors singled out making mistakes (Box 8.2), together with dealing with death and dying, relationships with senior doctors and overwork, as the most stressful events they had to deal with (Firth-Cozens 1987).

Box 8.2 Reactions to mistakes

(from Firth Cozens 1987, Wu et al 1991 and Christensen et al 1992)

'I missed the diagnosis of pulmonary embolism and treated the patient as a case of severe pneumonia until the day after. The patient's condition deteriorated and only then was the diagnosis put right. I felt guilty and lost confidence.'

'Missing a diagnosis of perforated peptic ulcer in a patient – at least she is now well and survived. It made me feel useless at my job though.'

'I was really shaken. My whole feelings of self-worth and abilities were basically profoundly shaken.'

'I was appalled and devastated that I had done this to somebody.'

'My great fear was that I had missed something, and then there was a sense of panic.'

'This case has made me very nervous about clinical medicine. I worry now about all febrile patients since they may be on the verge of sepsis.'

'It was hard to concentrate on anything else I was doing because I was so worried about what was happening, so I guess that would be anxiety. I felt guilty, sad, had trouble sleeping, wondering what was going on.'

In a series of eleven in-depth interviews Christensen and colleagues (1992) discussed a variety of serious mistakes, including four deaths. All the doctors were affected to some degree, but four clinicians described intense agony or anguish as the reality of the mistake had sunk in. The interviews also identified a number of general themes: the ubiquity of mistakes in clinical practice; the infrequency of self-disclosure about mistakes to colleagues, friends and family; the emotional impact on the physician, such that some mistakes were remembered in great detail even after several years; and the influence of beliefs about personal responsibility and medical practice.

After the initial shock, the clinicians had a variety of reactions that had lasted from several days to several months. Some of the feelings of fear, guilt, anger, embarrassment and humiliation were unresolved at the time of the interview, even a year after the mistake. A few reported symptoms of depression, including disturbances in appetite, sleep and concentration. Fears related to concerns for the patient's welfare, litigation and colleagues discovery of their 'incompetence'.

The Christensen study is rich in detail but confined to a small sample of potentially untypical individuals. Albert Wu and colleagues (1991) sent questionnaires to 254 interns in the US, asking the respondents to describe the most significant mistake in patient care they had made in the last year. A variety of types of error were reported, most frequently missed diagnoses (30%) and drug errors (29%). Almost all the errors had serious outcomes and almost a third involved a death. Wu found that accepting responsibility for the error was most likely to result in constructive changes in practice (i.e. learning from the error), although accepting responsibility was also associated with higher levels of distress.

Most of the mistakes were discussed with a clinical colleague, although only half with a supervisory clinician (who would have had overall responsibility for the patient). Only a quarter of mistakes were discussed with the patient or patient's family. Feelings of remorse, anger, guilt and inadequacy were common. Over a quarter of house officers feared negative repercussions from the mistake. A missed diagnosis by one young doctor made him reject a career in subspecialties that involve 'a lot of data collection and uncertainty'. This echoes the experience of Carlo Fonsecka (1996), who recounted the personal impact of mistakes in a remarkable personal paper that began 'Error free patient care is the ideal standard but in reality unattainable. I am conscious of having made five fatal mistakes during the past 36 years' (Fonsecka 1996 p 1640). Fonsecka wrote that, with hindsight, he believes that the impact of the first case was so great that he no longer felt able to carry on with clinical work and turned eventually to a laboratory-based career.

WHAT MAKES AN ERROR TRAUMATIC?

Clearly only a small proportion of errors are so traumatic. What singles out a mistake as being traumatic? There is no research on this issue to my knowledge, but some ideas can be put forward (Box 8.3). First, and most obviously, the outcome will be severe. Hindsight bias applies in this area, in that a bad outcome makes one more critical, and indeed more self-critical, of the care given. If you 'get away with it' the feeling is likely to be more relief than guilt. Second, it will be a clear departure from the clinician's usual practice, rather than a close call in a genuinely uncertain situation. The reaction of colleagues, whether supportive or defensive and critical, might be equally powerful. The reaction of the patient and his or her family can be especially hard to bear, particularly when the outcome is severe and if there has been a close involvement over a long period. For instance, psychologists or psychiatrists may find the suicide of a patient very hard to face if there has previously been a long therapeutic relationship.

Beliefs about the degree of control the clinician has will strongly affect the sense of personal responsibility for adverse outcomes and attitudes to mistakes. A certain degree of realism about the likelihood of mistakes, especially with increasing constraints on practice, pressure of work and the need to take short cuts at times, tempers reactions to individual mistakes and makes it less likely that someone will generalize from a single, regrettable mistake to a more general belief that they are incompetent (Box 8.4). In the study of the impact of suicide, discussed below, David Alexander and colleagues (2000) comment that psychiatrists have to strike a balance in their attitude to the suicide of their patients. If they regard suicide as unavoidable, they protect themselves and their profession but consequently end up in a position of therapeutic nihilism. If, on the other hand, they view every suicide as

---

Box 8.3 What makes a mistake hard to cope with?

- Bad outcome for the patient and family
- Anger or distress of patient or family
- Clear departure from usual practice
- Criticism and lack of support from colleagues
- Lack of support from family and friends
- Being very self-critical

> **Box 8.4 Contrasting beliefs about personal control and responsibility**
> (from Christensen et al 1992 and Alexander et al 2000)
>
> **In medicine**
> 'As I think about it, in medicine there's this element of control and responsibility that's infinite. There is no point at which you say comfortably, "Yeah, I did as much as I can and I couldn't do any more." You never reach that point.'
> 'I think that we over-estimate severely our supposed control over physiological events, . . . We may help people sometimes, we may help symptoms of the disease sometimes, but I think it's easy to have an exalted opinion of our power, . . . I don't think we change the date of death very much in most people.'
>
> **In psychiatry**
> 'There is a terrible sense of failure at having let down those who have put their trust in you.'
> 'As doctors we have high expectations of ourselves, and it is sometimes important to recalibrate those in terms of what we can realistically achieve.'

preventable, they lay themselves open to blame and guilt and would probably eventually be unable to continue their work.

Clinicians, like everyone else, vary in temperament, resilience and attitude to their own errors. Jenny Firth-Cozens (1997) has found that a tendency to self-criticism is predictive of stress; this tendency might be rooted in earlier relationships, which in turn might find an echo in relationships with senior colleagues. For a highly self-critical person, errors and mistakes will be particularly disturbing, causing further stress that might in turn make them more likely to make mistakes; in serious cases the clinician might enter a particularly vicious downward spiral of anxiety and shame. There is a fine balance to be struck between personal high standards and undue self-criticism. The high personal standards of excellent clinicians might in fact make them particularly vulnerable to the impact of mistakes. This tendency can be reinforced during medical training, in that the culture of medical school and residency imply that mistakes are unacceptable and, when serious, imply a failure of effort or character.

THE IMPACT OF LITIGATION

The impact of errors and mistakes is compounded and deepened when followed by a complaint or litigation, events that have become increasingly common in the last 20 years. Patients now demand much more of doctors and nurses, and can be less forgiving when their own expectations of outcome are not fulfilled, although they are right to be angry when no apology or explanation is given. Considerable media attention to medical catastrophes has also made the public much more aware of the potential for harm, as well as benefit from medical treatment.

The experience of being sued in a prolonged and difficult case is documented in Charles and Kennedy's (1985) book, *Defendant: a psychiatrist on trial for medical malpractice*. The psychiatrist in question described feeling utterly alone and isolated from colleagues, later finding that this was quite a common experience for those accused of malpractice. The case lasted 5 years, seemed to swallow up her life completely, demanded constant attention and made her anxious and insomniac. She felt she had lost her integrity as a person and as a doctor, again suggesting that these were common reactions (Charles & Kennedy 1985).

Charles and Kennedy's book broke new ground in bringing the experience of litigation into the open. We should nevertheless remember that 20 years have passed, our awareness of the extent of patient harm has been transformed, our understanding of its causes have also changed dramatically and, I think it is safe to say, that in many countries a claim for compensation is not necessarily seen as a shameful personal attack. That said, studies of the impact of litigation suggest that these experiences are by no means unique (Bark et al 1997', Charles 1984', Martin et al 1991', Shapiro et al 1989)'. Depression, anger and other nervous symptoms were common responses to litigation. In Martin et al's (1991)' study of 273 sued and non-sued physicians, anxiety, depression and traumatic responses were highest in the 2 years following litigation and gradually reduced thereafter, although not to the level of non-sued physicians. By contrast, feelings of shame and doubt, although prominent at an early stage, did return to ordinary levels, particularly in those who had won their case. Older physicians, however, seemed less affected and more able to put litigation into perspective, as a job hazard rather than an indictment of their ability. In Bark et al's 1997 study, the psychological effects on staff were often referred to and support from friends, colleagues, management and outside professionals was seen as important. Support groups and legal advice within the hospital system were often proposed, both as an information resource and for moral support. Over a quarter of doctors suggested the formal provision of a counselling service and nominated mentors to whom they could refer.

In a development of Charles' work, Shapiro et al (1989)' surveyed 171 matched pairs of doctors who had been sued and their patients who were taking action together with a sample of 100 doctors not involved in litigation. Sued doctors stated that they found the practice of medicine less rewarding and satisfying after legal action. Those who were more involved with their patients experienced more anger, tension, depression and sense of defeat as a result of legal action than those who were less involved, with 20% of sued doctors stating that such symptoms persisted for years. The results suggested that malpractice litigation is often preceded by difficulties in the relationship. Two-thirds of sued doctors thought that they had been open and honest with their patients but only one-third of patients agreed. Recent studies of obstetricians with high levels of litigation, compared with colleagues, suggest that those with litigation histories are distinguished not by the quality of their care but by different attitudes, insensitivity and poorer communication skills (Entman et al 1994, Hickson et al 1994).

Litigation can clearly be very unpleasant, and sometimes traumatic, but the impact of litigation should not be overstated. Often, when the case is clear cut and the harm not severe, or at least not permanent, it might be little more than tedious. In Britain at least, very few cases ever reach trial, almost all being settled by lawyers and risk managers, sometimes with little involvement of the clinical staff (which is sometimes welcome and sometimes not). We should just step back for a moment and reflect, from the perspective of both clinician and patient, why litigation has to happen at all. Although some people will always complain, and a few unpleasant or deluded characters delight in litigation, in fact very few patients sue; this is partly because, whatever the rights and wrongs of the case, it is a deeply wearing experience in which they constantly have to recall experiences they would much prefer to forget. When they do sue it is for explanations, apologies, to bring about change in the system and, to a widely varying extent, for money (Vincent et al 1994).

As was said earlier, for most of the deserving cases all of these things could be provided by proactive healthcare organizations without litigation and in fact without the need for legislation on no fault compensation. This in turn would make life a great deal easier for the staff involved; when care had been substandard, they would know the patients and family were being supported. When care had been satisfactory, and a case had to be defended, they would have the organization firmly on their side.

WHO CAN HELP?

Many of the doctors in Christensen et al's (1992) study had not discussed the mistakes or their emotional impact in depth with their colleagues. Fears of humiliation, litigation or punishment had prevented some from airing their feelings with other professionals, and they found it difficult to discuss the personal, rather than clinical, aspects of the case. When the case was discussed, it would be with close friends or colleagues whom they had come to trust over a long period. The doctors involved wanted the emotional support and professional reaffirmation, but their culture did not often permit such open discussions. However, this study reflected a very small number of interviews and it is hard to know how far to generalize these experiences. One might imagine that a very different atmosphere might prevail in, for instance, a primary care team that had worked closely together for many years. A larger study set in mental health sheds more light on who can be of most help after serious incidents.

The suicide of a patient under one's care is a particularly disturbing event. David Alexander and colleagues (2000) studied the impact on psychiatrists, who were asked to describe their most distressing suicide; 159 consultant psychiatrists provided information on suicides that had happened between 1 month and 20 years ago. Although the study does not specifically concern mistakes, any suicide by a patient in one's care raises the spectre of blame and personal responsibility, and anxiety about the critical reactions of both the patient's family and colleagues. The most common reactions were irritability at home, being less able to deal with routine family problems, poor sleep, low mood, preoccupation with the suicide and decreased self-confidence. Although none of the psychiatrists took time off work, the effects of the suicide were very persistent, with a number seriously considering early retirement. These experiences, not surprisingly, also affected their clinical management of suicidal patients, generally moving them towards more structured management, more use of suicide observations, more detailed communication about records, a greater willingness to intervene and a more cautious approach to suicide risk.

Team meetings were frequently held after the suicide, and discussion with colleagues in this format was generally very supportive. In mental health, whereas the psychiatrist might have overall medical responsibility, the sense of team responsibility for a patient is very strong; in a third of these suicides the patients managed to kill themselves while on a hospital ward. Critical incident reviews, presumably more analytic in tone, were held after about half the suicides and found to be helpful; we can speculate that exploring the full range of causes of such an event tends to put individual contributions, or omissions, in perspective. Legal and disciplinary proceedings, and fatal accident enquiries, with their judicial or quasi-judicial status, were, although uncommon, viewed as stressful and unhelpful.

Team members, other psychiatrists and the psychiatrists' own families and friends emerged as the most common and effective sources of help. Professional colleagues were particularly important, because they know what it is like to take such responsibility and their support mitigates the sense of professional isolation that can be felt. Family members, who themselves will be indirectly affected, provide a different kind of help. Talking it through with a colleague brings perspective, whereas talking it over with a husband or wife brings comfort. Patients' families could be very supportive but, understandably, sometimes critical, depending presumably on their own assessment of the care the patient had received and their own relationship with the person before the suicide. Psychiatrists felt that it was important that there was access to support and more formal methods of treatment, such as counselling or debriefing; however, they were adamant that these should simply be offered and no attempt should be made to push people into treatment.

STRATEGIES FOR COPING WITH ERROR, HARM AND THEIR AFTERMATH

Understanding that mistakes will always occur and that reacting to them is ordinary, and in fact necessary for learning, is a first step. Being understanding of others when they are in that unenviable position is a vital step towards a more open, indeed a safer, culture. Individual clinicians can do a great deal here, whatever their profession or seniority, to promote a more constructive and supportive approach to errors (Box 8.5).

There is no doubt that the wider organization and context play a large part in the way a healthcare professional will react to an error or harm to a patient. Just as systems thinking is needed to understand how harm comes about, its aim is to appreciate how things unfold afterwards. Many initiatives that are aimed to help patients, such as a policy of open disclosure, can also be a considerable help to staff. Supporting patients and supporting staff are not separate activities, but inextricably intertwined. Although there is little formal guidance, and almost no research on this topic, the following suggestions might be useful.

Box 8.5 Strategies for coping with error and disaster

- Be open about error and its frequency. Senior staff talking openly about past mistakes and problems is particularly effective.
- Accept that a need for support is not a sign of weakness. Clinicians have to be resilient but almost all are grateful for the support of colleagues when disaster strikes.
- Provide clear guidelines for discussion of error with patients backed up by a Board-level policy on open disclosure.
- Offer training in the difficult task of communicating with patient and families in the aftermath of an adverse event.
- Provide basic education in the law and the legal process, which should reduce some of the anxiety about legal action.
- Offer support to staff after major incidents. This might simply be informal support from a colleague.
- For a particularly profound reaction, perhaps to the death of a child, formal psychological intervention might be valuable.

Acknowledge the potential for error

First, the potential for error in medicine, as in other activities, needs to be recognized and openly acknowledged. Education about the ubiquity of error, its causes and likely consequences, would bring a more realistic attitude and constructive approach. During the student years, it might also be possible to identify those students who could be vulnerable to excessive reactions to errors, for example, those in whom tutors see signs of self-blame in clinical discussions. High self-criticism is a way of thinking, a cognitive style in which self-blame occurs whenever things go wrong; it could potentially be changed by teaching students how to allocate responsibility less destructively (Firth-Cozens 1997). In clinical medicine, open discussion of error, particularly by respected senior figures, is very powerful both at the time it happens and for future occasions because it provides a mandate for such discussions to occur at other times. In effect, the junior nurse or doctor learns that it must be acceptable to discuss errors and think about them, because their seniors do it. Modelling of behaviour, as the psychologists call it, is one of the most powerful influences on who we are and what we do.

Agreed policy on openness with injured patients

This has been discussed previously in relation to helping patients but it is equally important for staff. The openness and sensitivity of individual clinicians will be thoroughly and fatally undermined without an agreed policy of open disclosure. Some doctors are still torn between their own desire for a more open stance and the more cautious approach that they perceive to be demanded, rightly or wrongly, by managers, colleagues and medico-legal organizations. This can turn an already very difficult situation into a real conflict that is traumatic for staff and patient alike. This brings home the extent to which a different approach to error and adverse events on the part of clinicians must be mirrored by a similar shift in attitudes on the part of managers, lawyers, and indeed patients and relatives.

Education about medical law and the legal process

Part of the horror of a complaint or threat of litigation lies, for a young clinician at least, simply in ignorance of what is involved. The process varies from country to country but, in Britain for instance, there is no trial by jury for medical negligence and the great majority of cases are settled without a trial of any kind. Education in legal matters for all staff, together with specific information about the likely course of any complaint or claim, can reduce a great deal of unnecessary distress (Genn 1995). Many doctors act as experts in negligence cases and therefore have considerable experience of the litigation process and thus represent an important educative resource for their peers and for the junior staff. Through their experience of litigation procedures they can communicate practical information about what happens in the course of a negligence action (Hirst 1996).

Formal support and access to confidential counselling

Clinicians are resilient people but anyone can be vulnerable, because of personality, position or circumstance, to distressingly severe reactions. Whereas younger clinicians might be more vulnerable, anyone can be affected at any stage in their career, unless they have become so arrogant or damaged as to be insensitive to the impact of mistakes on their patients. Not everyone needs support after a serious mistake, but understanding and acceptance from colleagues is always important. Sometimes a private discussion will help, with a colleague or a senior figure. Some hospitals employ recently retired senior doctors as mentors. A link with a psychiatrist or psychologist, perhaps outside the hospital, might also be useful when the strain is severe or prolonged, as occurs when a member of staff feels responsible for a serious injury or death (Hirst 1996).

The range of potential support extends from a quiet word in a corridor to the offer of extended psychotherapy. Because the range is so wide, the choice of intensity must be left to the individual concerned, who should feel free to ask for a greater or lesser degree of involvement as time goes on. Managers tempted to provide 'stress counselling', especially from paid sources outside the organization, should remember that support from immediate colleagues is usually much more welcome and appropriate, and that some degree of anxiety is normal in times of stress (Hirst 1996).

Communication skills training

When things go wrong and a patient is harmed or disturbed in some way it is vital, for all concerned, that an explanation is given, an apology where appropriate, and remedial treatment and counselling instituted. Facing a patient harmed by treatment, or their naturally distressed and angry relatives, is a particularly difficult clinical situation for which little guidance or training is available. Both patients and staff will benefit if clinical staff have some training in communication skills for coping with, and helping dissatisfied, distressed, or injured patients and their relatives.

A personal assignment

Finally, a suggested personal assignment supplied by Albert Wu:

> Think back to your last mistake that harmed a patient. Talk to a colleague about it. Notice your colleague's reactions and your own. What helps? What makes it harder? Physicians will always make mistakes. The decisive factor will be how we handle them. Patient safety and physician welfare will be served if we can be more honest about our mistakes to our patients, our colleagues, and ourselves.
> **(Wu 2000 p 727)**

REFERENCES

Alexander DA, Klein S, Gray NM et al 2000 Suicide by patients: questionnaire study of its effect on consultant psychiatrists. British Medical Journal 320:1571–1574

Anderson M 1984 Facing our mistakes. New England Journal of Medicine 310:1676

Bark P, Vincent C, Olivieri L et al 1997 Impact of litigation on senior clinicians: implications for risk management. Quality in Health Care 6:7–13

Charles SC 1984 A different view of malpractice. Chicago Medicine 87:848–850

Charles SC, Kennedy E 1985 Defendant: a psychiatrist on trial for medical malpractice. Free Press, New York

Christensen JF, Levinson W, Dunn PM 1992 The heart of darkness: the impact of perceived mistakes on physicians. Journal of General Internal Medicine 7:424–431

Ely JW 1996 Physicians' mistakes. Will your colleagues offer support? Archives of Family Medicine 5:76–77

Entman SS, Glass CA, Hickson GB et al 1994 The relationship between malpractice claims history and subsequent obstetric care. Journal of the American Medical Association 272:1588–1591

Firth-Cozens J 1987 Emotional distress in junior house officers. British Medical Journal 295:533–536

Firth-Cozens J 1997 Predicting stress in general practitioners: 10-year follow-up postal survey. British Medical Journal 315:34–35

Fonsecka C 1996 To err was fatal. British Medical Journal 313:1640–1642

Gawande A 2002 Complications: a surgeon's notes on an imperfect science. Picador, New York

Genn H 1995 Supporting staff involved in litigation. In: Vincent CA (ed) Clinical risk management. BMJ Publications, London

Hickson GB, Clayton EW, Entman SS et al 1994 Obstetricians' prior malpractice experience and patients' satisfaction with care. Journal of the American Medical Association 272:1583–1587

Hilfiker D 1984 Facing our mistakes. New England Journal of Medicine 310:118–122

Hirst D 1996 Supporting staff during litigation – managerial aspects. Clinical Risk 2:189–194

Leape LL 1994 Error in medicine. Journal of the American Medical Association 272:1851–1857

Martin CA, Wilson JF, Fiebelman III ND et al 1991 Physicians' psychological reactions to malpractice litigation. Southern Medical Journal 84:1300–1304

Mizrahi T 1984 Managing medical mistakes: ideology, insularity and accountability among internists-in-training. Social Science & Medicine 19:135–146

Shapiro RS, Simpson DE, Lawrence SL et al 1989 A survey of sued and non-sued physicians and suing patients. Archives of Internal Medicine 149:2190–2196

Sutcliffe AG 2002 Death of a child. Lancet 359:2104

Vincent C, Young M, Phillips A 1994 Why do people sue doctors? A study of patients and relatives taking legal action. Lancet 343:1609–1613

Wu A 2000 Medical error: the second victim. British Medical Journal 320:726–727

Wu AW, Folkman S, McPhee SJ et al 1991 Do house officers learn from their mistakes? Journal of the American Medical Association 265:2089–2094

Culture and leadership for safety

9

> Join us in converting a culture of blame that hides information about risk and error into a culture of safety that flushes information out and enables us to prevent or quickly recover from mistakes before they become patient injuries.
> **(Leape et al 1998 p 1446)**

> A somewhat lethal cocktail of impatience, scientific ignorance and naïve optimism may have dangerously inflated our expectations of safety culture.
> **(Cox & Flin 1998 p 190)**

The term 'culture' is used in many different ways in discussions of safety in healthcare. Sometimes culture is just a lazy catch-all term for a whole mish-mash of practices that are somehow meant to combine to produce a coherent approach to safety. In this case, the flag waving and calls for a change in the culture are little more than feel-good messages offered as a substitute for meaningful action. When Lucian Leape and others talk about changing the culture however, they reflect a deeply held belief and commitment to a fundamental change in the way error and safety are approached and an equally deeply felt conviction that until the culture changes, nothing else will. The culture of an organization can be a major asset in the continuous struggle for safety or, conversely, a major obstacle to any meaningful change. However, there is precious little hard evidence that safety culture really does impact on safety. As Sue Cox and Rhona Flin (1998) point out, a naïve belief in the concept has far out-stripped the evidence for its utility.

THE MANY FACETS OF SAFETY CULTURE IN HEALTHCARE

Anyone who begins to examine the safety literature comes across a bewildering array of descriptors applied to the word culture, each of which is supposed to illuminate some essential facet of the all important safety culture. 'No-blame culture', 'open and fair culture', 'flexible', 'learning', 'reporting', 'generative', 'resilient', 'mindful' . . . the list goes on and on. In part, this reflects the fact that we are still in the early days of understanding safety culture and that people have not rallied around a single definition or set of

153

concepts. However, it also reflects the fact that there are a number of important facets to a culture of safety, as can be seen in the various examples of absent or inadequate safety culture (Box 9.1).

The examples of poor culture first show the importance attached to culture by experienced clinicians and safety experts. They also illuminate, to some extent, the different facets of culture and the different senses in which the word is used. The first two quotes are primarily concerned with the reaction to errors after they have occurred and the authors are rightly critical of unthinking, heavy-handed reactions both inside healthcare organizations and in the wider society; we are therefore concerned with the culture of both healthcare organizations and wider social mores. Another theme apparent here is that excessive blame prevents recognition of error, impedes learning and effective action to improve safety.

The principal theme of the third example, however, although also concerned with error, concerns anticipation rather than response. Here safety culture implies that the people concerned should maintain good standards of practice but also be alert to the possibility of error and take steps to reduce or eliminate that possibility.

The final example reveals another facet of safety culture, or rather its absence. In a deeply pathological culture, the difficulty is not so much blame as that problems are denied or not even acknowledged. As is sometimes said, the hardest problems to resolve are those where no one recognizes anything is

---

Box 9.1 Safety culture in healthcare

There is too often a blame culture. When things go wrong, the response is to seek one or two individuals to blame, who may then be subject to disciplinary measures or professional censure. That is not to say that in some circumstances individuals should not be held to account, but as the predominant approach this acts as a significant deterrent to the reporting of adverse events and near misses.
(Department of Health (DoH) 2000 p 77)

Increasingly, patients and physicians in the United States live and interact in a culture characterised by anger, blame, guilt, fear, frustration and distrust regarding health care errors. The public has responded by escalating the punishment for error. Clinicians and some health care organisations generally have responded by suppression, stonewalling, and cover-up. That approach has been less than successful.
(Leape et al 1998 p 1446)

Absence of safety culture. A young boy died after failing to recover from a general anaesthetic administered at a dental practice. A fatal accident enquiry concluded that the boy's death could have been prevented if a number of reasonable precautions had been in place. There was no agreement with a local hospital for rapid transfer of patients in emergencies, no heart monitor was attached when the anaesthetic was given, the anaesthetist lacked a specialist qualification and all staff lacked training in medical emergencies.
(DoH 2000 p 36)

A culture developed within the hospital that allowed unprofessional, counter therapeutic and degrading – even cruel – practices to take place. These practices went unchecked and were even condoned or excused when brought to the attention of the hospital. Some staff interviewed did not even recognise the abuse which had taken place as unacceptable practice.
(Commission for Health Improvement 2000 p 1)

wrong. Here the abuse referred to seems to have become normal, and therefore unnoticed by the staff concerned. Gradually, little by little, in a group isolated from mainstream clinical practice, behaviour that is unthinkable to begin with can become first tolerated, then routine and finally invisible.

All these examples supposedly concern the culture of safety; it seems to be a pretty broad, all-encompassing concept that is difficult to define with any precision. Does this matter? Well, yes it does. If our challenge is to change the culture, as so many commentators urge, then we need to understand what safety culture is, or at the very least decide what aspects to highlight, and bring as much precision to the definition as can be mustered. First though, we need to see how the concept emerged.

WHAT IS CULTURE?

Organizational culture

The word 'culture' has several different but related meanings. We are accustomed to thinking of culture in terms of the literary and artistic heritage of a people or the prevailing values and ethos of a particular nation. In medicine, culture has another meaning, as an environment in which bacteria or other organisms reproduce. This latter meaning could be seen as a metaphor for organizational culture – provide the right culture and the required attitudes and behaviours will flourish. Advocates of organizational culture in the business environment contrast their approach with the structural school of thought, which emphasizes the role of authority and rules in the functioning of organizations; the cultural perspective, on the other hand, considers attitudes, values and norms to be fundamental (Huczynski & Buchanan 1991). In the safety context, the contrast would be between relying on rules and regulations to produce safety and trying to engender a culture of safety.

Organizational culture has been studied for decades but it came to prominence as an explanatory concept during the 1980s, when it was put forward as an explanation of the excellent performance of some companies. Rather than look at the particular structures and management practices, management gurus such as Peters and Waterman (1982) emphasized the cultural attributes and the clear, guiding values of high-performance organizations. Given that quite a few of these companies have now gone to the wall, it might be that the importance of culture was over-stated, but nevertheless the concept of culture as a determinant of organizational performance remained. In healthcare, reflect for a moment on the experience of moving to a new hospital or a new ward to work. Very quickly one senses the differences in, for instance, how formal people are, how easy it is to speak up in meetings, the expectations of senior staff, the amount of help you can expect; all these reflect the culture of that particular organization or group.

The person who most clearly articulated the idea of organizational culture was Edgar Schein in his book *Organizational culture and leadership* (Schein 1985). The link with leadership will be discussed further below, but what interests us now is the clarity of Schein's conceptualization of culture. Karl Weick and Kathy Sutclifffe (2001) summarize this as follows:

Schein says that culture is defined by six formal properties: (1) shared basic assumptions that are (2) invented, discovered or developed by a given group as it (3) learns to cope with its problem of external adaptation and internal integration in ways that (4) have worked well enough to be considered valid and therefore (5) can be taught to new members of the group as the (6) correct way to perceive, think and feel in relation to those problems. When we talk about culture therefore, we are talking about assumptions that preserve lessons learned; values derived from those assumptions that prescribe how the organisation should act; and visible markers and activities that embody and give substance to the espoused values.

(Weick & Sutcliffe 2001 p 121)

So, in a healthcare setting, one basic assumption for all clinicians is that colleagues will always respond to a true emergency call; the priority of patient care in such situations is a core value, overriding all others. Locally, however, culture takes specific forms. The particular ways in which a crash team, for instance, organizes itself and works together might be based on national training but inevitably evolves over time and adapts as the members of the group develop a shared way of working together. In primary care, different practices organize themselves in different ways, with differing levels of availability to patients, differing degrees of shared responsibility and mutual support and so on. In short, culture is, as has often been said, 'the way we do things round here'.

Organizational culture and group culture

Culture, as noted above, is how we do things round here. Notice however, that 'here' can be a small group, part of an organization, a group of professionals or an entire, huge organization like the British NHS, the largest employer in Europe. (The Chinese army is apparently larger worldwide, although I do not have definitive figures.) Ideally, members of an organization share the same values and commitment, whether in a university, a business or a nuclear power plant. Safety, one would hope, would be a value on which everyone could agree and attitudes and values cohere. However, the safety culture within an organization can vary markedly in different areas and in different groups. For instance, in a survey of 1550 employees in the nuclear industry, Joan Harvey and colleagues (2002) found that managers had largely positive views of their own commitment to safety, personal involvement and saw themselves as taking responsibility for safety issues. Shop-floor workers, on the other hand, had generally more negative views about management commitment to safety, and about management's ability to listen and communicate. The divergence in views of managers and shop-floor workers might sound familiar to anyone who works in healthcare.

Healthcare is further complicated by the large number of professional groups, each with their own culture and ways of doing things. Nursing, for instance, tends to have a much stricter disciplinary code and harsher attitude to errors than medicine. Substantive nursing errors are often followed by formal warnings or sanctions, to a much greater extent than other professional groups.

National culture might also be influential, as Bob Helmreich's work has elegantly shown in the context of aviation (Helmreich & Merrit 1998). Efforts to train cockpit teams in more open styles of communication, for instance, have had to contend with widely varying cultural attitudes to seniority and hierarchy. Some cultures, particularly in Asian nations, have a much greater 'power gradient' than, for instance, the US and most European countries. With a steeper power gradient, there is greater deference to authority, an unwillingness to challenge senior figures not only in aviation but in the wider society; in this case cockpit attitudes reflect wider social mores. As we begin to explore the attitudes and experiences of patient safety in different countries, these differences are likely to emerge in healthcare.

SAFETY CULTURE

Safety culture did not spring up fully formed but emerged from organizational culture; when we talk of safety culture we are implicitly drawing on a wider academic context and also, implicitly, linking it with the wider culture of the organization. Recall the discussion in Chapters 5 and 6 about the organizational roots of many clinical incidents; here again we are linking safety issues to the priorities and values of the wider organization. In this section, we will define safety culture and consider some of the most important aspects, those relating to openness, blame, reporting and learning.

The UK Health and Safety Commission quotes the following definition in many of its documents, which was originally provided by the Advisory Committee on the Safety of Nuclear Installations (ACSNI). It nicely captures the essential features:

> The safety culture of an organisation is the product of the individual and group values, attitudes, competencies and patterns of behaviour that determine the commitment to, and the style and proficiency of, an organisation's health and safety programmes. Organisations with a positive safety culture are characterised by communications founded on mutual trust, by shared perceptions of the importance of safety, and by confidence in the efficacy of preventative measures.
> **(Health and Safety Commission 1993)**

The committee went on to say:

> In a safe organisation the pattern of shared assumptions puts safety high in its priorities. Whatever individual they affect then handles new events and decisions in the light of that priority. Thus the commitment to and the style and proficiency of an organisation's safety programmes matter as much as the formal definition of those programmes. This commitment and style are the produce of individual and group values, attitudes, competencies and patterns of behaviour.
> **(Health and Safety Commision 1993)**

A safety culture is therefore partly built of the attitudes and values of individuals and everyone contributes to the safety culture in their own way.

A strong organizational and management commitment is also implied; safety needs to be taken seriously at every level of the organization. The Chief Executive needs to provide clear and committed leadership, communicated throughout the organization, that gives the safety of patients and staff a priority. The cleaner on the wards must be conscious of infection risks, nurses need to be alert for potential equipment problems and drug hazards and managers must monitor incident reports. Finally, as the ACSNI committee indicates, producing and maintaining a safety culture is a long-term, systematic and continuing process. There is never a time when the job of enhancing and maintaining a safety culture is finished. Safety, like trust, is a highly perishable commodity with, as Richard Cook likes to say, the half-life of adrenaline.

An open and fair culture

The tendency for excessive, immediate and unreasoning blame in the face of patient harm, both from within and outside healthcare organizations, has led some to call for a 'no-blame' culture. This, if taken literally, would appear to remove personal accountability, and also many social, disciplinary and legal strictures on clinical practice. A culture without blame would therefore seem to be both unworkable and to remove some of the restrictions and safeguards on safe behaviour. A much better objective is to try to develop an open and fair culture, which certainly means a huge shift away from blame but preserves personal responsibility and accountability. An open and fair culture requires a much more thoughtful and supportive response to error and harm when they do occur.

After reflecting in several chapters on the nature of human error, we can see that the tendency to immediate blame, satisfying as it might be in the short term, is often unwarranted and certainly not in the long-term interests of patient safety. Yet it takes a very cool headed and thoughtful clinical leader or Chief Executive to take a systems view when faced with some awful incident, particularly when he or she might be under considerable pressure from relatives, the media and even government. Regulatory and professional bodies also face these pressures and equally have to decide whether a clinician's behaviour is deserving of censure and disciplinary action. It is no good simply appealing to systems thinking and a just culture; a call has to be made one way or the other and some action taken.

Assessing culpability: the Incident Decision Tree

To give form and structure to these decisions about culpability, the aviation firm Boeing developed a decision aid for maintenance error in which the psychological principles involved in the occurrence of such error were given flesh in the form of a step-by-step decision aid that examined the nature of the error, the influence of context and contributing factors, health and pressures and so forth. James Reason (1997) outlined a more general 'culpability matrix', which in turn was adapted by the UK National Patient Safety Agency (NPSA) in its 'Incident Decision Tree' (NPSA 2004a).

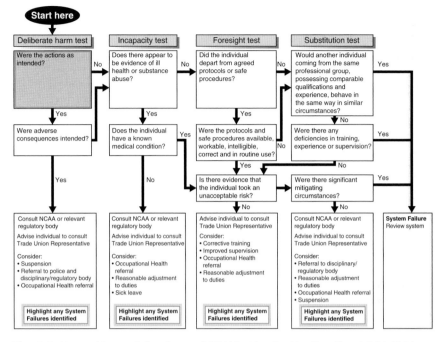

Fig. 9.1 National Patient Safety Agency (NPSA) Incident Decision Tree (from NPSA 2004a, © National Patient Safety Agency).

The structure of the NPSA's Incident Decision Tree is shown in Fig. 9.1. Essentially, after the incident has been investigated and some thought given to its causes, a series of questions is asked. Were the actions intentional? If, yes, was there an intention to cause harm or not? Is there any evidence of a medical condition? Was there a departure from agreed protocols, and so on. Consider the example in Box 9.2. The staff nurse did not set out to harm the patients. However, her actions were clearly intentional and the violation of protocols deliberate and without justification. In other cases, protocols and procedures might still have been ignored, but in circumstances that mitigate the error. The NPSA (2004a) gives the example of a midwife who failed to notice discrepancies in a fetal heart reading because she had been on duty for 15 hours without a break to cover absent colleagues. Finally, there are areas of particular difficulty when the 'correct' action is not clear cut, when a judgement must be made as to whether the risks outweigh the benefits. Generally speaking, any procedure or standard over-estimates the extent to which clinical practice, in fact any human behaviour, is routine and predictable. However, the decision aid commendably makes this an explicit issue:

> A surgical patient is receiving opiate analgesia via a syringe pump. A senior nurse, who has just come on duty, realises the pump has been set up to run much too fast and the patient's breathing is slow and shallow. The charge nurse urgently summons medical staff assistance but there is no response. The patient stops breathing. The nurse decides there is no

Box 9.2 Reckless behaviour in the care of the elderly

(adapted from NPSA 2004a p 21)

A staff nurse working on a care of the elderly ward reports to the sister that she has telephoned the senior house officer for diamorphine for a terminally ill patient in severe pain. She says the senior house officer has asked the nursing staff to administer the drug, saying that he will call in as soon as possible to write up a prescription retrospectively. The sister hands the drugs cabinet keys to the staff nurse without question and the patient is given the medication.

The following day it transpires that the staff nurse had not telephoned the doctor. Initially she lied about this, but subsequently admitted she had not even tried to call because 'You can never get hold of them.' The staff nurse said she did not regret her actions and had administered drugs without prescription before. She was fully aware that she was breaching protocols.

By contrast, the sister was shocked by the incident and mortified that she had accepted the staff nurse's explanation. She too realized she had breached protocols and volunteered to move to another ward while the investigation took place.

The Trust decided that both individuals have taken an unacceptable risk and that there are no significant mitigating circumstances. The staff nurse is suspended and subsequently dismissed, as it is believed her attitude toward the incident and her previous behaviour indicates an ongoing risk to patients. The sister is not suspended but is temporarily redeployed. She is subsequently disciplined but not dismissed.

option but to deliver a naloxone injection himself to try and save the patient's life. In doing so, he knowingly breached Trust protocols (which were generally clear, workable and in routine use) and his own profession's standards of accountability. However, the nurse was faced with a life or death situation and the risk to the patient of waiting for medical help was much greater than the nurse taking on what was properly a medical decision.

(NPSA 2004a p 41)

There is nothing very remarkable about any of these clinical scenarios. If they are not everyday occurrences, they are at least reasonably common, which does not necessarily make them any easier to interpret. Using the Incident Decision Tree requires an initial analysis of the case and some reflection on the web of causes and contributory factors and the intentions and circumstances of the people involved. Deciding whether someone should be supported, praised or disciplined is never easy but the Incident Decision Tree should make the process fairer, more explicit and more in the interests of future patients in that healthcare organization.

Reporting, understanding and learning

One my favourite aphorisms is that practice, in many different areas, is just 'one mistake after another'. This is partly a rueful acceptance of the humiliating and frustrating nature of the acquisition of any skill; learning the piano, for example, is inevitably an experience of fumbled notes, incomprehension and strident discords each time one advances to a more difficult piece. More importantly though, this phrase brings out the idea that people, and indeed organizations, learn through noticing and reflecting on errors. The total quality management gurus go as far as to say that every error is a treasure, which might be a step too far for some, but certainly errors can be highly informative. Organizations can advance and evolve by recognizing error or, conversely, can decay and become unsafe by suppressing information about error and safety, and adopting an ostrich-like 'head in the sand' approach to the landscape of error and hazard.

The nature and mechanisms of reporting systems were discussed in Chapter 4, along with some of the reasons why people do and do not report. Returning to this theme again we are more concerned, in the cultural context, with the attitudes and values that underlie a willingness to report and, more importantly, to reflect and learn. This means not just acknowledging error but sometimes even celebrating its successful resolution. There is a famous story about Werner von Braun, the rocket scientist (and inspiration for Dr Strangelove) presenting a bottle of champagne to a NASA engineer who had brought a major problem to his attention. Don Berwick provides a more recent example showing that this tradition continues (Box 9.3).

The key phrase for me in the story of the Titan rocket, the fulcrum on which it turns, is 'then you'll never be safe'. The attitude and understanding expressed here is that punishing people for honest error is not simply unfair and pointless; it is in fact, dangerous. Why is it dangerous? Because the effect of mindless sanctions is to suppress the very information you need to create and maintain a state

---

Box 9.3 The gold plated bolt

(adapted from Berwick 1998)

The Titan rocket was powered by liquid oxygen and hydrogen. The design of the rocket required great precision in the use of fuel – every drop had to be consumed before engine shutdown, completely emptying the tanks. To ensure the liquid emptied completely, four small metal baffles were placed at the bottom of the tank to stop the liquid swirling round the exit from the tank. Unfortunately, the fitted baffles were a little too big and an expensive, but necessary, fix was organized. The tanks were drained and a man lowered on a harness in a diving suit to trim the baffles. Four bolts and metal fragments had to be removed and collected in a cloth sack; if metal was left in the tank, it would be sucked into the high-pressure pump and the rocket would explode.

The problem arose when the engineer who did the trimming, Jerry Gonsalves, returned and emptied the cloth sack to find only three bolts. They went back to the tank and looked carefully for the missing bolt, could not find it and concluded that there must only have been three. That night, Gonsalves could not sleep thinking about the missing bolt. He returned to the tank and looked down to see if there were any places the bolt could be hidden. He found two and called the Director of Safety, Guy Cohen. The next morning they all assembled again, emptied the tank at huge expense, and lowered another engineer to check. He went to the first of the two hiding places Gonsalves had identified, and found the bolt.

Guy Cohen asked me a question at this stage in the story. 'Suppose it had been a nurse' he asked, 'and we were talking about a serious drug error. What would happen in one of your hospitals?' I knew the answer very well. 'An incident report,' I said. 'And the nurse would probably have had some sort of warning put in her file. If the patient had died, she would probably be fired or worse.'

'Then you'll never be safe,' he said. 'That's not what we did. We saved that bolt and had it gold plated and mounted on a plaque. And we had the NASA administrator come to the launch of that rocket a couple of days later. And in full view of everyone there, we gave the plaque to Jerry Gonsalves, and we dedicated the launch to him.'

of safety. The matrix of reward and punishment is handled entirely differently in the case of the nurse and the engineer; the nurse is punished for the error but the engineer is rewarded for his 'safety behaviour', in this case his continuing anxiety and honesty in the face of having made an error. The response of Cohen, and indeed the wider organization, was not to castigate him for the error but to act on the safety information and check the rocket once again.

In considering this example we return again to the reasons healthcare staff do and do not report, discussed in Chapter 4. The attitudes conveyed here are the converse of many of the reasons advanced for not reporting: fear of disciplinary action, the reactions of one's colleagues, not being listened to, it would make no difference and so on. But, in considering Don Berwick's story, we can see that the people involved are expressing something more than an operational policy of collecting error information. The organization is guided by a core principle that safety information must be valued, analysed, understood and communicated; this is the culture of understanding and learning.

FLEXIBILITY AND RESILIENCE: THE CULTURE OF HIGH RELIABILITY

Throughout this book we have used case studies of clinical scenarios to achieve a better understanding of the nature of error and safety. Case studies have also been used to bring a better understanding of the culture and practices of organizations, including those that, in the face of extraordinary levels of hazards, manage to achieve high levels of both safety and performance. These high-reliability organizations (HROs) include nuclear power plants, aircraft carriers and air traffic control; they have been examined rigorously by a mixture of observations, interviews, questionnaires and archival analysis (La Porte 1996, Roberts 1990). Many authors believe that the culture and practices of these organizations can inform the changing business and healthcare environments (Waller & Roberts 2003).

To begin with, we can get a flavour of life in an HRO from a US Navy veteran's description of life on board a carrier:

Imagine that it's a busy day, and you shrink San Francisco airport to only one short runway and one ramp and one gate. Make planes take off and land at the same time, at half the present time interval, rock the runway from side to side, and require that everyone who leaves in the morning returns the same day. Make sure the equipment is so close to the envelope that it's fragile. Then turn off the radar to avoid detection, impose strict controls on the radios, fuel the aircraft in place with their engines running, put an enemy in the air and scatter live bombs and rockets around. Now, wet the whole thing down with sea water and oil and man it with twenty-year-olds, half of whom have never seen an airplane close up. Oh, and by the way, try not to kill anyone.
(Weick & Sutcliffe 2001 p 26)

Weick and Sutcliffe go on to ask, in the context of addressing business leaders, 'Can you think of another environment that is quite this full of the unexpected?'

Well, yes, in healthcare maybe we can. Here is my paraphrase description of a central London Accident and Emergency department:

> Imagine that it's always a busy day and you shrink the entire hospital to one department and one entrance. Patients come and go every minute or two, wanting to be seen immediately. Any kind of illness may present, in a person of any age, physical and mental conditions; many patients do not speak the language of the doctors and nurses. Some are drug addicts, often HIV positive, posing real dangers to staff. Then impose severe constraints on the time available for diagnosis and investigation, the availability of back-up staff and beds, fill the area with dangerous drugs, add the threat of violence from a good proportion of the patients attending and the frequent presence of the police. Now, add a few cases of major trauma, staff the place with 25-year-olds who are completely new to this kind of environment and make sure the experienced staff are tied up with administration. Oh, and by the way, try not to kill anyone.

The similarities between HROs and some aspects of healthcare are at least superficially persuasive. Previous attempts to import lessons on quality and safety from manufacturing have sometimes been resisted because the routine, production-line processes seem to have little in common with the dynamic, hands-on, highly variable and adaptive nature of much work in healthcare. HROs seem to offer a better model because their procedures and practices have evolved specifically to deal with the dynamic, the variable and the unexpected. We should, however, inject some notes of caution here. First, much of healthcare is routine and largely predictable. Some aspects, such as pharmacy distribution or the supply of blood products, are much more like manufacturing processes than HROs. Second, HROs appear to be built very solidly on strict training, discipline and adherence to procedures, protocols and routine when conditions are routine. The qualities that are identified as particularly characteristic of HROs only come into play at certain times. Clinicians, by contrast, might be faulted for being unwilling to adhere to basic routines, introducing variability into practice when it is neither necessary nor desirable. Finally, it is perhaps worth remarking that there is a certain appeal in comparing one's own work to that of fighter pilots and those in operate nuclear carriers, but this can be over-played; much harder to think that healthcare might have something to learn from the communication and information systems at the local coffee shop franchise. (Although not always: Pat Croskerry, an emergency physician in Canada, laments that the technology used to support his morning coffee purchase is far superior to the imperfect systems he uses to keep his patients alive.)

The lessons of high-reliability organizations

Many of the HROs studied are military, or at least contain many military personnel (Reason 1997). There is a strong foundation of standard operating procedures, attempting to plan for every contingency, shared discipline and a commitment to working as a team. Although there are certainly hierarchy and discipline, sanctions and rewards, there are also shared values and attitudes that cannot be wholly engendered by rules and regulations. Weick & Sutcliffe (2001) argue that, as surveillance at all times by managers and senior staff is obviously impossible, shared understanding has to be mediated by culture, in essence by an acceptance of common ways of working and shared assumptions and values. Weick & Sutcliffe make the crucial point that the shared understanding and common view allows a flexible approach when it is required; in HROs the very acceptance and adherence to standardization and procedures is what permits a decentralized approach when necessary. Flexibility can be tolerated and utilized because when the need for it is over the organization can return to routine operation without being threatened by the temporary relaxation of hierarchy and procedure. The routine, discipline and standardization inherent in the HROs is not usually emphasized in healthcare, where people prefer the excitement of learning about dealing with crisis.

The aspect of HROs that has received most attention is their response to the unexpected, to crisis and change. Weick & Sutcliffe identify five hallmarks of HROs:

- preoccupation with failure
- reluctance to simplify interpretations
- sensitivity to operations
- commitment to resilience
- deference to expertise.

The relevance of each of these characteristics to healthcare could be examined in detail, but we can only pick out some key features here: by preoccupation with failure, Weick and Sutcliffe point to what James Reason refers to as chronic unease, ceaselessly watching for unexpected or disconfirming information. On a personal level, a clinician might become suspicious about a sudden rise in a patient's temperature; at an organizational level the risk manager might react to a flurry of reports about equipment from the ITU.

Sensitivity to operations also mirrors this concern with what is happening down on the wards, trying to keep a link between managers and senior clinicians and front line staff.

Reluctance to simplify is being willing, at an organizational level, not to accept the most obvious interpretation at face value. In an analysis of the failures at the Bristol Royal Infirmary, Weick identified a mindset in which poor results in cardiac surgery were explained away by reference to patient characteristics, rather than trying to see the more challenging and complex reality of a catastrophic breakdown in organizational and clinical processes.

The commitment to resilience is seen in the attention given to small errors and problems, in the knowledge that if not corrected they can lead to larger problems and an organization-wide attempt to deal with problems as they arise. It also encompasses an ability to anticipate and recover from error and crisis at both an individual and organizational level.

Deference to expertise is a most important concept and one with immediate and clear relevance to healthcare. Weick and Sutcliffe explain that, for various reasons, rigid hierarchies have their own special vulnerability to errors. If only senior staff are mandated to act, and those lower down have to wait for orders, this can be fatal in a fast-changing, hazardous situation. Junior doctors, for instance, are expected to act as best they can in an emergency if no senior help is available. Deference to expertise, however, is more subtle, allowing junior staff to take the lead even when senior staff are present. In hazardous, crisis situations senior commanders will defer to those with knowledge of the immediate environment and often, in the military, these people are non-commissioned officers or enlisted men. At these times, open communication and negotiation of differences of view, as opposed to a blind following of orders, become critical (La Porte & Consolini 1991).

This is a crucial issue in healthcare, where hierarchies within professions tend to be rigid and relationships between professions and specialties complicated by issues of power and status. Deference to expertise is a concept that, ideally, cuts across hierarchy to point to action in the patient's best interests. Will the senior physician visiting the ward on rounds rely on his or her own, necessarily brief, assessment of the patient or listen to the views of the young nurse who has watched the patient deteriorate through the night? Will a young doctor take advice from a senior nurse with 20 years more experience than he has? Will the psychiatrist be persuaded by her team that this patient is more dangerous than she had previously thought? Many of these negotiations and conversations happen successfully in medicine, being managed thoughtfully and without fuss by people who know and respect each other. What the HROs tell us is that we perhaps need to go further, that deference to expertise needs to be discussed, the circumstances in which it is necessary outlined, and a greater respect for informal communication inculcated.

We have only scratched the surface of the nature of HROs and their relevance to healthcare. This is a complex issue and, although these organizations display some fundamentally important characteristics, an uncritical adoption of high-reliability practices into healthcare could be a mistake in some settings. Most importantly, these organizations are already very safe, unlike many areas of healthcare, which are frankly dangerous. Rene Amalberti (2001) has pointed out, in the context of aviation, that the kind of safety measures needed in an organization relate to the degree of safety it has already achieved. Remember the extent of the proceduralization that underlies the flexibility of HROs; they can be flexible because they can also return to hierarchy and procedure. Trying to graft high-reliability characteristics into a healthcare organization that, at this particular point in its safety evolution, really needs better standards and procedures, could be destabilizing rather than safety enhancing. The wider cultural aspects of HROs have their counterpoint in individual behaviour, and we shall address both the need to follow rules and the need to depart from them in a later chapter.

MEASURING SAFETY CULTURE

Safety culture, as can be seen from our overview, has multiple facets and, less agreeably, seems to have multiple meanings. Sharpening the concept and assessing its validity requires, first, measuring it and, second, seeing if safety culture does indeed relate to other indices of safety, such as rates of error or incidents. In industrial settings, some progress has been made in both these objectives, although there is still no solid consensus on the key characteristics of safety culture. We should note that outside healthcare the term 'safety climate' is generally used when discussing measures of the underlying safety culture. The reasons for this are complex and relate to debates in organizational theory, but the basic idea is that safety climate is the surface manifestation of safety culture. A survey, whether by questionnaire or interview, can tell you only about the safety culture at that particular moment. As Cox and Flin (1998) express it, safety climate is a snapshot of the state of safety providing an indicator of the underlying safety culture of a work group, plant or organization. In healthcare people generally talk about measuring the safety culture, but the term safety climate is also used.

Rhona Flin and colleagues (2000) reviewed 18 different measures of safety climate in various industrial settings. Common features identified concerned management attitudes to safety, the presence of safety systems and policies, perceptions of risk and sometimes information on work pressures and competence: a fairly mixed bag of concepts variously subsumed under the general term safety climate. Some of these instruments had been validated, in that measures of safety climate had been related to accident rates, but it is not yet clear which aspects of safety climate are the crucial indicators of a safe or unsafe site. This group went on to examine 12 different instruments in use in healthcare, most of which did not meet basic psychometric standards for questionnaire design. A huge range of issues was covered, which varied between the different measures. Flin and Yule identified Nieva and Sorra's hospital survey on patient safety (Box 9.4) as one of the best-developed questionnaires, although this has not been used as widely as some other instruments. Some of these studies showed that ratings of culture were associated with clinicians' reports of safe behaviours but only two tried to relate safety culture to actual incidents, and only one of these concerned injuries to patients. For all the enthusiasm for safety culture there is, as yet, little hard evidence that a positive safety culture is indeed associated with reduced harm to patients.

The emphasis on the lack of evidence for safety culture being a key mediator of reductions in harm is a necessary caution against the wilder claims for

---

Box 9.4 Hospital survey on patient safety

(from Nieva & Sorra 2003)

42 items covering the following issues:
- Supervisor/manager expectations and actions promoting patient safety
- Organizational learning and continuous improvement
- Teamwork within units
- Communication and openness
- Feedback and communication about error
- Non-punitive response to error
- Staffing levels
- Hospital management support for patient safety
- Teamwork across hospital units
- Hospitals handoffs and transitions

culture. However, evidence of such a relationship will be difficult to obtain and might only emerge in time; for one thing, we have few valid measures or indices of error and harm against which to validate measures of culture. Useful findings are beginning to emerge, however, and measures of safety culture can be used practically to galvanize action on patient safety. Singer and colleagues (2003) surveyed 2989 employees in 15 Californian hospitals in an effort to assess basic safety-related attitudes and to see how they varied across different organizations. They classified responses that seemed to suggest a poor safety culture as 'problematic'. As Table 9.1 shows, a third of those responding said they were not rewarded for taking quick action to identify a serious mistake and 28% believed they would be disciplined if a mistake they made was discovered. A small but appreciable incidence of unsafe acts was noted, with many staff feeling that pressure of work and loss of experienced personnel had degraded safety; 39% had seen a co-worker do something unsafe in the past year and 8% admitted doing something unsafe themselves. Although all hospitals were taking action on patient safety, there was considerable variation between them; the average level of problematic responses varied from 13% to 22%. As happens outside healthcare, management tended to have much more positive attitudes and experiences than front-line clinical staff. The authors suggest this could be because front-line staff and middle managers tend to gloss over safety problems when briefing senior staff, which would make it very difficult for senior executives to understand the true state of their organizations and the extent of action needed on safety. Alternatively, the results could imply that senior executives have a genuine commitment to safety that is not being communicated to front-line staff. Either way, creating links between executives and front-line clinicians is a priority for improving safety.

Safety culture surveys have also been used simply to push forward the safety agenda and engage clinicians and leaders. Peter Pronovost and colleagues at Johns Hopkins University used short surveys of safety culture and strategies for leadership as a baseline for their attempts to improve patient safety (Pronovost et al 2003). Here again, senior managers perceived safety to be better developed than members of the patient safety committee, and front-line staff perceived that their immediate supervisors were more concerned with safety than were senior managers. The two surveys highlighted that senior leaders needed to become more visible to front line staff in their efforts to improve safety, that there was a need for much more proactive strategic planning and also a need to educate clinicians about patient safety. This prompted the development of such a strategy and a hospital-wide programme of action on patient safety.

CAN WE CHANGE THE CULTURE?

Mark Twain famously remarked, on the subject of the weather in England, that everyone complains about it but no one does anything about it. Is culture like the weather, something we have to tolerate and adapt to, or can culture be developed and changed over time? Organizational theorists of different

Culture and leadership for safety

Table 9.1 Problematic safety responses in Californian hospitals (from Singer et al 2003)

Illustrative questions	% Problematic	% Problematic or neutral
Organization		
Loss of experienced staff has negatively affected my ability to provide high quality patient care	51.8	70.0
I am rewarded for taking quick action to identify a serious mistake	33.1	64.0
I am provided with adequate resources to provide safe patient care	32.7	50.8
It is hard for doctors and nurses to hide serious mistakes	29.8	48.7
Senior management has a clear picture of the risk associated with patient care	20.9	37.3
Senior management has a good idea of the kinds of mistakes that actually occur in this facility	20.7	42.2
Good communication flow exists up the chain of command regarding patients safety issues	17.7	35.9
Senior management provides a climate that promotes patient safety	15.0	35.5
Senior management considers patient safety when programme changes are discussed	12.6	40.5
Department		
In my department, disregarding policy and procedure is rare	14.8	25.6
My department follows a specific process to review performance against defined training goals	14.7	37.1
Staff are provided with the necessary training to safely provide patient care	10.8	25.4
Compared with other facilities in the area, this facility cares more about the quality of patient care it provides	9.6	43.4
My department does a good job managing risks to ensure patient safety	7.8	18.6

Productions

I have witnessed a co-worker do something that appeared to me to be unsafe patient care	39.3	50.2
Compared to other facilities in the area, this facility cares more about increasing revenues or profits	21.4	60.8
I am asked to cut corners to get the job done	18.7	33
I have enough time to complete the patient care tasks safely	9.2	35.8
In the last year I have done something that was not safe for the patient	8.2	18.3

Reporting/seeking help

If people find out that I made a mistake, I will be disciplined	27.7	51.8
Reporting a patient safety problem will not result in negative repercussions for the person reporting it	11.3	24.7
I will suffer negative consequences if I report a patient safety problem	7.7	18.4
Asking for help is a sign of incompetence	4.1	7.8

Shame/self-awareness

Telling others about my mistakes is embarrassing	37.5	49.2
I have made significant errors in my work that I attribute to my own fatigue	7.2	17.1
I am less effective at work when I am fatigued	37.0	35.3

Adapted from Singer et al 2003 Quality and Safety in Health Care 12:112–118, amended and reproduced with permission from the BMJ Publishing Group.

Culture and leadership for safety

persuasions have different views on this question. Some, of a more anthropological orientation, see culture as a product of personal values and attitudes, deeply rooted in the history of a nation or an organization. Others, with a more business orientation, see culture as something that can be encouraged, developed and perhaps even manipulated. Changing national culture or the social mores of a society is a dangerous business and, arguably, an intrusion on personal freedom and values. Attitudes to safety and risky behaviour, however, can and do change, often for the better. Think, for instance, of attitudes towards driving while drunk, or wearing seat belts in cars, which have changed hugely, albeit slowly, in the last 20 years. With safety, we are hoping to change specific work-related attitudes and values rather than deeply held personal beliefs.

Rules, regulations, sanctions and rewards certainly play a part in defining a safety culture. If you are rewarded for reporting a safety issue, you are more likely to do it again next time than if you were disciplined. Above all, however, culture is socially mediated, a product of the relationships between people in the organization, particularly those who are influential in virtue of the position they hold or the respect they receive (ideally both). Karl Weick and Kathy Sutcliffe (2001), in discussing how leaders can encourage a mindful approach to high performance explain the emergence of a high-reliability culture as follows:

> What you need to do is to modify what people expect from each other. . . . This modification is not just a change in how people think, as important as that is, but a change in how people feel. You need people to absorb the lessons of mindfulness at an emotional level so that they will express approval when others hold certain beliefs and act in certain ways. For example, people need to feel strongly that it's good to speak up when they make a mistake, good to spot flawed assumptions, good to focus on a persistent operational anomaly. They need to expect praise for these acts when they do them, and they need to offer praise when they spot someone else doing them. Likewise you need to attach disapproval to people believing and acting in ways that undermine mindfulness. For example people need to agree among themselves and feel strongly that it's bad to refrain from asking for help, bad to let success go to their heads, bad to ignore lower-ranking experts. They need to express key values by making clear what is disapproved as much as by praising what is approved. When people make these kinds of changes, a new culture begins to emerge. The culture takes the form of a new set of expectations and a new urgency that people will live up to them.
> **(Weick & Sutcliffe 2001 p 119)**

Culture, therefore, is maintained and manifests in social processes and interactions. Everyone in an organization contributes, consciously or not, to its culture. What emerges might be positive and safety conscious or, over time, drift to a relentless negativity in which all manner of dangerous behaviour is tolerated or even encouraged. Maintaining a safety culture, indeed any kind of culture, requires ongoing work and commitment, which takes us to the crucial topic of leadership.

LEADERSHIP FOR PATIENT SAFETY

Leadership takes many forms and has many different functions. The leadership required during a crisis in the operating theatre differs from that required to lead a clinical department, which differs again from leadership in a management or executive role. Common features such as authority, clarity of objectives and purpose might be apparent but the style needs to change to match the context and the people being led. Although there might be agreement, within a hospital for example, on the people who have leadership qualities, it is not so easy to encapsulate exactly what abilities they share or what exactly marks them out as leaders. Theories of leadership abound and there is a vast literature; yet again patient safety draws us in to a complex area that many people spend a lifetime trying to master, whether as leaders themselves or as those trying to understand and teach leadership. We can only touch on a few aspects of leadership characteristics that might be especially important in promoting safety.

Leaders impact on safety in many ways. Think back to the analysis of accidents and clinical incidents discussed in Chapters 5 and 6. Organizational accident theory suggests that safety is influenced not just by people at the sharp end but also by decisions higher up the organization. Safety and quality in high-performing firms need not be seen as separate from financial and other matters, but as an integral part of productivity and profitability. When Paul O'Neill, who later became US Treasury Secretary, was Chief Executive of Alcoa, he made safety his 'signature issue', starting all Board meetings with that issue, always linking it to whatever was being discussed. Other people quickly learnt that paying attention to safety always engaged his attention, and the over-riding importance of safety permeated the culture of the company (Berwick 1998).

Senior leaders influence safety directly by setting up safety-related committees and initiatives and allowing staff time to engage in fundamental safety issues, such as the redesign of systems. Leaders also influence safety indirectly by talking about safety, showing they value it and being willing to discuss errors and safety issues in a constructive way. Safety is also strongly influenced by people in supervisory roles, such as a nurse in charge of a ward, both in the efficient management of processes and in the attitudes and values they foster in the people they manage. In turn, an individual nurse demonstrates her personal commitment to safety to trainees by attention to detail, by performing checks and by rigorous adherence to basic standards of care. Leadership, then, comes in many forms and is demonstrated at all levels of the organization. Can we find any characteristics that are particularly important for safety?

Rhona Flin and Stephen Yule (2004) outline a particular leadership theory that is of especial relevance to safety. The transformational leadership theory of Bass and Avolio (1994) distinguishes two broad types of leadership, both important for safety: transactional and transformational leadership.

Transactional leadership is, broadly speaking, an effective and efficient management style: set objectives, get agreement on what needs to be done, monitor performance and reward or sanction as appropriate. A theatre nurse, for instance, might set clear guidelines for behaviour and the standard of care he or she expects from the staff reporting to him or her.

By contrast, transformational leadership, which Bass and Avolio (1994) suggest is characteristic of high-performing teams, is more concerned with conveying a sense of purpose and vision, with empowering people in the team and treating people as unique individuals. Although the theory is not without its critics, there is evidence that transformational leadership is related to higher levels of performance, commitment and employee satisfaction than transactional leadership.

Flin & Yule (2004) review a variety of studies showing the importance of a transformational style for safety. For instance, supervisors who communicate effectively and frequently about safety with employees, and have a supportive leadership style, inspire a greater commitment to safety among the workforce. Involvement of employees in decision making about safety issues also promotes safety behaviour. Safety leadership higher up the organization is less well understood. However, Stephen Yule has found that transformational leadership at the top of the organizations does seem to be associated with lower accident rates. Key behaviours are: articulating an attainable vision of safety, demonstrating personal commitment to safety, engaging everyone with relevant experience and being clear and transparent when dealing with safety issues (Table 9.2).

Leadership in complex organizational settings, such as a hospital, requires other characteristics that are closely associated with the transformational leadership style. Ron Westrum (1997) calls such leaders 'maestros'. This wonderful image suggests that presiding over a large, complex organization that marries people and technology, is akin to being the conductor of a great orchestra. This notion of leadership might be far from the common image of great military or political leaders, but might be closer to the style required to

---

Table 9.2 Leadership behaviours for safety (adapted from Flin & Yule 2004)

	Transactional behaviours	Transformational behaviours
Supervisors	Monitoring and reinforcing workers' safe behaviours Participating in workforce safety activities (can also be transformational)	Being supportive of safety initiatives Encouraging employee involvement in safety initiatives
Middle managers	Becoming involved in safety initiatives (can also be transformational)	Emphasizing safety over productivity Adopting a decentralized style Relaying the corporate vision for safety to supervisors
Senior managers	Ensuring compliance with regulatory requirements Providing resources for a comprehensive safety programme	Demonstrating visible and consistent commitment to safety Showing concern for people Encouraging participatory styles in middle managers and supervisors Giving time for safety

Adapted from Flin & Yule 2004 Quality and Safety in Health Care 13:ii45–ii51, amended and reproduced with permission from the BMJ Publishing Group.

promote and maintain safe, high-quality care. When thinking of the wider organization, be it a clinical unit or an entire health system, the struggle for the aspiring maestro is to have the wider vision and to discern, predict and articulate the safety problems before they arise. The maestro should constantly watch for the weaknesses in the system and the conditions that might eventually combine to produce a catastrophe: the skills mix in the unit, the lack of information flow about safety issues and, in particular, problems at the interfaces with other departments and organizations.

What does this mean in practical terms? Sue Osborne and Susan Williams, Chief Executives of the National Patient Safety Agency, have brought together the key characteristics of patient safety leadership for chief executives in a pithy document that summarizes the key issues (Box 9.5). As an example of someone who put safety at the very forefront of his tenure as Chief Executive,

---

Box 9.5 Delivering safer healthcare: a leadership checklist for chief executives

(adapted from NPSA 2004b)

1. Build a safety culture
To help your organization learn about patient safety, you should create a culture in which staff share information freely because this is known to improve levels of safety. This can be fostered by:
- Undertaking a baseline cultural assessment of your organization and assessing whether it is open and fair.
- Having policies and procedures that support a culture in which:
  - staff can talk to colleagues and managers about incidents they have been involved in
  - reviews of incidents focus on why it occurred, not simply who was involved
  - staff are treated fairly and supported when an incident happens
  - tools such as the NPSA's Incident Decision Tree are used to determine the reasons behind an individual's actions.

2. Lead and support your staff
A safety culture requires strong leadership and a willingness to listen. The following three actions are known to make the biggest impact:
- Patient safety briefings by yourself or regular executive visits throughout an organization, meeting staff and patients to specifically discuss safety issues.
- Encouraging discussions around patient safety incidents and how they might be prevented.
- Developing communication and feedback mechanisms are vital so staff understand their contribution to safety and are encouraged to participate.

Additional clearly identified roles and responsibilities can also be helpful:
- Appoint patient safety champions for every part of the organization.
- Nominate a Board executive to oversee risk management and safety.
- Appoint someone sufficiently senior, with access to you, who is responsible for risk management, and ideally part of a central team taking an integrated approach.

3. Integrate your risk management activity
Safety is known to improve when organizations' leaders ask themselves the following:
- Is patient safety reflected in the organizational strategy, structures, functions and systems?
- Do patient safety objectives feature in the clinical governance strategy and plan?
- Are all clinical risk assessments for each specialty fed into the organizational risk register? Is this up to date, with action plans implemented, followed up and monitored?
- Are Board agendas structured to ensure that risk management and patient safety are on an equal footing with finance and performance targets?

Continued

Box 9.5 Delivering safer healthcare: a leadership checklist for chief executives—cont'd

4. Promote reporting

Reporting things that go wrong is fundamental for building a safer service for patients. Important actions are:

- To encourage all staff to report patient safety problems, particularly those groups that have low reporting levels.
- Aim to reduce the severity of incidents. You should receive reports and action plans for all deaths directly related to a patient safety incident.

5. Involve patients and the public

Open organizations are safer organizations. Patients and their carers need to know when harm has occurred and be involved in incident investigations. This can be done by:

- Producing an open disclosure policy.
- Obtaining Board-level support for the policy and then providing training for staff.
- Involving patients, their families and carers in investigations and informing them about recommendations made and the solutions developed following a patient safety incident.

6. Learn and share safety lessons

Healthcare will only become safer if we create a memory of things that go wrong both nationally and locally. This can be achieved by:

- Investigating and analysing incidents effectively using trained staff.
- You or your lead executive taking part in at least one case analysis each year.
- Analysing the frequency, type and levels of severity of incidents, and the lessons learned over time. Routinely report this work to the Board.

7. Implement solutions to prevent harm

Real progress will not be made in delivering safer healthcare unless necessary changes are implemented. The first steps should be:

- Review practice in relation to national recommendations and the findings of local, regional and national enquiries.
- Ensure recommendations are implemented and evaluated; assess what remains to be done; and feedback your organization's actions to national bodies.
- Establish a network that includes your and other organizations' patient safety champions to learn from those who have successfully implemented solutions.

we consider Jim Conway at the Dana-Farber Cancer Institute in Boston, who led a root and branch reform after a high-profile patient death in 1994. Jim Conway's reflections on the crucial elements of leadership for safety (Box 9.6) summarize and give life to the more academic treatment earlier in this section.

LEADERSHIP THROUGH POLICY AND REGULATION

This book is principally concerned with patient safety at the clinical and organizational level. Healthcare organizations of all kinds are profoundly influenced by the wider social environment, by regulation, and by political and financial imperatives and constraints. In day-to-day clinical practice the influence of these high-level factors is felt only indirectly, but year on year their influence is felt. We can address these issues only very briefly (Box 9.7), but should not neglect them altogether.

Box 9.6 Patient safety leadership in practice

(adapted from Institute for Healthcare Improvement 2004)

The leader's role is part strategic, part organizational and part cultural. First and foremost, leaders must: 'Provide focus, make patient safety not just another *program de jour* but a priority corporate objective. You must make everyone in the institution understand that safety is part of his or her job description.' This is more than a general pronouncement; executive leaders need to provide the human and financial resources to safety teams necessary for them to design and implement an integrated programme for identifying risks and reducing errors.

Along with the required technology and systems investment, an effective safety programme entails a leadership-driven cultural shift. 'You have to set the tone, provide a supportive, non-punitive environment for your staff. The goal is transparency – an atmosphere of open communication about safety concerns and incidents.' In more specific terms, this means leaders have to learn how to listen and start talking about safety concerns continually – with front-line staff and at the highest levels of the organization. 'If you're not hearing about errors, don't assume they're not happening.' He urges leaders to 'Go looking for trouble, probe your staff, ask people "What feels unsafe?" Your staff is incredibly worried about safety. You must provide opportunities for conversations.' At the other end of the spectrum, leaders must involve the board, trustees and executive committee in safety discussions. This can take a variety of forms: sharing adverse event reports, being included in root cause analysis meetings, hearing patient stories

Patients are very much at the centre of the safety mission. Conway speaks passionately about the rewards of forming partnerships with patients in the safety drive. 'Patients and their families can make unbelievable contributions,' he says. 'That errors happen and patients are at some risk when they come to your institution for treatment is no secret to them,' he adds, and the atmosphere of silence is outdated and counterproductive. Hearing their experiences is 'sobering but incredibly useful. Again and again I hear from patients and families that they want to find leaders in the hospital who will talk to them about safety. They want opportunities for conversations.'

Many of the most powerful drivers of patient safety lie outside healthcare organizations. Reports from government and professional organizations, social, legal and media pressure all contributed to the emergence of patient safety. Pressure for continued progress and reform is driven partly by clinical will and patient participation, but also externally by regulatory and other agencies. In the US, for instance, JCAHO sets specific safety targets and mandates certain safety-related activities, and many other countries have similar healthcare regulatory bodies. Box 9.7 gives some examples of JCAHO's hospital patient safety targets for 2005. Professional organizations run conferences, introduce safety-related training and the topics of risk management and safety into interviews for senior clinical posts. The UK is unusual, and fortunate, in having a national organization, the National Patient Safety Agency, that is dedicated to enhancing safety. The World Health Organization (WHO) has now passed resolutions on patient safety, which promise in due course to link the programmes WHO already has on such subjects as the safety of blood products, chemical safety and injection safety. The WHO programme will be given further impetus by the World Alliance on Patient Safety, proposed and led by Sir Liam Donaldson, UK Chief Medical Officer. Large organizations and major programmes of this kind often move slowly, but are vital to keeping the momentum of patient safety and, crucially, providing leadership, direction and political influence to ensure that the safety of healthcare remains a priority.

Box 9.7 JCAHO: examples of the 2005 hospitals' national patient safety goals

(from JCAHO 2005)

Goal: improve the accuracy of patient identification
- Use at least two patient identifiers (neither of which should be the patient's room number) whenever administering medications or blood products, taking blood samples and other specimens for clinical testing, or providing any other treatments or procedures.

Goal: improve the effectiveness of communication among caregivers
- For verbal or telephone orders, or for telephonic reporting of critical test results, verify the complete order or test result by having the person receiving the order or test result 'read back' the complete order or test result.
- Standardize a list of abbreviations, acronyms and symbols that are not to be used throughout the organization.

Goal: improve the safety of using medications
- Remove concentrated electrolytes (including, but not limited to, potassium chloride, potassium phosphate, sodium chloride > 0.9%) from patient-care units.
- Standardize and limit the number of drug concentrations available.
- Identify and, at a minimum, annually review a list of look-alike/sound-alike drugs and take action to prevent errors involving the interchange of these drugs.

Goal: improve the safety of using infusion pumps
- Ensure free-flow protection on all general-use and patient-controlled analgesia (PCA) intravenous infusion pumps used in the organization.

Goal: accurately and completely reconcile medications across the continuum of care
- Develop a process for obtaining and documenting a complete list of the patient's current medications when the patient is admitted to the organization; involve the patient in this. This process includes a comparison of the medications the organization provides to those on the list.
- A complete list of the patient's medications is communicated to the next provider of service when the patient is referred or transferred to another setting, service, practitioner or level of care within or outside the organization.

REFERENCES

Amalberti R 2001 The paradoxes of almost totally safe transportation systems. Safety Science 37:109–126

Bass B, Avolio B 1994 (eds) Improving organizational effectives through transformational leadership. Sage, New York

Berwick DM 1998 Taking action to improve safety: how to increase the odds of success. Rancho Mirage, California

Commission for Health Improvement 2000 Report following an investigation into physical and psychological abuse of elderly patients. HMSO, London

Cox S, Flin R 1998 Safety culture. Philosopher's stone or man of straw. Work and Stress 12:189–201

Department of Health 2000 (DoH) An organisation with a memory: learning from adverse events in the NHS. The Stationery Office, London

Flin R, Meams K, O'Connor P 2000 Measuring safety climate: identifying the common features. Safety Science 34:177–192

Flin R, Yule S 2004 Leadership for safety: industrial experience. Quality and Safety in Health Care 13:ii45–ii51

Harvey J, Erdos G, Bolam H et al 2002 An analysis of safety culture attitudes in a highly regulated environment. Work and Stress 16:18–36

Health and Safety Commission 1993 Organizing for safety, ACSNI Human Factors Study Group (report no. 3). HMSO, London

Helmreich RL, Merrit AC 1998 Culture at work in aviation and medicine: national, organisational and professional influences. Ashgate, Aldershot

Huczynski A, Buchanan D 1991 Organisational behaviour, 2nd edn. Prentice-Hall International, Hemel Hempstead, UK

Institute for Healthcare Improvement (IHI) 2004 Health care leaders leading: a Dana-Farber Cancer Institute executive describes the crucial role of leadership in driving patient safety. Online. Available at: http://www.ihi.org/IHI/Topics/PatientSafety/MedicationSystems/Literature/HealthCareLeadersLeadingADanaFarberCancerInstituteexecutivedescribesthecrucialroleofleadershipindriv.htm

Joint Commission on Accreditation of Healthcare Organizations (JCAHO) 2005 National patient safety goals. Online. Available at: http://www.jcaho.org/accredited+organizations/05_npsg_guidelines_2.pdf

La Porte TR 1996 High reliability organisations: unlikely, demanding and at risk. Journal of Contingencies and Crisis Management 4:60–71

La Porte TR, Consolini PM 1991 Working in practice but not in theory: theoretical challenges of high reliability organisations. Journal of Public Administration Research & Theory 1:1–21

Leape LL, Woods D, Hatlie M et al 1998. Promoting patient safety by preventing medical error. Journal of the American Medical Association 280: 1444–1447

National Patient Safety Agency (NPSA) 2004a Incident decision tree. Online. Available at: http://www.npsa.nhs.uk

National Patient Safety Agency (NPSA) 2004b Delivering safer health care. Online. Available at: http://www.npsa.nhs.uk

Nieva VF, Sorra J 2003 Safety culture assessment: a tool for improving patient safety in healthcare organizations. Quality and Safety in Health Care 12:ii17–ii23

Peters TJ, Waterman RM 1982 In search of excellence. Harper and Row, New York

Pronovost P, Weast B, Holzmueller CG et al 2003 Evaluation of the culture of safety: a survey of clinicians and managers in an academic medical center. Quality and Safety in Health Care 12:405–410

Reason JT 1997 Managing the risks of organisational accidents. Ashgate, Aldershot

Roberts KM 1990 Some characteristics of high reliability organisations. Organisation Science 1:160–177

Schein B 1985 Organization culture and leadership. Jossey Bass, San Francisco

Singer SJ, Gaba DM, Geppert JJ et al 2003 The culture of safety: results of an organization-wide survey in 15 California hospitals. Quality and Safety in Health Care 12:112–118

Waller MJ, Roberts KH 2003 High reliability and organizational behavior: finally the twain must meet. Journal of Organizational Behavior 24:813–814

Weick K, Sutcliffe K 2001 Managing the unexpected. Assuring high performance in an age of complexity. Jossey Bass, San Francisco

Westrum R 1997 Social factors in safety-critical systems. In: Redmill R, Rajan J (eds) Human factors in safety critical systems. Butterworth-Heinemann, Oxford

9

Culture and leadership for safety

Making healthcare safer: clinical interventions and process improvement

10

'How do you get good enough to go to the moon'? Guy Cohen had no one-liners to offer me. He didn't say 'report cards' or 'market forces' or 'incentive pay' or even 'accountability.' In fact, as I recall, not one of those words came up in the time we spent together. His view of human nature, organisations, systems, and change would not permit one-line answers.
(Berwick 1998 p 1)

Guy Cohen was Director of Quality, Safety and Reliability at NASA until the mid-1990s. Don Berwick, then working on improving the quality of healthcare in the Harvard Community System, had asked how to improve healthcare faster and more effectively; in one 5-hour meeting Cohen had barely started telling him what he had learned about quality and safety (Berwick 1998).

In healthcare, we are just beginning to understand how difficult the safety problem is, in cultural, technical, clinical, and psychological terms, not to mention its massive scale and heterogeneity. We have seen, in the analysis of individual incidents, just how many factors can contribute to the occurrence of an error or bad outcome. Yet still, at safety conferences, you will hear people saying 'it's the culture', 'the key is strong leadership', 'team building is the answer', 'if we just had good professional standards all would be well', 'we know we've got a problem, lets just get on and fix it' and so on. Of course, all these things are important, and there are some things that can and should be 'just fixed', but one of the greatest obstacles to progress on patient safety is, paradoxically, the attraction of neat solutions, whether political, organizational or clinical. First, we must understand what a complex problem this is; only then will we be able to tackle all aspects of it effectively.

Healthcare is an extremely diverse enterprise and the causes of harm, and the associated solutions, will differ according to the process under consideration. Some factors, such as leadership, culture and attitudes to safety, are generic and important in all environments. However, the kinds of specific solutions required to ensure high reliability in, for instance, blood transfusion services, will obviously differ from those aimed at reducing in-patient suicides in mental health. Improving safety is therefore likely to require some generic, cross-organizational action, coupled with some specialty- and process-specific activities. The way in which the specific and generic might combine (or interfere) has not yet been established and many of these interventions are underpinned by radically different philosophies of clinical work and safety.

At the clinical level, safety can be elusive, for all the specialist knowledge and experience available. There are multiple possibilities and lines of attack. Should we rely on team building, vigilance and awareness of hazards? Should we attack the numerous process problems, inefficiencies and frustrations that beset clinical staff, sapping their morale and precipitating error and patient harm? Perhaps, as in so many other industries, technology is the answer – getting the human being out of the loop? Or perhaps patient harm is best prevented by clinical innovations, for instance the development of new drugs and procedures to counteract the hazards of hospital acquired infection? All of these approaches are likely to be useful but, as yet, we have little idea how much weight to give to any one of them in any specific circumstance. This chapter and Chapters 11 and 12 will examine examples of many different approaches, with the aim of showing their essential features, advantages and limitations. At least we will then have a menu of possibilities, which will steer us away from the quick fixes, and permit a more considered and ultimately more effective approach to safety. First it is useful to sketch out the territory and consider some of the underlying assumptions. We will outline some of the broader features of the different approaches and examine some of the implicit, often unspoken, assumptions underlying them.

MAKING HEALTHCARE SAFER: APPROACHES AND ASSUMPTIONS

A wealth of different techniques and approaches are available for the quest for safer healthcare, variously supported by theory, evidence and common sense, and it can be very difficult to discern underlying themes and directions. To begin with, the scope of safety interventions depends to some extent on how widely one defines patient safety. If one takes the reasonable view that the target is preventing any harm to patients from healthcare, then any therapy or technique that reduces complications of any kind falls within the remit. This was essentially the approach taken by the Agency for Healthcare Research and Quality (AHRQ) reviewers in their massive and comprehensive report on patient safety practices (Shojania et al 2001; discussed below), which highlighted many evidence-based practices that should, but often are not, used to make healthcare safer. For some people, however, this clinical approach does not quite capture the essence of patient safety. Patient safety, at its heart, is not so much about the development or evaluation of therapies (vital though that is) but about the failure of people and systems to use these therapies effectively and safely. Thus, although we will discuss the important AHRQ report, our focus in this and the following chapter will be more on the latter question. Here we can distinguish two broad approaches, which have links to the safety paradigms discussed in Chapter 5. These two visions of safety are seldom explicitly articulated, but are ever-present themes in debates and discussions about patient safety.

Two visions of safety

The term 'technology and standardization' summarizes one vision of safety, which is closely linked to the engineering safety paradigm discussed in

Chapter 5. In this view, human fallibility is to the fore and the aim is to improve basic clinical processes and reduce reliance on people or at least offer as much support as possible in those tasks for which people are necessary. Process improvement approaches are discussed in this chapter and the role of technology in Chapter 11. 'People create safety' encapsulates the second broad approach, discussed in Chapter 12. Woods and Cook (2002), following Rasmussen (1990) and others, have argued for an alternative to the rigid, proceduralized, technology-driven view of safety that more truly reflects the realities of clinical work. Underlying these two visions are two contrasting views of human ability and experience, the one stressing error and fallibility, the other stressing adaptability, foresight and resilience (Table 10.1). Adopting one or other of these positions, whether acknowledged or not, will determine the kind of practical steps taken to improve safety and so has important practical consequences. In practice, elements of both approaches might be needed to resolve particular problems, but distinguishing them is important because many discussions and debates about safety revolve around these two positions.

Technology and standardization

Many approaches to quality improvement in healthcare are rooted in a basic industrial model, in which the solutions to errors and defects rest in an increasing standardization usually coupled with a reliance on technology. Ideally, the human contribution to the process of care is reduced to a minimum as in industrial production or commercial aviation. Careful design of the basic processes of care and appropriate use of technology overcomes human fallibility, vulnerability to fatigue and environmental influences. Examples of safety measures within this broad framework would include: simplification and standardization of clinical processes, computerized medication systems, electronic medical records and memory and decision support, whether computerized or in the form of protocols, guidelines, checklists and *aides memoires*. Note that even systems that explicitly acknowledge human fallibility, such as decision support systems, still require human ingenuity and expertise to use them. For instance, although decision support systems assist clinicians by reminding them of actions to be taken and helping with complex decisions,

Table 10.1 Two visions of safety	
Replace or support human beings	**Practitioners create safety**
Emphasizes fallibility and irrationality	***Emphasizes expertise and skill***
Hindsight bias & memory failure	Flexibility and adaptability
Extreme overconfidence	Experience and wisdom
Vulnerable to environmental influences	Anticipation of hazards
Lack of control over thought and action	Recovery from error
Technical and procedural interventions	***New and enhanced skills***
Design and standardization	Culture of high reliability organizations
Protocols & guidelines	Mindfulness & hazard awareness
Information technology	Training in anticipation and recovery
Technical solutions	Teamwork and leadership

they can be useful only if the clinician has the expertise to extract relevant information from the patient, use the system appropriately and so on. You need expertise in order to use decision support effectively.

We also need to distinguish two broad types of standardization and proceduralization. The first relates to systems that attempt to improve on existing systems of communication, such as the electronic medical record. There is no doubt that an electronic record could have immense advantages in terms of access to information, reliability of coding, standardization of information recorded and linkage to other systems. However, from the clinician's viewpoint, such systems might introduce other problems, for instance problems of access when hardware fails, slowness of response, and other unanticipated problems. Nevertheless, most clinicians would agree that it is desirable to bring hospital information systems up to the standard of, for instance, the average supermarket chain.

A more important and contentious issue relates to the standardization of clinical practice itself, in the form of guidelines, protocols, decision support and structuring of tasks and procedures. Clinicians are sometime suspicious of these initiatives, suspecting that standardization is being imposed not to improve healthcare but to regulate, cut costs and otherwise constrain clinicians in their work. However, while accepting that these pressures exist, such approaches are potentially a support to the clinician in the sense that they make care more reliable and predictable and reduce the cognitive load on clinical staff – thus freeing them for more important clinical tasks that require human expertise.

People create safety

Proponents of the 'people create safety' view are, rightly, extremely impressed by how often outcomes are good in the face of extreme complexity, conflicting demands, hazards and uncertainty. Making healthcare safer depends, according to this view, not on minimizing the human contribution but on understanding technical work and how people overcome hazards. Cook et al (2000) remind us how reliant safety is on clinicians and others looking ahead, bridging gaps, managing conflicts and, in effect, creating safety. A good illustration of this approach is in their recommendation that researchers study 'gaps' – discontinuities in the process of care – which might be losses of information, losses of momentum or interruptions in the delivery of care. They suggest that safety will be increased by understanding and reinforcing practitioners' normal ability to bridge gaps.

Although clinicians' ability to anticipate, react and accommodate to changing circumstances is crucial to effective and safe healthcare, there is a danger in assuming that safer care will be achieved by greater reliance on these human qualities. The difficulty comes in devising solutions and safety enhancements. To begin with, this reliance on human expertise places an additional burden on those at the sharp end, returning us – oddly – to a reliance on training that systems thinking sought to free us from. True, it is training of a different kind (anticipation, flexibility) but training nevertheless. More importantly, it seems an odd response to gaps. Why should we not try to reduce the number of gaps in the first place, with more efficient systems and better design? This depends, of course, on the nature of the gaps and other problems that practitioners need to anticipate and address; there will undoubtedly always be gaps of some kind in any system. A sudden change in the patient's condition, a sudden emergency that places an additional burden on staff, require all the qualities that Woods and Cook (2002) rightly highlight. Anticipation is also used, however, to resolve organizational deficiencies, as when a surgeon has to improvise because notes are not available at the start of an operation, or telephones ahead to double-check that equipment is available. However, notes and equipment that reliably turned up would reduce, if not obviate, the need for such anticipation. The real problem is to find a way to marry the two approaches, standardizing and proceduralizing – where this is feasible and desirable, while knowing that this can never be a complete solution and simultaneously promoting human resilience and the 'creation of safety'. Before developing this theme however, we will discuss the clinical approach as exemplified in the AHRQ report.

CLINICAL PRACTICES TO IMPROVE SAFETY

The first Institute of Medicine Report on patient safety, *To err is human* (Kohn et al 1999), called on all parties in healthcare to make patient safety a priority. To this end the Institute recommended that the AHRQ determine which patient-safety practices were effective and produce a report to disseminate to all clinicians. The resulting report, written by Kaveh Shojania and colleagues at the Evidence-based Practice Center in San Francisco, with the assistance of numerous US experts, is a massive, wide-ranging compendium of patient-safety practices and an invaluable resource of clinical practices that reduce the complications of healthcare (Shojania et al 2001). The review followed, wherever possible, a standard approach to reviewing the literature on a specific topic, making a formal assessment of the strength of evidence available. For each safety practice, the authors of the relevant section were asked to examine:

- prevalence of the problem targeted by the practice
- severity of the problem targeted by the practice
- the current use of the practice
- evidence of efficacy and/or effectiveness of the practice
- the practice's potential for harm
- data on cost if available
- implementation issues.

Shojania and colleagues acknowledged that this approach, more usually applied to specific clinical interventions, was difficult to apply to generic safety interventions, such as information technology or human factors work. Many of these practices were drawn from areas outside medicine and often little researched in healthcare. Some generic practices, such as clinical decision support, were separated out and described as techniques for promoting and implementing safety practices. The final list of 79 selected practices was roughly

---

Box 10.1 Most highly rated patient safety practices from the AHRQ report

(adapted from Shojania et al 2001)

- Appropriate use of prophylaxis to prevent venous thromboembolism in patients at risk.
- Use of peri-operative beta-blockers in appropriate patients to prevent peri-operative morbidity and mortality.
- Use of maximum sterile barriers when placing central intravenous catheters to prevent infections.
- Appropriate use of antibiotic prophylaxis in surgical patients to prevent peri-operative infections.
- Asking that patients recall and restate what they have been told during the informed consent process.
- Continuous aspiration of subglottic secretions to prevent ventilator-associated pneumonia.
- Use of pressure-relieving bedding materials to prevent pressure ulcers.
- Use of real-time ultrasound guidance during central line insertion to prevent complications.
- Patient self-management for warfarin to achieve appropriate outpatient anticoagulation and prevent complications.
- Appropriate provision of nutrition, with a particular emphasis on early enteral nutrition in critically ill patients.
- Use of antibiotic-impregnated central venous catheters to prevent catheter-related infections.

---

grouped according to the strength of evidence for each one and promising areas were highlighted for future research. Eleven practices (Box 10.1) were singled out as having very strong evidence of efficacy. A further 14 had good evidence for efficacy; these included such practices as using hip protectors to prevent injury after falls, localizing surgery to high-volume centres, use of computer monitoring to prevent adverse drug reactions, improving information transfer at time of discharge, and multi-component programmes to tackle pain management and hospital-acquired delirium. In the summary, the authors emphasize that their report was a first attempt to organize and evaluate the relevant literature, which they hope will act as a catalyst for future work and will not be seen as the final word on the subject.

Preventing venous thromboembolism

As an example of a safety practice with good evidence, we will consider the important topic of preventing thromboembolism. Venous thromboembolism (VTE) refers to occlusion within the venous system, and includes deep vein thrombosis (DVT). VTE occurs frequently in hospital patients, with risk of VTE depending on multiple factors including age, medical condition, type of surgery and duration of immobilization. Without prophylaxis, DVT occurs after approximately 20% of all major surgical procedures and over 50% of orthopaedic procedures. Measures to prevent VTE can be pharmacological (heparin, warfarin, aspirin) or mechanical (elastic stockings, pneumatic compression). The authors of this section of the AHRQ report present extensive evidence for the efficacy, safety and cost-effectiveness of prophylaxis in a wide range of conditions and procedures. For instance, pooled results of

46 randomized trials have established that low-dose unfractionated heparin (LDUH) reduces the risk of DVT after general surgery from 25% to 8%. Prophylaxis is by no means always effective though; in a review of 384 patients with VTE at Brigham and Women's Hospital in the US, over half had received prophylactic treatment but still suffered an embolism.

VTE is frequent, painful, dangerous, wastes time and resources and is sometimes fatal; it is, in many cases, preventable. Despite this, prophylaxis is often under-used or used inappropriately. Surveys of both general and orthopaedic surgeons in the US, for instance, have found that over 10% never use VTE prophylaxis, with rates of prophylaxis varying widely for different procedures. The use of appropriate prophylactic measures is undoubtedly a valuable clinical practice. The mystery is why, when the evidence is so strong, is it so often not used or used inappropriately. The authors comment that the reasons for this under-use have not been completely elucidated and nor have we succeeded in finding out how to improve rates of prophylaxis, although various strategies have been tried in a small number of studies. Educational programmes promoting guidelines and computerized decision support, both separately and in combination, improved the use of prophylaxis, which the authors suggest reflects a lack of awareness and knowledge of prophylaxis measures amongst staff.

If staff are unaware of such a basic practice it is alarming, to say the least, but, as we have seen, the reasons for failure and error are many and various. From our point of view, the most important point at this stage is that an evaluation of a clinical practice has led to questions of a psychological nature and towards core patient safety issues of error and human behaviour. These themes emerge more strongly in the next section, which addresses some criticisms of the report's approach to patient safety,

EVIDENCE-BASED MEDICINE MEETS PATIENT SAFETY

Following the publication of the AHRQ report, Lucian Leape, Don Berwick and David Bates (2002) wrote a powerful critique in which they argued that the report had in various respects missed the point of patient safety. We will review their arguments, not to dismiss the undoubtedly useful report, but to highlight important issues about the nature of patient safety and the directions it should take in improving the safety of care.

In the first place, Leape and colleagues recalled that in the original Harvard study only about one-third of adverse events were not preventable with current practice. The remainder were due to error or more general problems in the process of care. The AHRQ report, they suggested, was targeting new therapies and techniques and to some extent side-stepping the thorny issues of error and poor quality care. The primary reason for this, they suggested, was not that the AHRQ authors were reluctant to tackle these issues but simply that they followed the evidence and concentrated on areas where there was a substantial body of research. The upshot of this was that the report was heavily weighted towards individual safety practices and therapies, and gave insufficient weight to the factors that determine what care patients actually receive. This is well expressed in the following section of the paper:

Achieving safer care has three agendas, all of which are necessary for success: identifying what works (efficacy), ensuring that the patient receives it (appropriate use) and delivering it flawlessly (no errors). The relationship amongst these factors is well illustrated by the practice given the no. 1 rating in the report: prophylactic anticoagulation for venous thromboembolism . . . Anticoagulation is efficacious. However the practical patient safety issues for practitioners are: (1) how to ensure that every patient who needs anticoagulation receives it and (2) how to ensure that the medication is delivered flawlessly – on time, in the right dose, every time, without fail. Such systems are at the heart of patient safety but not addressed by the report.
(Leape et al 2002 p 504)

Leape and colleagues went on to argue that many established safety practices (such as sponge counts after an operation) had been omitted simply because they are well established and, more importantly, that many promising avenues, such as systems for reducing medication errors, had not been given sufficient attention. They further questioned whether the standard evidence-based approach was necessary where practices had obvious face validity or where sufficient evidence had accumulated in other environments (such as the impact of fatigue on performance and judgement).

Why were Leape and colleagues so concerned about the direction taken by this report? Essentially, it seems, because it might set a direction for patient safety that they regarded as misconceived. Even though the report does give some attention to human factors and systems issues, the weight given to specific clinical practices might suggest that the problems of patient safety could be effectively addressed with new therapies and careful evaluation. In fact, most patient safety practitioners are much more concerned about the fragmented, chaotic state of most healthcare systems and the frankly abysmal safety record in many areas. Resolving this requires a tenacious attempt to improve the basic processes and systems of healthcare, as well as engaging all who work in healthcare in the endeavour. The remainder of this book addresses the various ways in which this colossal task is being attacked, beginning with the key issues of simplification and standardization.

SIMPLIFYING AND STANDARDIZING THE PROCESSES OF HEALTHCARE

Manufacturing industries have made huge gains in safety, efficiency and cost-effectiveness by close attention to the design, maintenance and performance of the processes used in factories. Much of the impetus for these improvements stemmed from W. Edwards Deming's system of profound knowledge, a name of which is more suggestive of esoteric spiritual practices than the science of quality improvement. Deming's intention, however, and the approach he describes, is resolutely practical. Deming, Joseph Juran, Kauro Ishigawa and others have described and documented the successful application of these approaches since the 1950s in Japanese and American industries (Langley et al 1996).

Healthcare, in comparison, has little standardization, comparatively little monitoring of processes and outcome, and few safeguards against error and other quality problems (Bates 2000). Most healthcare processes were not designed, but just evolved and adapted to circumstances. The process of prescribing, ordering and giving drugs is a good example of this; successful for the most part but error prone and not designed for reliable operation. David Bates gives an example of the problems that he observed in his own hospital before a sustained attack on medication error and adverse drug reactions:

> Take for example the allergy detection process used in our hospital several years ago, which was similar to that used in most hospitals at the time. Physicians, medical students and nurses all asked patients what their allergies were. This information was recorded at several sites in the medical record, though there was no one central location. The information was also required to be written at the top of every order sheet, although in practice this was rarely done. The pharmacy recorded the information in its computerised database, but it found out about allergies only if the information was entered into the orders, and often it was not. Checking by physicians, pharmacy and nursing staff was all manual. This information was not retained between the inpatient and outpatient settings, or from admission to admission. Not surprisingly, about one in three orders for drugs to which a patient had a known allergy slipped through.
> **(Bates 2000 p 788–789)**

Reading this description it is hard to understand why, even before technological advances, this system had been allowed to continue for so many years. Multiple sites of information; numerous, possibly conflicting sources of information; excessive reliance on human vigilance and memory; excessive complexity and potential for error at every stage – if you had been trying to design a system to produce errors you could hardly have done better. When you work in such a system, and we all do in one way or another, it is hard to step back and see the whole process and understand its flaws. Furthermore, in healthcare, very often no one person has responsibility or oversight of the whole system, which makes both monitoring and improvement very difficult.

The system Bates describes has now been replaced by one in which all allergies are noted in one place in the information system, drugs are mapped to 'drug families' (for example penicillin) so that they can be checked more easily, information is retained over time and checking for allergies is routinely performed by computers, rather than tired and fallible human beings. Many healthcare systems, however, have not benefited from such an overhaul. Ordering and reading of X-rays, communication of risk information about suicidal or homicidal patients, informing patients and their family doctors about abnormal test results, booking patients in for emergency operations, effective discharge planning; all these and many more are vital for safe healthcare, yet day-to-day experience tells patients and staff that they are far from error free.

A particular problem is that many healthcare processes are both long and complicated. Simply mapping the process that currently exist can be a major task, and performing a failure, modes and effects analysis on that process can be immensely time consuming, as we have seen. As Don Berwick points out, complex systems break down more often than simple ones because there is more opportunity:

> The statistics are quite simple. Imagine a system with, say, 25 elements each of which functions properly – no errors – 99% of the time. If the errors in each element occur independently of each other, then the probability that the entire system of 25 elements will function correctly is $(0.99)^{25}$ or about 0.78. With 50 elements, it is 0.61; with 100 elements, it is 0.37. Make the reliability of each element higher, say 0.999, and the overall success rates are 0.98 for 25 elements, 0.95 for 50 elements and 0.90 for 100 elements. We can, indeed, improve the reliability of a system by perfecting its parts and handoffs, but reducing complexity is even more powerful. **(Berwick 1998 p 4)**

Designing and building simpler, standardized processes that rely less on human vigilance is therefore a powerful way of making at least some parts of healthcare much safer, as well as cheaper and more efficient. How is this to be done? The Institute for Healthcare Improvement (IHI), which Don Berwick leads, has pioneered quality improvement in healthcare, drawing together ideas and practical experience from healthcare and many other sources. We will use its approach to reducing medication error as an overall framework to illustrate the potential of process improvement, addressing the particular role of technology in a later section.

REDUCING MEDICATION ERROR

The IHI has led a number of collaborative projects to bring about rapid reduction in medication errors, drawing on the work of Lucian Leape, David Bates and many others and, importantly, also drawing heavily on the knowledge and expertise of people within the institutions taking part. These are genuine collaborative projects, not simply consultants coming in to advise or, at worst, 'asking to see your watch and then telling you the time'.

There are three basic elements to improving the safety of a medication process:

- design the system to prevent errors occurring in the first place
- design the system to make errors more visible when they do occur
- design the system to limit the effects of errors so that they do not lead to harm.

Preventing errors is, broadly speaking, achieved by reducing the complexity of information that healthcare staff need, reducing the opportunity for mixing up different medications and trying to limit errors that occur because staff are trying to do too many things at once (Table 10.2). Errors can be made more visible by using a variety of additional checks, both by people (staff and patients) and by computers. For instance, having a pharmacist reviewing orders before dispensing, asking staff to repeat-back verbal orders and careful use of laboratory monitoring systems are all means of detecting errors that might have occurred.

Table 10.2 Principles for reducing medication error (adapted from Berwick 1998)

Principle	Action
Reducing errors due to information complexity	Provide an information system that allows access to patient information for all staff and allows electronic prescribing
	Limit hospital formularies to essential drugs and doses
	Pharmacists on ward rounds to monitor and advise
	Briefing at handover and shift change on circumstances that increase risk of error, such as an unfamiliar disease, new staff or unusual drug regimens
Reducing errors due to complex or dangerous medication	Remove high-risk medications, such as concentrated electrolyte solutions, from patient-care areas
	Label high-risk drugs clearly to indicate their danger
	Remove or clearly differentiate look-alike or sound-alike drugs
Reducing errors due to multiple competing tasks	Wherever possible, reallocate tasks such as calculating, drawing up and mixing doses to pharmacy or the manufacturer
	Establish standard drug administration times and avoid interruptions at those times
	Assign one person who does not have other duties at that time to perform the necessary double-checks; use double-checks sparingly and make them properly independent
	Standardize equipment and supplies, such as intravenous pumps, across all units
	Involve patients in active checks such as identifying themselves, checking drugs and allergies

Even with all these checks and system improvements, errors will sometimes occur, if only because of the enormous numbers of drugs given. The final protection is to always be ready to mitigate the effects of any error, to assume in fact that errors will occur and to prepare for it. Anticipating error is a sign of a safe, rather than unsafe, system. In this case, keeping antidotes for high-risk drugs on hand at the point of administration is a key defence against harm to patients; staff also need to train and rehearse treatment of serious adverse reactions, such as anaphylaxis. Rehearsal of such routines is especially important if such reactions seldom occur, because that is when such skills are lost.

These, then, are the general principles derived in years of experimentation, evaluation and practical application with many organizations. Let us see how this works in practice.

Reducing medication errors and adverse drug events at St Joseph's Medical Centre

St Joseph's medical centre is a 165-bed hospital in the heart of Illinois, providing a variety of services including open-heart surgery and trauma care. The hospital has established a number of safety projects backed by a strong commitment to cultural change and backing from senior executives (Haig et al 2004).

In June 2001, a survey of records suggested an ADE (adverse drug event) rate of 5.8 per 1000. Flowcharting of the medication process proved it to be complicated, labour intensive and involving multiple members of staff from the time the order was written to the point when the patient received the medication. Common sources of errors included unavailable patient information, unavailable drug information, miscommunication of medication orders, problems with labelling or packaging, drug standardization, storage, stocking and process flaws. By May 2003, ADEs were running at 0.50 per 1000, a tenfold reduction, and the process of medication delivery had been hugely simplified and standardized. How was this achieved?

A broader commitment to safety, open reporting and discussion of errors provided the foundations for the programme. Some very specific process improvements were the key to solid change, however, as summarized in Box 10.2. One of the most important was the introduction of a medication reconciliation process. Medication reconciliation is the process of comparing the medications the patient has been taking with the medications currently ordered. This allows the staff member to identify medications that might need to be continued/discontinued, adjust frequency or dose as necessary and also check for errors that occurred during the patient's journey through the system. A common problem, for instance, is that when patients are discharged from hospital they do not return to the medication appropriate to their life at home. Medication reconciliation tackles this and related problems in three phases: on admission the home medications are compared to initial clinician's orders; on transfer between units, the medications on the previous unit are compared with those on the current unit; on discharge, hospital medication is compared with clinician orders for discharge medication and, if necessary, prescriptions from the general practitioner or family doctor. Any variances are then 'reconciled' by the nurse and pharmacist. In this thoughtful strategy, we can see first, a mapping of the steps in the patient journey when errors might occur, second, the assumption that errors can and will occur, and third,

---

Box 10.2 Reducing medication errors in St Joseph Medical Centre

(adapted from Haig et al 2004)

- Added an adverse drug event hotline leading to a 10-fold increase in reporting of adverse drug events and medication errors.
- Monthly reporting of medication data to hospital quality council.
- Implemented use of a single heparin/enoxaparin nomogram.
- Developed pre-printed heparin/enoxparin orders based on the nomogram.
- Developed a single form that could be used for reconciliation of medications at both admission and discharge.
- Separated sound-alike and look-alike medications in the pharmacy and on the nursing units.
- Implemented daily rounds by a clinical pharmacist who compares medication orders to laboratory values.
- Standardized intravenous drip concentrations.
- Decreased the amount of stock medications kept on patient care units.
- Eliminated the use of high-risk abbreviations.
- Changed process for non-standard doses so that all are prepared and packaged in pharmacy.
- Standardized epidural pumps and use yellow coloured tubing with these pumps.

a structured, standard process of checking to identify errors and problems and prevent actual patient harm.

Standardization of processes was a major feature of this programme, with particular attention paid to high-risk medications. For instance, all adult intravenous medications were standardized and a single, weight-based, heparin nomogram was developed and used throughout the hospital. A particularly popular intervention was increasing the availability of pharmacists on nursing units to review and enter medication orders. This had the double benefit of saving nurse time, although at the cost of increased pharmacist time, and giving the pharmacist the opportunity to inspect drug orders to identify potential dosage errors, drug interactions and so on. Finally, the patients themselves were engaged in the process. Each patient admitted to the hospital is given a Medication Safety Brochure that provides advice for them and a form on which to list their current medication. The patients then carry the form with them to allow any clinician to check current medication. Patients are also actively encouraged to check with staff if they have been given unfamiliar medication. Technological innovations, in the form of automated medication dispensing machines, formed the next phase of the drive to further reduce errors.

Whereas medication errors and medication processes have received most attention, achievements have not been confined to medication safety. Boxes 10.3 and 10.4 show examples of similarly sustained and radical change in the

---

Box 10.3 Reducing errors made by emergency physicians in interpreting radiographs

(adapted from Espinosa & Nolan 2000)

When Espinosa and Nolan began their initial improvement efforts, the average rate of clinically significant errors was 3%, consistent with findings from a number of studies. Long delays in processing films were common. At this time, four separate radiology systems were in place, with the process and responsibility for interpreting varying with time of day and between weekdays and weekends. Initial improvement efforts left the basic system untouched but brought a much stronger focus on reducing error. All staff reviewed clinically significant discrepancies at monthly meetings; a file of clinically significant errors was kept and used for training; study of this file was made mandatory for all new staff; patterns of errors for each physician and for the department as a whole were routinely reviewed and discussed. Over the subsequent 2 years the error rate fell to 1.2% (Fig. 10.1), essentially by a sustained focus on training, attention to error and collaborative work by the team.

To further reduce delays and errors, a more fundamental redesign of the process was carried out by an interdisciplinary team. A system was developed for interpreting radiographs that would be followed regardless of the day of the week or time of day. All standard radiographs were brought directly to the emergency physician for immediate interpretation; a radiologist provided a further interpretation within 12 hours as a quality check, with rapid recall of patients if necessary. The primary responsibility was clearly assigned to the emergency physician, reducing the confusion and ambiguously defined responsibilities of the previous system. A new form was designed to provide feedback to the physicians about significant discrepancies, which was sent direct to the emergency physician concerned, embedding feedback and training into the day-to-day running of the department. These further changes reduced the error rate to below 0.5%. In commenting on their success, the authors stress the importance of cooperation between professional groups and the systemic nature of the intervention, relying both on individual and team effort and process improvement.

Continued

Box 10.3 Reducing errors made by emergency physicians in interpreting radiographs—cont'd

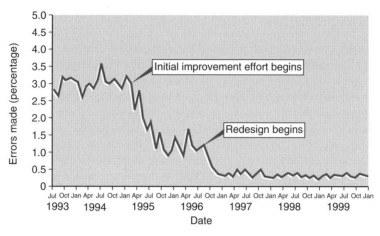

Fig. 10.1 Reduction in radiographic errors (from Espinosa & Nolan 2000 British Medical Journal 320:737–740, amended and reproduced with permission from the BMJ Publishing Group).

Box 10.4 Reduction in errors in laboratory test reports using quality improvement techniques

(adapted from Banning et al 1993)

The department of Clinical Chemistry, Westmead Hospital, operates 24 hours a day and processes 175,000 specimens a year. It issues the same number of final pathology test reports and many interim pathology reports. At the time the study began, all pathology requests were transcribed manually and entered into the computerized information system from handwritten request forms; all test reports were printed in the department and despatched by internal mail, courier or post. The biggest problem, causing much delay and additional work, was wrongly or inadequately addressed test reports. In the initial assessment the prevalence was 1.3% (average 44 per week) sometimes rising to 3.5% or 118 reports per week, delaying diagnoses and treatment for large number of patients each year. Previous repeated attempts to address this problem with memos, directives and massed mailings had utterly failed, with the base error rate being seen as a 'fact of life'.

The team used a combination of standard quality improvement techniques allied with failure modes and effects analysis to examine the main causes of the problem. The unsatisfactory nature of the current process was brought starkly to light by an attempt to map it on a flow chart. The process was so complicated, extending to multiple avenues and side branches, that the team abandoned the attempt to even describe it in favour of completely redesigning it. In addition to simplifying the basis process, three specific solutions were imposed: revision of the computer system to ensure it recognized valid addresses; graphical feedback to staff on the daily error rate; training for staff on correct location of barcode labels (so addresses are not obscured), handwriting recognition and basic procedures. These measures brought the error rate to 0.08% within 6 months, a 17 fold reduction in error, combined with an overall reduction in the time taken to process reports.

interpretation of radiographs and laboratory processes. As so often, healthcare processes had evolved and adapted over time, rather than being designed to produce a certain standard of care. Looking at the examples quoted so far in this chapter, common themes emerge: data collection, defining the process, identifying weak points, simplification, standardization. We might also note that all these improvements took time, commitment and patience. An important lesson that healthcare needs to learn is that safety and quality require a much bigger investment of time and resources than it has been given so far. Producing major changes to systems might start with a few enthusiasts fitting in meetings around their other work, but sustained safety and quality requires committed staff with dedicated time and resources.

REFERENCES

Banning J, Brown J, Hooper L 1993 Reduction of errors in laboratory test reports using continuous quality improvement techniques. Clinical Laboratory Management Review 7:424–436

Bates DW 2000 Using information technology to reduce rates of medication errors in hospitals. British Medical Journal 320:788–791

Berwick DM 1998 Taking action to improve safety: how to increase the odds of success. Rancho Mirage, California

Cook RI, Render M, Woods DD 2000 Gaps in the continuity of care and progress on patient safety. British Medical Journal 320:791–794

Espinosa JA, Nolan TW 2000 Reducing errors made by emergency physicians in interpreting radiographs: longitudinal study. British Medical Journal 320:737–740

Haig K, Wills L, Pedersen P et al 2004 Improvement report: reducing ADEs per 1,000 doses. Online. Available at: http://www.ihi.org/IHI/Topics/PatientSafety/MedicationSystems/ImprovementStories/ImprovementReportReducing ADEsper1000Doses.htm

Kohn L, Corrigan J, Donaldson ME 1999 To err is human. National Academy Press, Washington, DC

Langley GJ, Nolan KM, Nolan TW et al 1996 The improvement guide: a practical approach to enhancing organizational performance. Jossey Bass, San Francisco

Leape LL, Berwick DM, Bates DW 2002 What practices will most improve safety? Evidence-based medicine meets patient safety. Journal of the American Medical Association 288:501–507

Rasmussen J 1990 The role of error in organising behaviour. Ergonomics 33:1185–1199

Shojania KG, Duncan BW, McDonald KM 2001 Making health care safer: a critical analysis of patient safety practices. Evidence Report/Technology Assessment No. 43:2001. Agency for Healthcare Research and Quality (AHRQ), Rockville, MD. Online. Available at: http://www.ahcpr.gov/qual

Woods DD, Cook RI 2002 Nine steps to move forward from error. Cognition Technology and Work 4:137–144

Using information technology to reduce error

Everyone complains about their memory, but no one complains about their judgement.
(Francois, Duc de la RocheFoucauld, *Maximes* 1666)

Memory is also knowledge in the world.
(Norman 1988 p 72)

Modern healthcare is hugely reliant on technology. Most technology is aimed primarily at improving existing practice or developing new diagnostic techniques or treatments. For instance, the advent of PET, CAT, MRI and fMRI scanners allows unprecedented diagnostic access in ways that were unthinkable 20 years ago. Some technologies, particularly information technology, are directly targeted at the reduction of error and the improvement of safety. Of course, the principal motivation for their introduction might be cost control and greater efficiency, but safety is an increasingly important driver.

The use of information technology is inevitably accompanied by some degree of standardization and reduction in the variability of provision provided by human beings. Such standardization, when in the form of guidelines and protocols, can be criticized as being overly prescriptive and not taking a patient's particular circumstance and constellation of symptoms into account. However, when provided with the appropriate information, computers can completely tailor their guidance or information provided to the individual patient. In other, less complex industries such as computer manufacturing, this is referred to as 'mass customization', the efficient and reliable customization of a product to fit the specification of the individual consumer. Thus technology potentially provides a marriage between the need for standardization with the clinician's necessary insistence that treatment is tailored to the individual patient.

Bates and Gawande (2003) identify a number of ways in which information technology can reduce error: improving communication, making knowledge more readily accessible, prompting for key pieces of information (such as the dose of a drug), assisting with calculations, monitoring and checking in real time, and providing decision support. We will examine the role of information technology in medication safety and then consider some other specific examples. Be aware, however, that this is a very limited discussion of an enormous topic. Before we turn to the information technology and its potential for enhancing safety, it is worth reminding ourselves why we need it with a brief discussion of the respective strengths and fallibilities of computers and human beings.

MACHINES AND PEOPLE

The sheer quantity of medical information, even within a single specialty, is often beyond the power of one person to comprehend. People, that is the human brain, simply cannot cope with the amount of information that they need to function safely and effectively. For instance, more than 600 drugs require adjustment of doses for multiple levels of renal dysfunction; an easy task for a computer but one that will inevitably be performed poorly by a person (Bates & Gawande 2003). Machines can therefore act as a kind of extended memory, which we can access at will, to overcome the transience and limitations of human memory storage. However, these are not the only problems of memory; other limiting factors are not always appreciated.

The fallibility of memory

In his review of memory's strengths and imperfections, Daniel Schachter (1999) identified 'seven sins' of memory, each of which has application and relevance to clinical work. The first three involve different types of forgetting– essentially sins of omission: (i) transience, meaning that information fades over time, or is at least less accessible; (ii) absent-mindedness, meaning inattention and consequent weak memory traces; and (iii) blocking, temporary inaccessibility of memories, the so called tip of the tongue phenomenon. The next three involve distortion or inaccuracy – essentially sins of commission: (iv) misattribution involves attributing a recollection or idea to the wrong source, such as thinking that a particular scene from one film came from another with a similar theme; (v) suggestibility refers to memories that are implanted as a result of leading questions or comments during attempts to recall past experience; studies of eye witness testimony have shown that we easily, and unknowingly, adjust our memories to accord with new information provided by other people and become convinced that our new 'memories' are veridical; (vi) bias involves retrospective distortions and unconscious inferences that are related to current knowledge and beliefs; in effect we adjust our memory of, for instance a relationship, to accord with our current experience, whether good or bad. Finally, the seventh sin – persistence – refers to pathological memories: information or events we wish we could forget but cannot however hard we try.

Our memory then, while generally highly effective and efficient in daily life, can lead us astray in a number of ways. Examples of how each of these seven sins might affect clinical work are shown in Box 11.1 and a real example of an instance in which relying on memory led to disaster is shown in Box 11.2.

There are, of course, multiple lessons to be taken from this story of wrong site surgery, particularly about the communication between junior and senior staff; the fallibility of memory however is a core theme. Relying on

---

Box 11.1 Seven sins of memory

Transience
Forgetting your patient has poor renal function.

Absentmindedness
Reading and remembering 5000 when the label says 500.

Blocking
Being unable to recall the dosage even though you have given the drug many times.

Misattribution
Clearly remembering details of a medical history that in fact apply to a different patient.

Suggestibility
Unintentionally convincing your patient that they certainly did have an angiogram (even though they did not).

Bias
Remembering, incorrectly, that a cancer patient showed early signs of the disease consistent with your current diagnosis.

Persistence
The distressing memory of your worst mistake that comes back to you at unexpected moments.

Box 11.2 Hemivulvectomy for vulvar cancer: the wrong side removed

(adapted from Vincent 2003)

A 33-year-old female with microinvasive vulvar carcinoma was admitted to a teaching hospital for a unilateral hemivulvectomy. After the patient was intubated for general anaesthesia, the trainee reviewed her chart and noted that the positive biopsy was from the left side. As the trainee prepared to make an incision on the left side of the vulva the attending surgeon stopped him and redirected him to the right side. The trainee informed the attending surgeon that he had just reviewed the chart and learned that the positive biopsy had come from the left. The attending physician informed the trainee that he himself performed the biopsies and recalled that they were taken from the right side. The trainee complied and performed a right hemivulvectomy.

The next day the Chief of Pathology called the trainee to inquire about the case. The specimen he received was labelled 'right hemivulvectomy' and did not reveal any evidence of cancer. The preoperative biopsies the pathologist had reviewed had been positive but they were labelled 'left vulvar biopsy'. He wondered if there had been a labelling error.

The trainee informed the pathologist that the right side had been removed, and then informed the surgeon about the alleged error. The attending surgeon denied that any error had been made; he insisted that the original biopsies had been mislabelled. The surgeon did not inform the patient of the error. When the patient returned for routine follow-up the surgeon performed a vulvar colposcopy and biopsied the left side. Microinvasive cancer was noted in the biopsies. Shortly thereafter, the patient underwent a second hemivulvectomy to treat her vulvar cancer.

---

remembering that the biopsy was taken from the right side, in the face of evidence from the medical record that it came from the left is, to put it charitably, not entirely sensible. However, Schachter points out that we should not necessarily conclude that memory is hopelessly flawed. Most of the features that make us fallible in some circumstances are also adaptive. Forgetting unnecessary information, such as where you parked your car the day before yesterday, is highly adaptive. Jorge Luis Borges story, *Funes the memorious*, imagines a man who forgets nothing; Funes is paralysed by reminiscence. Real-life examples exist of mnemonists with perfect recall who are unable to function at an abstract level through being inundated with detail. A perfect memory in a computer is marvellous; in a person it could be a liability.

Judgement and decision making

The fallibility of memory is an everyday experience, which is generally not too embarrassing to admit. Using devices to compensate, whether a shopping list, a diary or a computer, comes easily to us. Our judgements and decisions, however, are more precious to our self-esteem and there is much more resistance to allowing guidelines and protocols, whether on paper or instantiated in software, to take over human decisions. In other spheres, such as navigation, judgement has given way to measurement and calculation and now to computation. My grandfather, flying in the First World War, navigated by compass and flying along railway lines, dipping down to inspect the countryside from time to time. My father, flying a Catalina flying boat in the Second World War, made careful calculations of direction, wind speed and compass bearing, taking into account the discrepancy of true and magnetic north and the error introduced in the compass reading by the metal hull of the airplane. Today, an onboard computer just sorts it all out.

Research on judgement (weighing the options) and decision making (choosing between the options) has yielded different perspectives on human abilities. On the one hand, the naturalistic decision-making school, most powerfully and persuasively represented by Gary Klein (1998), has shown how experts can rapidly assess a dangerous situation and, far from analysing and choosing, seem to just 'know' what to do. A firefighter can just see that the fire is in the basement and the building above is about to collapse; a physician takes one look at a patient and sees that he or she is dangerously hypoglycaemic. Klein describes this as 'recognition primed decision making' – rapid, adaptive and effective. This is the classic image of the expert physician who assesses a complex set of symptoms and immediately perceives the correct diagnosis. It is difficult, but not impossible, to imagine replacing this kind of intuitive brilliance with the stolid, systematic approach of a computer. In principle at least this thought process could be handled by a machine; in practice the time spent entering the relevant data might be the most limiting factor.

Consider, however, some other common medical scenarios, such as assessing the risk of suicide. A psychiatrist must consider past history, diagnosis, previous attempts at self-harm, declared intention and family support available, then weigh all these factors and decide whether the patient can return to the community. Or, consider a paediatric cardiac surgeon weighing up the risks of operating on a young baby: anatomy of the heart, pulmonary artery pressure, findings from the echocardiogram and a host of other features will be considered to assess the likely short- and long-term outcomes for the child of operating now, operating in 6 months or not operating at all. Both of these decisions involve complex calculations, weighing of different factors and combining them to produce a judgement between two or more choices. People must assemble the information, but would a machine or an algorithm make a better decision? In fact, numerous studies have shown that we vastly overestimate our power to make such judgements and that we also overestimate the number of factors that we take into account. Using statistical methods and models is nearly always superior to using unaided human judgement (Box 11.3) (Hastie & Dawes 2001). This phenomenon – of the superiority of statistical over clinical and other expert judgement – was first documented by Paul Meehl in 1954, and he has seen no reason to revise his opinion as the number of studies has increased. The most recent update of his findings Meehl (Grove & Meehl 1996) concluded that empirical comparisons show that the mechanical (statistical, whether computer or calculated) method is almost invariably equal or superior to the clinical method (global expert judgement).

The field of judgement and decision making is vast and the issue of human ability and fallibility much debated. My intention is simply to show that, in some instances at least, there is good reason for thinking that the computational aspects of some medical decisions might be more consistently and accurately carried out by a computer than by a person, however expert. Decision support therefore might, if used appropriately, have a major impact on patient safety.

We do not yet have a good understanding, in healthcare at least, of how to marry human abilities with the reliability and dependability of machines. As David Bates and colleagues (2001) point out, human beings are erratic and err in unexpected ways, yet we are also resourceful and inventive and can recover from errors and crises. In comparison, machines, at least most of those currently in use, are dependable but also dependably stupid. An almost perfect instruction, quite good enough for any human operator, can completely disable a machine. With increasing computational power we can envisage that machines will become increasingly adaptable and flexible, but human beings will always be important because of our capacity to respond to an 'unknown unknown', that is an event that could not have been predicted (Bates et al 2001).

Box 11.3 Clinical and statistical prediction

(adapted from Hastie & Dawes 2001)

Thirty experienced psychologists and psychiatrists predicted the dangerousness of 40 newly admitted psychiatric patients. The experts were provided with 19 cues, mostly derived from the judgements of psychiatrists who interviewed the patients on admission. The human judges predicted the likelihood of violent assault on another person in the first week of hospitalization with an accuracy of 0.12; the most accurate human judge scored 0.36. By contrast, a linear statistical model achieved an accuracy of 0.82 with the same data.

A world expert on Hodgkin's disease and two assistants rated nine characteristics of biopsies taken from patients and assessed `overall severity' as a predictor of longevity. In fact, judgements of severity by human beings were associated with patients living slightly longer; the judgement trend was in the wrong direction. By contrast, a multiple regression model based on the same nine characteristics showed a clear, although not strong, reliable association with longevity.

One of the key problems for the future then will be to assess which aspects of the clinical process will be more effectively carried out by machine. At the moment it seems safe to say that computers, memory and decision aids of all kinds are grossly underused and there is excessive reliance on human memory and other fallible processes. The boundaries of the human–machine interface will change over time as we develop more powerful and sophisticated systems and, equally important, accept that clinical expertise, essential though it is, does not necessarily bring reliability and consistency to routine operations. In some areas, however, there have been considerable advances; the best developed is the use of computerized systems in the process of medication administration.

USING INFORMATION TECHNOLOGY TO REDUCE MEDICATION ERRORS

Medication errors arise from a variety of causes. Almost half result, in some degree, from clinicians lacking information about the patient or the drug. This might be simply because they do not know the information themselves, because test results are not available or because other patient- or drug-specific information is not available. Other common problems are that handwritten orders are illegible, do not contain all necessary information, are transcribed incorrectly or contain errors of calculation (Bates 2000). Several medication technology systems have been addressing these and other problems, operating at various stages of the medication and delivery process (Fig. 11.1). They show great promise but, as David Bates warns, are not a panacea:

> Information technologies . . . may make some things better and others worse; the net effect is not entirely predictable, and it is vital to study the impact of these technologies. They have their greatest impact in organizing and making available information, in identifying links between pieces of information, and in doing boring repetitive tasks, including checks for problems. The best medication processes will thus not replace people but will harness the strengths of information technology and allow people to do the things best done by people, such as making complex decisions and communicating with each other.
> **(Bates 2000 p 789)**

The system that has probably had the largest impact on medication error is computerized physician order entry (CPOE), in which medication orders are written online. This improves orders in several ways. First, they are structured, so they must include a drug, dose and frequency; the computer, unlike a person, can refuse to accept any order without this information. They are also always legible and the clinician making the order can always be identified if there is a need to check back. Finally, all orders can be routinely and automatically checked for allergies, drug interactions, excessively high or low doses and whether the dosage is appropriate for the patient's liver and kidney function.

Bates and his colleagues (1998) have shown that the introduction of a computerized order entry system resulted in a 55% reduction in medication errors.

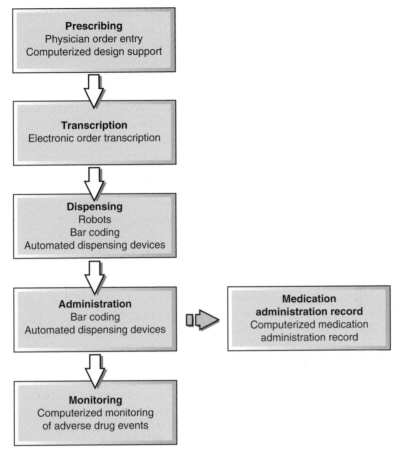

Fig. 11.1 Role of automation at each stage of the medication process (from Bates 2000 British Medical Journal 320:789; amended and reproduced with permission from the BMJ Publishing Group).

This system provided clinicians with information about drugs, included appropriate constraints on choices (dose, route, frequency) and assistance with calculations and monitoring. With the addition of higher levels of decision support, in the form of more comprehensive checking for allergies and drug interactions, there was an overall reduction of 83% in medication errors. A variety of smaller studies of more basic systems have shown, for instance, improvement of prescribing of anticoagulants, heparin and anti-infective agents and reductions in inappropriate doses and frequency of drugs given to patients with renal insufficiency (Kauschal et al 2003). In a review of CPOE, however, Kauschal et al (2003) caution that whereas these systems show great promise, most studies have examined 'home-grown' systems and have only considered small numbers of patients in specific settings. Much more research is needed, particularly with major commercial systems, to compare different applications, identify key components, examine factors relating to acceptance and uptake and anticipate and monitor the problems that such systems may induce.

Looking further ahead (Box 11.4) it is possible to envisage the use of many other technologies in the process of medication delivery. Most of these are in the early stages of development, are relatively untested and sometimes delayed by external constraints. Bar-coding for instance, widely used in supermarkets, could be enormously useful but cannot be implemented until drug manufacturers have agreed common standards (Bates 2000).

FORCING FUNCTIONS AND COROLLARY ORDERS

Recent studies of the quality of care, reviewed in Chapter 3, have shown that large numbers of patients do not receive standard investigations and treatment for clearly identified conditions (McGlynn et al 2003). Staff, who rely largely on memory to order investigations and treatment, fail to provide about half of indicated investigation and treatment. Many of the investigations and treatment required are relatively clear cut but are somehow missed. Frequently, part of the correct treatment is given but not the whole, implying that staff knew what should be done but somehow failed to follow through.

Forcing functions are reminders or constraints that suggest or require a certain response from the person using the machine. When you use your debit card to obtain money from a cash machine, the screen prompts you to remove your card before issuing any money (Nolan 2000). This is a classic use of design to overcome human absent mindedness and the previously common situation of removing the cash, which is the focus of your attention, and leaving the card in the machine. You meant to take the card but you were talking to your friend, took your money, turned away and left the card in the machine. Similarly, clinicians placing certain drug orders usually intend, but quite often forget, to order the necessary tests that routinely accompany the medication.

Overhage and colleagues (1997) call these basic medical decisions corollary orders. Ordering gentamicin should, almost always, trigger ordering gentamicin levels; angiotensin-converting enzyme (ACE) inhibitors require serum creatine levels; insulin means blood glucose monitoring and so on. Although the decision to carry out a corollary order is simple, they are frequently

---

Box 11.4 The medication system of the future

(from Bates 2000)

In future physicians will write orders online and get feedback about problems like allergies and decision support to help them choose the best treatment. The orders will be sent electronically to the pharmacy, where most will be filled by robots; complex orders will be filled by pharmacists. Pharmacists will be much more clinically oriented and focus on promoting optimal prescribing and identifying and solving problems. Automated dispensing devices will be used by nurses to provide drugs to patients. All drugs, patients and staff will be bar coded, making it possible to determine what drugs have been given to whom, by whom and when.

missed. Various strategies have been used to combat these omissions, such as monitoring adherence using chart review and mounting educational programmes. These can be successful but are difficult to maintain in the long term. Paper-based reminders placed in the chart are partially effective but not always available to the clinician at the time he or she writes the order. A computerized reminder, however, linked to an electronic medical record system, allows an immediate prompt. Overage et al (1997), in a 6-month trial, showed that clinicians ordered the suggested corollary orders in 46% of cases when prompted, compared with 22% in a control group. Clinicians discriminated among the suggested orders, rejecting some and accepting others, and it is reasonable to assume that the additional orders were necessary ones that the clinicians, once reminded, considered important.

These examples concern a specific corollary order but the general principle of reminders might have a wider application. Volpp and Grande (2003) suggest that standardized, evidence-based order sets could be used in many common situations, such as ruling out myocardial infarction, and would ensure that the optimum procedure is followed. Well-designed order sets, with modular components for use in specific situations, could reduce errors, particularly omissions, and reduce the time taken to write multiple sets of similar orders. These order sets could be paper based, but ideally would be computer generated. Such a grouping of orders would greatly simplify the investigation and treatment of common conditions, reducing the number of steps in the decision-making chain. This in turn would reduce the mental load on the clinician and, in a sense, reduce human involvement in the routine aspects of care delivery. Clinicians might argue that patients require individual care and one cannot just bundle groups of tests for all occasions. This argument loses its power, however, if the bundle is simply the default option, which clinicians can vary as they deem necessary. A greater worry is that clinical staff would reflect less on unusual presentations, relying on order sets and broad-brush clinical intervention. Order sets are certainly not meant to be a substitute for clinical acumen and reflection. However, with many patients receiving only half the treatment they should have, corollary orders and order sets seem greatly preferable to relying on memory, even at the risk of some over standardization.

COMMUNICATION AND ALERTS

The introduction of an effective electronic medical record should improve basic communication of all patient information. Staff would have access to a common database of medical information, including the results of investigations and tests, notes on outpatient visits and hospitalizations, records of drug allergies and recent medical history. Although the technological and standardization problems of implementing such systems are formidable, particularly when covering a whole healthcare system such as the British NHS, there is clearly scope for massive increases in efficiency, avoidance of duplication of investigations and treatment, and reduction of errors caused by crucial information not being available.

A particularly dangerous time for loss of essential information, particularly for patients who are very sick and whose condition is fluctuating, is at the handover, or sign-out, when one member of staff takes over from another. Handover, when verbal, is frequently rushed, casual and sometimes absent altogether.

> I just got called by the nurse about Ms Davis, who is hypotensive. All I know about her is that she is an 82-year-old woman with a urinary tract infection who is due to go home tomorrow.
> **(Volpp & Grande 2003 p 852)**

At the Brigham and Women's Hospital in Boston, a computerized sign-out system automatically includes up-to-date information on drug allergies, current medications, results of recent tests and relevant medical history. Doctors covering the wards are expected to update the medical history each day with details of changes in clinical condition and current treatment plan. All this information is available to other clinical staff. Furthermore, the electronic process of sign-out and the transfer of pagers ensures there is no ambiguity about who is on duty at any one time.

Information technology can also detect and transmit information about laboratory abnormalities as soon as the result is available. For instance, a dangerously low serum potassium level requires urgent action, but the information might be delayed while a ward clerk sorts the results and might not reach the relevant doctor until some time later after he has finished other duties. With an alert system coupled to a hand-held PDA or mobile phone, an instant alert can be generated and transmitted. In a controlled trial, such a system reduced response time by 11% and reduced the duration of dangerous conditions in patients by 29% (Bates & Gawande 2003).

DECISION SUPPORT

Decision support encompasses a vast range of tools with different names, foci and outputs and with widely differing levels of technological input. For example, an automatic prompt, in a sense, supports clinical decision making by reminding the clinician to make a particular decision to order a test. Clinicians have used decision support in some form for many years, in the form of pocket guides to drugs, personal lists and reminders of ward practices and so on. Decision-support systems include paper-based guidelines and protocols giving general guidance and objectives, more specific paper-based algorithms that assist diagnosis or calculations of appropriate drug dosages, computer-based systems of prompting possible diagnoses right through to systems that could potentially supplant human judgement (Morris 2000). In practice, all systems allow the clinician to override them, but some are sufficiently sophisticated as to be clearly superior to human judgement; the one, absolutely crucial, exception is when the clinician has access to information that the machine cannot take into account. This might be clinical information or, perhaps even more importantly, knowledge of the particular values and preferences of the patient and his or her family. We will return to this theme at the conclusion of this section.

Computer-based decision support has a major advantage over almost all paper-based general protocols and guidelines: it can be patient specific to a degree that is almost impossible to achieve in a paper-based guide. A computer-based system can remind you when to act, suggest courses of action, perform necessary calculations, monitor the output and take any number of patient specific clinical variables into account. Far from being cookbook medicine, this opens up the possibility of treatment being individualized and customized to a much greater degree. A full decision-support system does, of course, standardize clinical decision making in the sense that it follows specific, evidence-based decision-making rules; standardization in this sense simply means being explicit about how the treatment is being customized. Whereas human beings will resort to (generally successful) heuristics to make rapid, clinically informed decisions, the computer can, in many circumstances, achieve a perfect consistency in diagnostics and patient management. As yet, most systems are prototypes, being tested and evaluated in particular local circumstances and have not yet achieved full clinical integration. Increasingly, however, systems are being developed that have not only been shown to improve decision making but have been adopted as an essential part of routine practice (Box 11.5).

Whereas technology has enormous potential to support, and sometimes supplant, human decision making, the importance of clinical judgement and intuition should not be underestimated. Rather, it is a question of discovering

---

Box 11.5 Some examples of computerized decision support

Computerized mechanical ventilation protocols for acute respiratory distress syndrome

(adapted from Morris 2000)

In the intensive care unit at LDS Hospital in Salt Lake City, all nine intravenous pumps and the monitor above the bed are directly wired to the decision-support system. Data on such factors as intravenous flow, intravenous drug administration and physiological monitoring are sampled automatically, with other data entered by the clinician at a keyboard. In a trial in 10 hospitals, physicians objected to only 0.3% of generated suggestions for action over 32,000 hours of application. When the system was compared with ordinary care in two groups of patients, survival was comparable in the two groups but barotrauma was significantly less in the group that received standardized decisions from the computerized protocol.

Acute myocardial infarction detected by neural networks

Artificial computer-based neural networks are first provided with output from an electrocardiograph (ECG) and the classification of the relevant measurements, which in this case would include a decision on the presence or absence of myocardial infarction. These networks learn over time to associate the training examples with the given classification for each case. In a comparison of 1120 ECGs from patients admitted to a coronary care unit and 1120 controls, the neural networks showed higher sensitivities and discriminant power than cardiologists. The authors concluded that:

Artificial neural networks could be used to improve automated ECG interpretation for acute myocardial infarction. The networks may be useful as decision support even for the experienced ECG readers.

(Heden et al 1997)

205

Continued

Box 11.5 Some examples of computerized decision support—cont'd

Implementing antibiotic practice guidelines through computer-assisted decision support (from Evans et al 1998)

At the LDS Hospital, Salt Lake City, practice guidelines, developed by staff, were embedded in decision-support programmes as rules, algorithms and predictive models. Decision-support programmes now manage all prophylactic antibiotics before surgery and those used for the treatment of suspected and confirmed infections. These programmes continually track and assist physicians in managing each patient treated with antibiotics. For instance, in the treatment of infections, the programmes will provide information on the presence of resistant pathogens, untreated infections, an incorrect dose, route or interval; the absence of renal function data; the need for serum levels; population-based probabilities of infections in relation to specific patient variables and cost-effective alternatives to current treatment. In a study of over 63,000 patients over a 7-year period, the proportion of patients receiving antibiotics increased from 31.8% in 1988 to 53.1% in 1994, although overall costs decreased. Treatment with appropriate prophylactic antibiotics before surgery increased from 40% to 99.1%, with the average number of dosages per patient decreasing from 19 to 5.3 doses. Antibiotic-related adverse drug events decreased by 30% in the period of the study.

where technology can help and where we need to assist human judgement. In emergency medicine, for example, clinicians are faced with an extraordinarily dynamic and changing environment. One can imagine using computerized decision aids to assist in the diagnosis of a myocardial infarction once the possibility has been identified. However, someone has to talk to the patient when he or she first comes in, understand the story, the possible language problems, the distress and human response, and decide whether this is a bad case of indigestion or an atypical myocardial infarction. Human beings are certainly needed here, but there are myriad ways in which human beings can be led astray in these circumstances by the very heuristics that might be helpful on other occasions (Croskerry 2002). As a simple example, the recency bias means that we tend to recall and be unduly influenced by recent apparently similar cases; an atypical myocardial infarction last week, very nearly missed, might lead the clinician to err on the side of caution and admit a patient who could safely be sent home. In the emergency department, and in other settings where rapid clinical decisions are needed, training in decision making and the judicious use of simple decision aids and guides might be the way forward. The evidence is mixed on how far people can improve their judgement and decision making, and there is disagreement about how best to achieve this. There is, however, some evidence that a knowledge of the nature of decision making, an understanding of heuristics and biases and systematic exposure and feedback on a range of different cases may assist in the development and optimization of clinical judgement and decision making (Bornstein & Emler 2001).

How will patients react to the increasing use of decision support? The computer by your intensive-care bedside monitoring your physiology and the drugs you receive could be seen as a support, even a comfort, to a patient, perhaps allowing the nurses more opportunity to care for very sick and vulnerable people. But would you want to go to your surgeon and find that they use a computer to decide whether to operate or not? Would the use of a computer destroy trust and degrade the doctor–patient relationship? Decision support will probably become more important to patients as they increasingly participate in treatment decisions and have to face the same complexities as clinicians. Do you watch and wait with possible prostate cancer and put up with the symptoms? Do you opt for radiotherapy and its attendant risks or for radical surgery, a potential complete cure but with possible loss of sexual function? In part, this decision will depend on the weighing of options and in part on personal values and preferences, and the key to the proper use of decision support lies in separating these two aspects. Decision support can, and should, be placed at the service of the doctor–patient relationship, handling what one might call the 'calculative' aspects of the decision and allowing the doctor and patient to explore the human side, the personal and emotional consequences of each course of action. The preferences of the patient, and the doctor, are separated from the preferred mode of judgement and decision making and no longer conflated as they are in a more traditional clinical scenario. Doctor and patient first explore what the patient feels is most important, the doctor has assessed the clinical factors and the full clinical interview is still conducted; the machine, or other decision aid weights the options on the basis of the information and presents the likely outcomes. In the end though, the patient still decides (Dowie 2001).

PROBLEMS AND BARRIERS

The increasing use of technology, and the rapid increase in computer power, has allowed many systems to operate with little or no intervention from human beings. The classic exemplar of such systems is the flight deck of a modern commercial airliner, in which the pilot's role has, apparently at least, progressively been diminished. The aircraft of the future, so the story goes, will be flown by a single pilot and a dog; the dog is there to bite the pilot if he touches anything. In fact, pilots need greater skills with such a highly automated system; they must be able to both fly the plane and understand the automated systems, which becomes steadily more difficult as automation increases.

Such systems are always vulnerable to both hardware and software breakdowns, but their very sophistication and level of automation produces new problems for the human operator and new vulnerabilities. These are, in Lisanne Bainbridge's elegant phrase, the 'ironies of automation' (Bainbridge 1987). In a classic paper she outlined some of the principal ironies, summarized here as follows:

- Many systems successfully automate the routine elements of a process yet leave the supposedly unreliable human operator to carry out tasks that the designer could not think how to automate – most notably recovering from system breakdown.
- In highly automated systems, the main task of the human being is to monitor the systems and check for any abnormalities. Yet vigilance and monitoring over long periods are notoriously difficult for human beings

- When systems break down only rarely, the human operators have little chance to practice recovering from the breakdown or of using their own skills to take over control. Skills such as these degrade when not used, which inevitably happens when a machine takes over.
- The systems that are most highly automated paradoxically require the highest level of skill and training to deal with their complex, sometimes opaque modes of operation.

Few healthcare systems are near this level of automation, although it might apply to some laboratory processes. Bainbridge's cogent analysis does, however, point to the fact that we can expect the increasing use of information technology, even if clearly beneficial overall, to produce its own problems. Can we detect any early signs?

Studies of the problems associated with technology in healthcare are few and far between, although anecdotes are easy to come by. The shutdown of an automatic drug dispensing system in an Emergency department for instance, led to delays in giving urgent drugs and a near disaster; subsequently nurses took to carrying adrenaline around in their pockets in case the problem recurred. In another example, staff took to sticking reminder notes on the computer screen because the software did not allow them to input the reminders they needed. These classic 'workarounds', although understandable, clearly create the potential for other kinds of error. They stem not so much from technology *per se*, but from technology designed and implemented without sufficient understanding or regard for the way clinical work is actually carried out.

Ash and colleagues (2004), in a paper entitled *The unintended consequences of technology*, have begun to outline some of the principal forms of error that technology precipitates. For example, computer interfaces with easy, pull-down menus or other quick ways of entering data can lead to substitution errors, especially when people are distracted:

> I was ordering Cortisporin, and Cortisporin solution and suspension comes up. The patient was talking to me and I accidentally put down solution, then realized . . . I would not have made that mistake if I had been writing it.

> Patients were getting the wrong orders for medications. You would order it on one patient and, because of the vagaries of the light-pen system, it was really ordered for somebody else and the wrong patient got the medication.
> **(Ash et al 2004 p 106)**

Computerized systems can also be simply inflexible, insufficiently adaptable to the complexities of real, individualized patient treatment; if urgent medication is required, and cannot be released before the full authorization and data input, dangerous delays might be introduced; transfers from Emergency to a ward can similarly be delayed while the admitting system demands key information that is not available. More serious problems can arise through failing to study the nature and flow of the work prior to implementation. In one British hospital, laboratory results were telephoned to the wards, direct to physicians, thus allowing rapid communication of urgent results. When this system was replaced by entering results into a computer system, physicians had to remember to log on and check the laboratory results; the new system had advantages in terms of clinical workload and time management but it led to delays in receiving urgent information and some results that were missed entirely (Ash et al 2004).

In a careful qualitative study of the introduction of a bar-coding system for medication, Emily Paterson and colleagues (Patterson et al 2002) noted five main types of unanticipated side effect of the system. First, there were occasions where the nurses were simply confused by the system, particularly when it dropped medication orders simply because they had been delayed. Second, it sometimes led to a decrease in communication between physicians and nurses; physicians would previously have a quick glance at the (paper) medication records, but would not check the computer system unless there was a query because it was slower. Third, there were problems with scheduling activities because the system demanded very precise timings, delaying other clinical work that should have taken priority. Fourth, there were difficulties in entering unusual, non-standard medication regimens. Finally, they observed the ingenuity of the nurses in getting round the system with workarounds when they were short of time or otherwise pressured. Rather than scan the wristband on the patient's wrist, they might type in the code number, scan the patient ID card instead or take the wristband off and scan it on the table. Scanning of multiple medications at the same time saved time, as did delaying documentation of medications that would not scan at the time. In all these workarounds we can see the trade-off between needing to get things done and bypassing the systems at the cost of a greater likelihood of making a mistake by, for instance, typing in a code number rather than scanning the bar code.

A final problem relates to the achievement of very high levels of safety in any system. When errors and problems occur all the time, then people become used to dealing with them, are continually on the lookout for error and develop ways of recovering. The more errors we make, the more skilled we become at recovering from them. Conversely, when errors are very rare we can become lulled into a false sense of security, particularly with apparently 100% reliable technology. David Bates and colleagues (2001) quotes an example of this phenomenon in healthcare concerning radiation therapy. Macklis and colleagues (1998) examined the safety record of a system that double-checked radiation treatments. The system had an error rate of only 0.18%, and all the errors that did occur were minor in nature. However, about 15% of the errors that occurred related to the way operators used the system. Because they believed it was so reliable they tended to believe 'the machine had to be right' even in the face of conflicting evidence. Thus over-reliance on technology, indeed on any highly reliable system, can increase the possibility of certain kinds of errors through reduced vigilance.

Information technology, especially computerized decision support, is still not widely accepted and not in routine use. Many barriers remain to be overcome: some financial, as considerable investment is needed for large-scale change; some practical, such as the lack of standards for representation of data; and some cultural, in that both the research and the use of decision support is still slightly suspect in both academic and clinical circles (Bates & Gawande 2003). Nevertheless, harking back to the discussion of human memory and decision making, it is clear that much greater use of information technology is needed if healthcare is ever going to attain even reasonable standards of reliability and safety. The fact that the implementation of technological solutions can lead to errors and unanticipated hazards does not mean that we should stop implementing information and other technology to improve safety. Rather, we need to be alert in design, implementation and usage to the unanticipated consequences and side effects. This said, even with much more reliable basic processes we will still be ultimately reliant on people to anticipate, monitor and respond to the unexpected, which is the subject of the next and final chapter.

REFERENCES

Ash JS, Berg M, Coiera E 2004 Some unintended consequences of information technology in health care: the nature of patient care information system-related errors. Journal of the American Medical Informatics Association 11:104–112

Bainbridge L 1987 The ironies of automation. In: Rasmussen J, Duncan K, Le Plat J (eds) New technologies and human error. Wiley, London

Bates DW, Cohen M, Leape LL et al 2001 Reducing the frequency of medication errors using information technology. Journal of the American Medical Informatics Association 8:299–308

Bates DW, Leape LL, Cullen DJ et al 1998 Effect of computerized physician order entry and a team intervention on prevention of serious medication errors. Journal of the American Medical Association 280:1311–1316

Bates DW 2000 Using information technology to reduce rates of medication errors in hospitals. British Medical Journal 320:788–791

Bates DW, Gawande AA 2003 Improving safety with information technology. New England Journal of Medicine 348:2526

Bornstein BH, Emler C 2001 Rationality in medical decision making: a review of the literature on doctors' decision-making biases. Journal of Evaluation in Clinical Practice 7:97–107

Croskerry P 2002 Achieving quality in clinical decision making: cognitive strategies and detection of bias. Academic Emergency Medicine 9:1184–1204

Dowie J 2001 Decision analysis and the evaluating of decision technologies. Quality and Safety in Health Care 10:1–2

Evans RS, Pestonik SC, Classen DC 1998 A computer assisted management program for anti-biotics and other anti-infective agents. New England Journal of Medicine 338:232–238

Grove WM, Meehl PE 1996 Comparative efficiency of informal (subjective impressionistic) and formal (mechanistic, algorithmic) prediction procedures: the clinical – statistical controversy. Psychology, Public Policy and Law 2:293–323

Hastie R, Dawes RM 2001 Rational choice in an uncertain world. The psychology of judgement and decision making. Sage Publications, California

Heden B, Ohlin H, Rittner R et al 1997 Acute myocardial infarction detected in the 12-lead ECG by artificial neural networks. Circulation 96:1798–1802

Kauschal R, Shojania KG, Bates DW 2003 Effects of computerized physician order entry and clinical decision support systems on medication safety: a systematic review. Archives of Internal Medicine 163:1409–1416

Klein G 1998 Sources of power. How people make decision. MIT Press, Boston

Macklis RM, Meier T, Weinhaus MS 1998 Error rates in clinical radiotherapy. Journal of Clinical Oncology 16:551–556

McGlynn EA, Asch SM, Adams J et al 2003 The quality of healthcare delivered to adults in the United States. New England Journal of Medicine 348:2635–2645

Morris AH 2000 Developing and implementing computerized protocols for standardized clinical decisions. Annals of Internal Medicine 132:373–383

Nolan TW 2000 System changes to improve patient safety. British Medical Journal 320:771–773

Norman D 1988 The design of everyday thinks. Doubleday, New York

Overhage JM, Tiernery WM, Zhou X et al 1997 A randomized trial of 'corollary orders' to prevent errors of omission. Journal of the American Medical Informatics Association 4:364–375

Patterson ES, Cook RI, Render ML 2002 Improving patient safety by identifying side effects from introducing bar coding in medication administration. Journal of the American Medical Informatics Association 9:540–553

Schachter DL 1999 The seven sins of memory. Insights from psychology and cognitive science. American Psychologist 54:182–203

Vincent C 2003 Hemivulvectomy: the wrong side removed. Online. Available at: http://www.webmm.ahrq.gov/

Volpp KGM, Grande D 2003 Residents' suggestions for reducing errors in teaching hospitals. New England Journal of Medicine 348:851

Using information technology to reduce error

People create safety

> If we do not concern ourselves with problems we do not have, we soon
> have them.
> **(Dorner 1996 p 52)**

Safety is, as is often said, a property of the whole healthcare system. Making
healthcare safer will require clinical innovation, process improvement, information technology and cultural change. However, the people who work in an
organization are part of that system and each brings their own contribution to
safe, high-quality care. Clinical staff, in addition to simply doing their jobs
well, actively create safety as they work. Atul Gawande expresses this well
when discussing the limits of a systems view:

> It would be deadly for us, the individual actors, to give up our belief in
> human perfectibility. The statistics may say that some day I will sever
> someone's main bile duct, but each time I go into a gallbladder operation
> I believe that with enough will I can beat the odds. This isn't just
> professional vanity. It's a necessary part of good medicine, even in
> superbly 'optimized' systems. Operations like that lap chole have taught
> me how easily error can occur, but they've also showed me something
> else: effort does matter; diligence and attention to the minutest detail can
> save you.
> **(Gawande 2002 p 73)**

Although there is a certain amount of work in industry on safety behaviours
and attitudes, comparatively little attention has been paid in the patient
safety movement to the precise ways in which individuals, whether singly
or in teams, can contribute to safer healthcare. People partly create safety by
being conscientious, disciplined and following rules; however, they also create safety by going beyond the rules when circumstances dictate. This does
not involve breaking rules but recognizing when one must think beyond
standard procedures. This theme reappears in the discussion of the particular ways in which teams of individuals can create safety, which is also a balance between disciplined, regulated behaviour and necessary flexibility.
There is, however, one other individual who plays a role in creating safety.
Before thinking about what healthcare staff can do, we consider that much-
neglected person in patient safety – the patient, and of course his or her
friends and family. What role can patients play in ensuring their own and
others' safety?

A PRIVILEGED OBSERVER WITH A KEEN INTEREST IN SAFETY – THE PATIENT

Patient safety, you would think from the name, had the patient's interests at heart, and so it does in many respects. However, this has seldom extended to actually involving the patient in the quest for safer care. Safety is addressed and discussed in multiple ways, lessons are sought from all manner of other industries and experts, from the disciplines of psychology, ergonomic, engineering and many others. Yet the one source of experience and expertise that remains largely ignored is that of the patient.

One might argue that patients do not have much to contribute; after all, many people fly but aviation safety does not rely on the passengers for safe operation. In healthcare, however, unlike aviation, the patient is a privileged witness of events both in the sense that he or she is at the centre of the treatment process and also in the sense that, unlike clinical staff who come and go, the patient observes almost the whole process of care. Patients might not, of course, understand the technical and clinical issues at stake, but they do observe and experience the kindnesses, the small humiliations, the skilfulness of a line insertion, the inconsistencies in care, the errors and, perhaps, the disasters. In the case of people with chronic illnesses they become experts not only on their own disease but on the frailties, limitations and unintentional cruelties of their healthcare system. The trouble is that, for all this potential knowledge and insight into the frailties of the healthcare system, they find it astonishingly difficult to make their voice heard, particularly where errors and safety are concerned.

Even experienced senior doctors can find it hard to make their voice heard when dealing with hospital staff caring for themselves or their family. Don Berwick has movingly described his experiences of being with his wife, Ann, during her treatment for a serious autoimmune spinal cord problem (Box 12.1). In his account, Don stressed the good will, kindness, generosity and commitment of the healthcare staff but, even after two decades of grappling with the quality and safety of healthcare, he was appalled at the operation of the healthcare systems. Notice especially his last remark about migrating to the edge of being a difficult patient; drawing attention to the deficiencies in your care does not necessarily make you popular and the last thing any patient wants to do, in hospital at least, is alienate the staff who might – literally – have your life in their hands.

Patients as active participants in their care

Patients are usually thought of as the passive victims of errors and safety failures, but there is considerable scope for them to play an active part in ensuring their care is effective, appropriate and safe. Angela Coulter (1999) has argued that instead of treating patients as passive recipients of medical care, it is much more appropriate to view them as partners or co-producers with an active role in their care. For instance, patients have a vital role to play in providing an accurate and relevant clinical history. Unfortunately, they are often not able to present their story. In a recent study in the US, patients were

Box 12.1 Being and feeling unsafe in hospital

(adapted from Berwick 2003)

Above all we needed safety; and yet Ann was unsafe... The errors were not rare; they were the norm. During one admission, the neurologist told us in the morning, 'By no means should you be getting anticholinergic agents' and a medication with profoundly anticholinergic side effects was given that afternoon. The attending neurologist in another admission told us by phone that a crucial and potentially toxic drug should be started immediately. He said 'Time is of the essence.' That was on Thursday morning at 10.00 a.m. The first dose was given 60 hours later. Nothing I could do, nothing I did, nothing I could think of made any difference. It nearly drove me mad. Colace was discontinued by a physician's order on day 1 and was nonetheless brought by the nurse every single evening throughout a 14-day admission... I tell you from my personal observation: no day passed – not one – without a medication error. Most weren't serious, but they scared us.

We needed consistent, reliable information, based, we would have hoped, on the best science available. Instead we often heard a cacophony of meaningless and sometimes contradictory conclusions. Drugs tried and proven futile in one admission would be recommended in the next as if they were fresh ideas. A spinal tap was done for a test for Lyme disease but the doctor collected too little fluid and the test had to be repeated. During a crucial phase of diagnosis, one doctor told us to hope that the diagnosis would be of a certain disease, because that disease has a benign course. That same evening, another doctor told us to hope for the opposite because that same disease is relentless, sometimes fatal. Complex, serial information on blood counts, temperature, functional status and weight – the information on the basis of which risky and expensive decisions were relying – was collected in disorganized, narrative formats, embedded in nursing notes and narrative forms. As far as I know, the only person who ever drew a graph of Ann's fevers or white blood cell count was me, and the data were so complex that, short of a graph, no rational interpretation was possible. As a result, physicians often reached erroneous conclusions, such as assuming that Ann had improved after a specific treatment when, in fact, she had improved before it or not at all.

The experience of patient-hood, or patient-spouse-hood, as the case may be, was one of trying to get the attention of decision makers to correct their impressions or assumptions. Sociologically, this proved very tough, as we felt time and again our migration to the edge of the label 'difficult patient'.

allowed to speak for only 23 seconds before being interrupted by their doctor with the result that important information was often missed (Marvel et al 1999). When allowed to speak without interruption, and with simple encouragement, most people in outpatient consultations only seem to need about 90 seconds to present their story before spontaneously saying something like 'That's all, doctor' (Langewitz et al 2002).

At most stages of patient care there is the potential for patients to contribute to their own care through provision of diagnostic information, participation in treatment decisions, choice of provider, the management and treatment of disease and the monitoring of adverse events (Vincent & Coulter 2002). This requires that healthcare professionals encourage and support a more active stance from patients, but also that patients are prepared, where possible, to take more responsibility for their health and their care. The degree to which patients can be involved will vary considerably from specialty to specialty and will depend on the nature and complexity of the treatment and the degree of technical knowledge required to understand the treatment process. Most importantly, it will depend on the extent to which patients feel willing and able to play a more active part, which undoubtedly varies enormously from person to person. At the one extreme are those people who prefer, whether from temperament or custom, to leave all decisions to their doctor and take a passive role. At the other are those who wish to be involved in the minutest details of their treatment. Both these approaches can be appropriate in particular circumstances: for an acute medical emergency the sensible patient does indeed leave decisions to the treatment staff. In the case of a long-term chronic illness, the actively involved, enquiring patient is more likely to receive appropriate treatment and to cope more effectively.

There are some impressive examples of patients being actively involved in the management of a hospital, entirely changing the nature and tone of the usual patient clinician relationships. At Dana-Farber Cancer Center in Boston, for example, patients are member of several important hospital committees and regarded as an essential voice in the re-design or improvement of services. By involving patients, the hospital learnt that patients with neutropenia (a reduction in white blood cells occurring in many diseases) often experienced long, wearying waits in emergency departments, seriously delaying the start of treatment. Telephone screening and direct admission to appropriate wards transformed this process and reduced the risk of infections and other complications.

The patient's role in patient safety

Many medication errors could be avoided if communication with patients was improved and they were encouraged to speak up when they notice unexplained changes in their medication. Patients who are given full information about the purpose of medicines and their likely effects, including side effects, are more likely to take them as recommended, leading to better health outcomes. Unfortunately, patients are often not given crucial information about their drugs, which is a major cause of non-compliance with treatment recommendations (Vincent & Coulter 2002). Patients should be encouraged to report postsurgical complications promptly so that swift action can be taken if necessary. Unfortunately, lack of information about what to watch out for after discharge from hospital is a very common complaint. In a postal survey of patients discharged from hospital, 31% of respondents said they weren't given a clear explanation of the results of their surgical procedures, 60% weren't given sufficient information about danger signals to watch out for at home and 61% weren't told when they could resume their normal activities. If greater attention was paid to providing this type of information, it could lead to a reduction in the rate of complications and readmissions (Coulter 2001).

To encourage patients to take a more active stance, some organizations are now producing leaflets setting out what patients can do to make their own care safer. The American Joint Commission on Accreditation of Healthcare Organizations (JCAHO), for instance, has campaigned for patients to speak up to prevent errors in their care. This is a very interesting development and as yet we have little idea what the consequences will be, or how such campaigns will be received by the public. The openness about the possibility of error and the active involvement of patients in some specific activities must certainly be welcomed; asking patients where they expect to have surgery is clearly an important check in the process and beneficial to all concerned. Encouraging patients to ask questions about their medication to make sure they understand, not to take medication unless they are clear about its purpose and to be responsible for their own contribution to their treatment seem reasonable and useful precautions (Box 12.2) although, if followed to the letter on all occasions, they could take up a great deal of staff time.

Encouraging patients to ask questions is straightforward enough and would be accepted by most patients and staff, although attitudes to such questioning vary considerably in different countries. Much more difficult is the suggestion that patients might actively challenge a health professional.

Box 12.2 Speaking up

(adapted from JACHO 2004)

Speak up if you have questions or concerns, and if you don't understand, ask again. It's your body and you have a right to know:

- Don't be afraid to ask about safety. If you're having surgery, for example, ask the doctor to mark the area that is to be operated on, so that there's no confusion in the operating room.
- Don't be afraid to tell the nurse or doctor if you think you are about to receive the wrong medication.

Pay attention to the care you're receiving. Make sure you're getting the right treatments and medications. Don't assume anything:

- Notice whether your caregivers have washed their hands. Hand washing is the most important way to prevent the spread of infections. Don't be afraid to gently remind a doctor or nurse to do this.
- Make sure your nurse or doctor confirms your identity, that is checks your wristband or asks your name before he or she administers any medication or treatment.

Educate yourself about your diagnosis, the medical tests you are undergoing and your treatment plan:

- Ask your doctor about the specialized training and experience that qualifies him or her to treat your illness.
- Write down important facts your doctor tells you, so that you can look for additional information later. And ask your doctor if he or she has any written information you can keep.

Ask a trusted family member or friend to be your advocate:

- Ask this person to stay with you, even overnight, when you are hospitalized. You will be able to rest more comfortably and your advocate can help to make sure you get the right medications and treatment.
- Review consents for treatment with your advocate before you sign them and make sure you both understand exactly what you are agreeing to.

Know what medications you take and why you take them. Medication errors are the most common healthcare mistakes:

- If you do not recognize a medication, verify that it is for you. Ask about oral medications before swallowing and read the contents of intravenous (i.v.) fluids. If you're not well enough, ask your advocate to do this.
- If you are given an i.v. drip ask the nurse how long it should take for the liquid to 'run out'. Tell the nurse if it doesn't seem to be dripping properly (that is, too fast or too slow).

Patients are meant to observe whether their identity band has been checked, tell the staff if they think they might be being confused with another patient and remind nurses and doctors to wash their hands. Although well intentioned, this is a considerable extension of the patient's role and, arguably, an abdication of responsibility on the part of healthcare staff. Trying to involve patients in safety problems, such as poor hygiene and infection, might well be very worthwhile. However, it remains to be seen to what extent sick people, or their advocates, are able and willing to do this, and how it will be received by staff.

CREATING SAFETY BY FOLLOWING RULES AND PROCEDURES

Clinical work is founded on tried and tested ways of diagnosing and treating patients; being willing to follow procedures is fundamental to being a good clinician. Running an outpatient clinic for chronic asthmatics or diabetics, for instance, while still requiring much clinical acumen, requires good organization, clear procedures, good communication and reliable information technology delivering tried and tested, evidence-based care. Much flexibility in healthcare stems not from necessary adaptation to changing circumstances but from unnecessary, casual and inappropriate departure from good clinical practice. One way in which people create safety therefore is observing rules and by boring, conscientious following of standard procedures.

Organizational intention and individual action

Fiona Moss is a chest physician and was, for 10 years, editor of the journal *Quality and Safety in Healthcare*. In her last editorial for the journal she chose to focus on an intractable issue that she sees as fundamental to improving the safety of healthcare, which is the fact that clinicians routinely break rules and ignore basic and reasonable organizational procedures and practices. As Moss puts it, there is a chasm between organizational intention and individual action (Moss 2004).

Recall the death of Wayne Jowett described in Chapter 6, in which several staff departed from standard procedures, and then consider this extract:

Learning to buck the system is a frequent early learning experience for many doctors. For example, hospitals in the UK do not allow house officers to prescribe or administer cytotoxic chemotherapy. Although this 'organisational rule' has been in force for several years, we sometimes find that it has been broken. This usually happens at night, when a patient has not been given chemotherapy; the person who should give it is no longer on duty and the 'covering' doctor is called. Although this very inexperienced doctor and the nurse may both be aware that the doctor should not give the chemotherapy, neither perceives any real danger as the action needed is simply to attach an infusion bag to an already sited drip; both are concerned that the patient get the treatment

and so the treatment is given. An organisational rule is broken. Nothing happens, no one knows. A culture that ignores the system of the delivery of care is enforced and the system becomes a little more dangerous.
(Moss 2004 p 406)

Notice first that there are many plausible reasons there are for breaking this rule. The patient needs the treatment and it would probably be time consuming to call another doctor with the authority to administer the treatment. The other doctor might in any case be off site or dealing with an emergency elsewhere; there might be good reasons for breaking the rule on at least some occasions. But in healthcare the fact that it is sometimes necessary to think beyond rules very easily shades, by sleight of hand, into simply ignoring rules because it is inconvenient for some reason and then the system really does become that little bit more dangerous. Once ignoring rules is socially, if not organizationally, sanctioned the system becomes a little more dangerous, then more dangerous still, and so on until there is a major disaster. Within healthcare organizations there are some rules that are never broken, others more on the margins, and some that are routinely flouted. These shifts in what is acceptable are known as migrations, in the sense that an individual or a team steadily drifts from behaviour that is, if not optimal, at least reasonable in the circumstances towards serious violations of procedures and behaviour that is frankly dangerous (Polet et al 2003).

Hand washing and hospital-acquired infection

Hand washing is an example of a rule that is routinely flouted; studies have found that average levels of compliance have varied from 16% to 81% (Pittet 2001), although compliance is probably much higher in high-risk environments such as the operating theatre where the routine of getting scrubbed is solidly embedded. Some have thought to excuse the low level of compliance by arguing that there is no proven link between poor hand hygiene and hospital-acquired infection. The causes of infection are undoubtedly complex and there are various routes of transmission. However, contamination through hand contact is a major source and hand hygiene a major weapon in the fight against infection (Burke 2003). Despite this, it has proved extraordinarily difficult to persuade healthcare workers to wash their hands.

Previous interventions to change clinicians' behaviour have included education, feedback, financial rewards and penalties, and administrative changes. The history of research into hand washing has been a litany of failure, in the sense that most interventions have shown only small or transient effects; however this has been coupled with a steadily increasing sophistication in understanding of the many factors that influence this behaviour and of the need for multifaceted interventions (Larson et al 1997). The lack of washing facilities at the patient's bedside, skin problems through frequent washing and shortage of time are all important barriers to hand washing for busy clinicians. Didier Pittet and colleagues (2000) solved these problems by introducing a fast bedside procedure of hand disinfection with an alcohol-based rub. In a 4-year intervention in the University of Geneva hospitals, they improved compliance from 48% to 66%; in the same period the prevalence of nosocomial infection reduced from 16.9% to 9.8% and the transmission rates of MRSA halved. The intervention involved a massive and continuing educational campaign, regular surveys and observations and the backing and involvement of all professional groups at all levels of the hospital. Compliance increased most markedly for nurses and nursing assistants but they were at a loss to explain, or at least would not publicly state, why compliance remained poor among doctors. There is now considerable political and regulatory pressure in many countries for improvements in both rates of nosocomial infection and hand hygiene, but it remains to be seen whether the improvements demonstrated in Geneva can be replicated more widely.

CREATING SAFETY THROUGH HAZARD AWARENESS, ANTICIPATION AND PREPAREDNESS

The safety of healthcare is such a huge problem and the causes so diverse and complex that it might seem as if the individual clinician can do little to influence the overall safety of care. Changes are needed at many different levels; many require action at senior management level, and some by governments. But at the coalface, minute-by-minute, safety can either be eroded by the actions and omissions of individuals or, conversely, created by skilful, safety-conscious professionals.

For a doctor, treating a patient with a complex, fluctuating clinical condition requires thinking ahead, instructing the nurses to call you when observations fall outside specified ranges and being prepared to adjust treatment as the condition changes; nurses have, in their turn, to anticipate changes in the patient's condition and the likely need for support or medical assistance. Safety in these circumstances requires anticipation, awareness of hazards, preparedness, resilience and flexibility, the qualities that those studying high-reliability organizations have sought to capture and articulate. We will never be able to rely entirely on standardization, rules and procedures, indeed no organization can. When thinking about safety, however, we are also calling on a broader vision in which the clinician is anticipating not only the disease but the functioning of the organization in which he or she works, assessing the hazards emanating from the organization as well as the patient. What are the particular qualities and attributes of the safe practitioner? Rather 'What are the qualities of the practitioner who can create safety?', for this is not a static quality but an ability to look ahead and respond to circumstances.

Personal responsibility and professionalism

Safety clearly requires solid professional competence. Healthcare relies on the contributions of numerous professional groups, all of whom need to be well trained, reasonably conscientious in their duties and fulfil their commitments. Given the emphasis on systems thinking in patient safety it is worth pointing out that taking a systems view of medical error in no way implies that the individuals within the system should abdicate responsibility; they too are part of the system, in fact its key component. Professionalism and personal responsibility are fundamental.

Graham Neale (2004) has emphasized the importance of a sense of responsibility in his examination of the case of Wayne Jowett. Although accepting the importance of the organizational context and the absolute need to make systems as fail safe as possible, he points out that in clinical practice the risks, by the very nature of the enterprise, will always be high. Clinical work depends on heavily engaged staff, often inadequately resourced, making decisions in real time on the basis of incomplete evidence. In the case of Wayne Jowett, death might have been avoided if individual members of staff had taken responsibility:

> If the appropriate person in the Department of Health (who had known of the problems for many years) had taken real responsibility; if Wayne and his family had accepted the need to adhere to appointments; if the consultant had provided a fail-safe means of contact and insisted that he alone had the skills necessary to ensure safe administration of chemotherapy; if the pharmacy technician had been made to feel that he was more than a provider; if the unit managers had insisted that no one would be allowed on the unit without adequate induction; and if the SHO and registrar had striven to know how to safely administer chemotherapy, Wayne would be alive today.
> **(Neale 2004 p 196)**

In considering this case again from another perspective, we are not seeking to again criticize those involved. However, the case, usually used to illustrate systems failure, equally illustrates the role of personal responsibility as a key factor in the erosion, or creation, of safety.

Awareness of error and human fallibility

Does reading about safety, researching safety and reflecting on the ways things can go wrong make any difference to clinical practice? Consider the findings summarized so far in this book. Patients are frequently harmed, often preventably; errors are common in every area of medicine yet examined; although people are resourceful, there are certain limitations to human cognition that markedly increase the chance of error; healthcare systems and processes have evolved, rather than been designed, and tend to be long, unnecessarily complex, uncoordinated and prone to failure; the working conditions of many healthcare professionals are far from ideal, thus increasing the chances of error. Anecdotally, being involved in safety research and practice does seem to influence clinical work. When I asked some of my clinical colleagues if their engagement in safety research had influenced their practice, their response was that it certainly had (Box 12.3).

Generally we do not reflect or study our working environment because we have to just get on with the work. And yet, where safety is concerned, a reflective attitude and some anticipation of potential problems is an essential fundamental attitude. The first step towards safety for the healthcare professional

Box 12.3 Safety in clinical practice

'Being more vigilant in terms of errors that occur in day-to-day practice, which I may have missed in the past. Being willing to address loose ends rather than say this is not part of my problem.'

'Involving the patient in their care. For example always asking the patient which side they thought they were having the operation.'

'Being more explicit about my instructions, discussing everything I think or intend to do with the patient and gaining opinion of other colleagues.'

'At handover always summarizing the situation, outlining the plan and being absolutely clear about what to monitor and at what point I want to be called.'

'Ensuring documentation of everything.'

'I do not undertake any procedure unless I am sure I am competent in performing it or have adequate supervision.'

'Senior clinicians say they want their juniors to err on the side of safety yet many younger clinicians do not follow that principle for fear of seeming weak. I make a point to reminding myself day after day that I want to be safe first, and brave afterwards.'

'Spending longer with patients explaining and discussing the risks and benefits of treatment.'

'Being obsessive about hand washing. I am now very aware of why we are asked to do this and so less irritated about the time it takes.'

'Having enough humility to recognize when you are out of your depth and being willing to ask for help.'

is to understand the nature of error and safety and then to consider how it applies in one's own environment. Which are the most dangerous processes on the ward? Which are most prone to error and failure? What are the peak times at which errors are most likely to occur? What are the principal forms of harm that can afflict patients in this environment? The next step is openness about error and a willingness to discuss the hazards and dangers of the environment, as a team is much more likely to be able to monitor and prevent error than an individual. Anyone at any level can foster an openness about error and hazard. A nurse running a ward can make it clear that it is acceptable to discuss the possibility of error, can constantly reinforce the possibilities for error, the need for anticipation and cross checking. The most junior nurse can steer a new doctor away from a hazardous situation. All of this is crucial, safety-conscious behaviour.

An understanding of error and its causes can help one become error aware, in the sense of heightening one's vigilance in error prone situations. James Reason (2004) has suggested a simple but memorable way of doing this: the three-bucket model. This provides a simple way of assessing when alarm bells should be ringing in your head. The three buckets correspond to three factors that affect performance and the likelihood of error: yourself, the context and the task you are carrying out. If, for instance, you are carrying out a new procedure for the first time unsupervised, you are tired and hungry and the environment is noisy and distracting then all three buckets are full and you should be very wary. (You can decide for yourself what the buckets are full of, conjuring up your own particular image.) When conditions are particularly bad, particularly error prone as it were, it is best to step back if at all possible to see if the procedure can be delayed until conditions are more favourable, such as when you have had a chance to get some food, get some help or deal with some of the distractions. This is a much more skilful approach to hazardous environments than just ploughing on regardless with an impregnable belief in one's own abilities and a trusting assumption that things will turn out all right. Whether approaches of this kind can be learned and applied as a particular error skill remains to be seen.

Caution and hazard awareness

Safe practice is understood intuitively by many experienced clinicians, whose youthful enthusiasm and willingness to have a go has been tempered by the experience and observation of countless errors of judgement and a few disasters. A degree of caution and circumspection are useful qualities in any potentially dangerous situation, provided they are coupled with a willingness to act decisively when the situation demands. A lack of caution and hazard awareness can have serious consequences for the patient as the example in Box 12.4 shows.

Caution in this sense does not imply hesitancy or dithering, more a cool deliberation and a weighing of risk and benefit. (Weighing risks and benefits takes place in every area of medicine and it is curious, to say the least, that the subject of risk *per se* hardly features in the medical and nursing curricula.) Spinal surgeons, for instance, might have to resist pressure from patients to operate and take away their back pain, because they have a more realistic view of what the potential gains and risks are; moderate pain relief against

---

Box 12.4 Lack of hazard awareness

An elderly woman developed an irregular bowel habit with attacks of diarrhoea that responded to constipating drugs. She was referred to a gastroenterologist who arranged for numerous investigations, including barium studies of the gut, upper and lower gastrointestinal endoscopy, and scanning of the abdomen by ultrasound and CT. The body of the pancreas was described as atrophic. Routine blood tests showed no abnormality. It was decided to investigate by undertaking ERCP (endoscopic retrograde cholangio-pancreatography) on the grounds that the patient might have cancer of the head of the pancreas or chronic pancreatitis. After ERCP the patient developed severe pancreatitis (a fairly common complication, especially in patients with narrow ducts) and a nasogastric tube was left in situ for 3 weeks to allow the inflammatory process to settle. The nasogastric tube led to inflammation that caused stricturing of the oesophagus (a rare but recognized complication). The oesophagus required repeated dilatation and the patient was never be able to eat normally again.

In this case the risks of investigation clearly outweighed any possible benefit. The investigation carried substantial risks and was very unlikely to produce useful diagnostic information. Surgical intervention would not have been indicated with either diagnosis. Furthermore, if the symptoms were due to pancreatic insufficiency this could have been established by examination of stools and treatment with oral pancreatic enzyme supplements. In fact, the patient was subsequently diagnosed as having an irritable bowel. Thinking ahead to the possible hazards of the investigations and reflecting on their purpose of the investigations would have led to a more considered approach very much more in the patient's interests.

the risk of paralysis might be a gamble the patient would live to regret. In primary care, doctors are constantly judging who needs to be referred for further investigation by other specialists. One might think that they too should be cautious and err on the safe side; however, in Britain at least, if doctors in primary care behaved like this the health system would be rapidly bankrupted by a flood of unnecessary investigations. Safety in the strict sense of absolute caution has to be balanced by a concern for the use of resources and the dangers of unnecessary investigations.

Anticipation and vigilance

Anticipation is a key component of expertise in many areas. In a study of the control of fighter aircraft, Amalberti and Deblon (1992) found that in pre-mission planning, which often took longer than the mission itself, pilots spent a great deal of time analysing each part of the route for possible threats, whether from hostile aircraft, personal factors, weather or technical breakdown. During the flight itself, pilots devoted over 90% of the time when they were free to think to anticipation; typically they developed a 'tree' of events that might occur, which became more or less salient over the course of the flight.

Anticipation and vigilance lie at the heart of all clinical work, in the sense that the clinician must always anticipate the likely course of the disease, have strategies ready for eventualities and be flexible about responding to developments, whether positive or negative. Experts are constantly thinking ahead and looking to the future. For instance, Cynthia Dominguez showed surgeons a video of an operation involving an 80-year-old woman with an infected gall bladder that needed to be removed. She used the video as a prompt to ask the surgeons how they prepared for such an operation and what they would be thinking at each stage. She found that experienced surgeons made more predictions about likely problems than their junior colleagues. In particular, they predicted, and were thus prepared for, difficulty in dissecting and identifying the surrounding structures because the gall bladder and surrounding areas would be swollen and inflamed. Second, they predicted a higher risk of complications, such as an injury to nearby structures or tearing of the gall bladder itself, thus releasing bile and increasing the chance of abdominal infection (Dominguez et al 2004). With these predictions in mind they were therefore mentally prepared for the hazards that lay ahead; like the fighter pilots they mentally mapped the route and anticipated likely hazards along the way.

With safety, though, we need to add an additional dimension to this anticipation; we not only have to anticipate the course of the disease but also anticipate the behaviour and response of colleagues and the wider organization. If error and harm to patients is caused partly by organizational and system factors, then being safe requires thinking ahead and having strategies in place to deal with these factors too. Clinicians get very used to dealing with these kinds of problems; yet again the notes are not available and one resorts to asking the patient to repeat as much of their history as they can remember. Vigilance means anticipating the disease but also the vagaries of the organization and the possibility that others may not check as assiduously as you would wish. My colleague Ros Jacklin expresses this clearly:

> I feel that one of the keys to being a safe practitioner comes down to vigilance – looking for problems before they happen, when they still are in the brewing stage. For instance, if you are on call, find out who has been operated on that day, and have a brief look at them before you go to bed, whether or not anyone specifically asks you to. If the patient looks dry, you might check that there's nothing to suggest bleeding, and increase their fluids a little overnight. Otherwise, no one notices that they are dry until their urine output has dropped. If that were to happen, you can probably easily rectify the patient's fluid status with i.v. fluids at this stage, but if for any reason there is a delay, the patient may find themselves in established renal failure.

In addition to being vigilant oneself, the clinician looking ahead at potential problems will also be assessing how vigilant the staff on the next shift are likely to be. Sometimes a clinician will end a shift knowing that he or she has left the patients in safe hands; at other times, if a less than conscientious person takes over, nagging anxiety remains and a few additional checks and enquiries might be warranted.

Strategies, algorithms and preparedness

Having tried to anticipate all possible threats and hazards, the pilots in Amalberti and Deblon's study would then mentally simulate a response to see if it would resolve the problem; if not they would see if they could adjust the flight in some way so that they could deal with all contingencies. A key component of the pilots' expertise lay in predicting and avoiding dangerous situations. Expertise is not so much an ability to improvise and escape danger (their improvised solutions were often quite poor) but the ability to stay within an envelope of safe operation and have prepared strategies to deal with problems. Similarly, expert clinicians do not rely on their brilliance at escaping from dangerous situations but on trying to avoid them in the first place and having solid routines to fall back on when a crisis does emerge. As Bob Wears, an emergency physician, reminded me that when a crisis occurs one does not so much rise to the occasion as fall back on one's training.

Note that these strategies of recovery are rehearsed routines, not intuitive on-the-spot improvisation. They can be rehearsed physically, in actual practice or simulation, or mentally. Running through in your mind what you will do if some particular problem occurs is a powerful way of preparing yourself for the eventuality. Box 12.5 gives an example of a senior surgeon discussing a strategy for dealing with operative bleeding. Clinicians will pick up these strategies and routines from more experienced colleagues; they are seldom formally taught. Clinicians are taught what to do, but much less attention is given to how to recover from disaster.

> **Box 12.5 Anticipation and preparedness in surgery**
>
> You need to have a strategy ready when there is bleeding: cold, automatic responses to a hazardous situation ingrained in your mind so that it can be done without stress and strain. What to do if the groin starts to bleed is one of the worst situations. When teaching I give them a list of things they're going to do. I get them to repeat it to me over and over again so that when it does happen to them, and it will eventually, they don't need to think, they just go into autopilot.
>
> The first thing is to put a pack in which stops the bleeding. The second thing is to ask for some extra help; you need another person to use the sucker, because often you're on your own with the theatre sister. Third, you need to tell the anaesthetist you've got some bleeding. You then need to elevate the foot of the bed, which lessens the amount of bleeding, and to extend the wound without moving the pack. Once you've got it controlled you can get everything else you need sorted out. Make sure you've got the right instruments, the right support, the anaesthetist knows what's going on and you have everything ready, so when you take the pack out you have help and suction and view and all the things you need to deal with the situation. The sucker will show you where the bleeding's coming from and you deal with it. When they know all this by rote then dealing with the problem becomes routine.

TEAMS PROTECT SAFETY

A team in a formal sense is a group of individuals with a shared, common goal who, although they each have defined individual tasks, achieve the goal by working interdependently and cooperatively. Teams are sometimes little more than a group of individuals brought together by chance, haphazardly struggling to work together; alternatively they might work seamlessly, fluidly and, with few words, communicate, anticipate and respond to each other and to the ebb and flow of the work. Healthcare teams vary hugely in size, complexity, the mix of skills, professions involved and seniority of members. They include, for instance, surgical teams, nurses running a ward, management teams, primary care groups and mental health rapid response teams who deal with acute psychosis across wide geographical areas. In this section the discussion is limited to surgical and emergency medicine teams.

Teams and the management of error

Teams, like individuals, can erode or create safety. A group of people has many opportunities to miscommunicate and get things wrong. For instance, in their study of communication in the operating theatre Lorelei Lingard and colleagues (2004) classified about a quarter of the specific operation-relevant communications they observed as communication failures because they were made too late or too early, because essential content was missing, because they were addressed to the wrong person or because the purpose was simply unclear. The nurses and anaesthetist, for instance, discussed the positioning of the patient for surgery without consulting the surgeon, resulting in wasted time and interpersonal friction later in the case. A team that is not working effectively multiplies the possibility of error. Conversely, when working well, teams have the possibility of being safer than any one individual because a team can create additional defences against error, by monitoring, double-checking and backing each other up; when one is struggling, another assists; when one makes an error, another picks it up.

Patient safety has been particularly influenced by aviation teams and the use of simulation in pilot training; this approach has been particularly important in anaesthesia, and latterly in surgery and emergency medicine (Cooper & Taqueti 2004). Crew resource management (CRM) is the term usually used to describe the training of cockpit teams and other aviation teams. One of the reasons that CRM has been such an important influence is that the detection and management of error has always been a central component of the more successful training programmes (Helmreich & Merrit 1998). The CRM training includes instruction in human vulnerability to stressors, the nature of human error, and error counter-measures. The objective of the training is to reduce the risk that crews will make a series of important errors because they failed to foster teamwork, solve problems, communicate and manage their workload effectively (Risser et al 1999).

A particularly influential and important model of error in the aviation and medical environments was developed by Helmreich and colleagues at the University of Texas Human Factors Project (Fig. 12.1). Helmreich's model (Helmreich 2000) aids the identification of errors committed, for example, deficiencies in training and knowledge, ineffective error detection strategies, error management strategies, threat detection and systemic threats. Immediate threats include such factors as fatigue, communication or patient-related

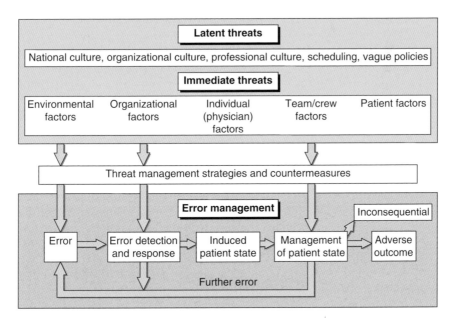

Fig. 12.1 The Helmreich model of threat and error management (from Helmreich 2000 British Medical Journal 320:781–778; amended and reproduced with permission from the BMJ Publishing Group).

People create safety

factors, such as a difficult intubation, whereas latent threats concern organizational matters such as shift patterns and staffing. Of particular importance is the attention given to the process of error observation, detection and recovery being an attempt to study not only the occurrence of error, but the process of recovery from error.

As so often in patient safety, we are looking at a small corner of a vast area. There is a substantial literature on teams in many different kinds of organization, and research from a variety of psychological, sociological and management perspectives (Paris et al 2000). Notwithstanding the importance of crew resource management, it is important to realize, first, that aviation will only be a good parallel for some healthcare teams and, second, that, as patient safety matures as a discipline, we should be drawing on a wider range of models, research literature and methods of training.

A shared understanding of the task and team

Underlying a number of specific team skills, such as prioritizing tasks, monitoring each other's work and communicating effectively, is the idea that the team has a common understanding of the task in question and the nature of team work. This is sometimes referred to as a 'shared mental model', analogous to the mental models of the world that each of us has as individuals. From a leadership and training standpoint this would imply that one of the key tasks is to ensure that 'everyone is on the same page' both during the training of teams and when actually working together. One tends to assume that everyone else in the team has the same understanding as you do about what is happening, but this might be far from the case. Think back again to the catastrophic role played by assumptions about competence and supervision in the death of Wayne Jowett. Effective, safe teams continually check each other's assumptions so that they never drift too far from a common understanding of the task in hand and their own role in it. This is the reason for, in highly skilled and effective teams, constant team briefing and exchange of information.

A good first step towards a shared understanding is a team briefing. At Orange County hospital in the US, theatre teams have introduced a routine preoperative briefing (Box 12.6; Leonard et al 2004). An interesting sideline on the development of the briefing was the way in which it revealed discrepant assumptions between professions. For instance surgeons, not unreasonably, thought that nurses' priority would be to know about the procedure and what equipment was needed; in fact the nurses' priority was to know whether the surgeon was on call and whether they needed to answer his or her pager during the operation, a potentially very disruptive influence. Looking at the perioperative briefing checklist we can see that a number of the key themes we have discussed are embedded into it; the team first sets out exactly what will be happening, prioritizes tasks as either standard or non-standard procedure, considers whether this procedure presents any particular threats (long operation, hypothermia, other potential problems), looks ahead to the possible need for other services and inputs, and allows each member of the team to review the information given by the other.

Box 12.6 Team briefing in surgery

(adapted from Leonard et al 2004)

Surgeon
- Identify patient and site
- What type of surgery and how long will it take?
- Any special equipment needed
- Is this a standard procedure or are there special needs?
- Are there any anticipated problems?
- Are there any special intraoperative requests, e.g. hypothermia?

Circulating nurse
- Identify patient site and marking
- Allergies?
- Verification of medication on the back table
- X-ray available and other special services?
- Blood available?

Scrub nurse
- Do we have all the instruments?
- Are there any instruments missing from the tray?
- Are all the instruments working?
- What special instrumentation do we need?
- Do they have any questions about instruments?

Anaesthetist
- What type of anaesthesia will be used?
- Risks?
- Should we anticipate any problems?
- Any special needs – positioning, medication?
- Any special lines needed because of anaesthesia

Most importantly, the very fact of a briefing in which all team members take part embeds the idea of open communication from the beginning of the operation, whether or not the team members have worked together before. Implicit in the fact of the briefing is the idea that everyone in the team has a right, in fact a responsibility, to communicate and to speak up if they foresee or notice any errors or problems. Such briefings, whether formal or informal, are certainly not confined to surgery. Wards, for instance, which have a regular daily meeting at which all patients are reviewed with both nurses and doctors present, are building in checks against false assumptions, miscommunication and errors of all kinds. This might not be the declared purpose of the meeting but it will certainly be a major benefit from the gathering of staff, exchange of information and anticipation of potential problems.

EMERGENCY MEDICINE: TEAM TRAINING TO REDUCE ERROR

In emergency medicine, the MedTeams Consortium has drawn heavily on crew resource management but has also founded its training on the findings of research on emergency medicine teamwork failures. In a review of malpractice claims, it found frequent instances of poor coordination of care, when individual team members did not share a common understanding of the plan of action, of failure to prioritize tasks, failure to speak up, and the failure of team members to monitor colleagues' work as well as their own. These problems are well illustrated in a case described by Risser and colleagues (1999) (Box 12.7).

From reviews of cases such as this, Risser and colleagues identified some key team behaviours that would protect and defend against errors; these overlap with other key error-prevention and team-enhancement strategies fostered in other high-risk environments, such as navy teams (Box 12.8). Implicit in these strategies is an acceptance that errors will always occur, that no one can function effectively all the time and that the environment will always present unexpected threats. Individuals can respond to these threats and challenges to some extent, but a team has a better chance of bringing a patient through a critical phase if members constantly watch each other, communicate openly and effectively and back each other up when necessary. Team skills require an outward focus, an awareness of others and a strong sense of how one's own work fits into the overall work process; these skills are not strongly emphasized in healthcare training, which tends to be highly individualistic and professionally based. Enhancing team performance is

---

Box 12.7 Failures in teamwork and the death of a patient

(adapted from Risser et al 1999)

A 39-year-old woman with a history of documented coronary artery disease came to the emergency department complaining of increased frequency of anginal chest pains over the past 2 weeks. She was triaged as 'urgent', the second highest triage category in a four-tier triage system, even though she had abnormal vital signs and a history that should have placed her in the highest category. The emergency department was extremely busy and almost 1 hour elapsed before she was evaluated by a medical student. At that time she complained of chest pain and was found to have weak-to-absent peripheral pulses.

Ninety minutes after she arrived, a reassessment of her vital signs showed her blood pressure to be 61/32 mmHg, but this was not communicated to the medical student or the physician. To relieve the patient's chest pain, the physician ordered sublingual nitroglycerin. Later the nurse reported on a written statement that she was uncomfortable giving nitroglycerin, a drug she knew could lower blood pressure, to a hypotensive patient but assumed that the physician 'knew what he was doing'. The patient continued to complain of chest pain and shortness of breath; morphine sulfate was given and a nitroglycerin drip was started. Finally, almost half an hour after the initial hypotensive episode, her low blood pressure was noted by the physician, the nitroglycerin infusion was discontinued and an internal medicine specialist was called, who arrived a further half hour later. The patient remained hypotensive, short of breath and continued to have chest pain. Finally, she became extremely bradycardic, lost her blood pressure and a 'code' wascalled. Advanced cardiac resuscitation was carried out including adrenaline (epinephrine), atropine, defibrillation, external pacing and pericardiocentesis. However, this was unsuccessful and the patient was pronounced dead 3 hours and 10 minutes after entering the department.

This case demonstrates a chain of errors in which poor organizational climate, lack of team structure, poor task prioritization, poor communication, lack of cross-monitoring (team members checking each other's actions) and lack of assertiveness within the emergency department contributed to a catastrophic patient outcome. The consequences of this team failure were dramatic: the patient died, the family was devastated, the staff was distressed and demoralized, the hospital's reputation was harmed.

sometimes reduced to going out drinking together in the hope that alcohol-induced team bonding will be an acceptable substitute for the learning of highly specific professional skills.

In strong contrast, the MedTeams Consortium training programme (Morey et al 2002) is focused on teaching core team skills underpinned by an understanding of the nature of team work and how it impacts on clinical practice. Led by a doctor and a nurse, the teamwork training involves groups of about 16 clinical staff who complete 8 hours of formal instruction on the fundamentals of team training and on specific behaviours with direct clinical application in the emergency department. Once this is completed, the team training is taken into clinical settings with the deliberate formation of specific teams at the start of each shift, additional instruction in specific team behaviours for each member of staff and coaching and mentoring of teamwork behaviours by staff during normal working hours.

The MedTeams Consortium has carried out a formal evaluation of the training in nine emergency departments. Team training produced significant improvements on standardized team measures as assessed by observers in the emergency department. These observers also monitored a sample of cases in each department, recording overall teamwork and any specific errors. For instance, in one case an intern discussed a case with a senior physician but failed to mention a raised blood pressure; none of the technicians or nurses who were present mentioned this and nor did they re-check the blood pressure. In another case, a technician did an electrocardiograph on a patient with chest pain; he prepared the patient but neglected to tell anyone and the patient was left unobserved for 25 minutes. Following team training there was a substantial reduction of errors of this kind. Clearly there are many

People create safety

Box 12.8 Team behaviours to prevent, detect and recover from errors

(adapted from Risser et al 1999 and Ilgen 1999)

- Identify the protocol to be used or develop a plan. It must be clear to everyone on the team what protocol or plan is being used.
- Prioritize tasks for a patient. Team members must understand the plan and how their individual tasks fit into the overall task.
- Speaking up. The healthcare professional must speak up when a patient is at risk; team leaders must foster a climate in which this can occur.
- Cross-monitoring within the team. Team members should watch each other for errors and and problems; this needs to be seen not as criticism but as a support to other team members and an additional defence for the patient.
- Giving and accepting feedback. Feedback is not restricted to team leaders; any member of the team can provide feedback to any other. Implicit in this is that team members understand each other's roles.
- Closed loop communications. Messages and communications are acknowledged and repeated by those who receive them; often the senders of these messages will again repeat them. This is seen as an additional check and defence.
- Backing-up other team members. Team members are aware of other's actions and are ready to step in to support and assist.

questions to be asked about the impact of such training on a wider scale, the extent to which enhanced team performance would be maintained and so on. Nevertheless, the overall programme, targeted specifically at clinical practice and clinical errors, produced impressive benefits.

TEAM LEARNING: HOW DO TEAMS TRAIN THEMSELVES?

The MedTeams project was based on an initial formal training programme but clearly relies for its eventual success on the adoption of these practices and the fact that members of each team then foster and develop them. A few hours of training by itself would have little direct impact; rather it acts as a catalyst for the team to develop itself.

An intriguing study Amy Edmondson and colleagues (2001) examined 16 cardiac surgery teams who were learning a new procedure. The basic coronary bypass operation is well established but teams were learning to carry out these procedures endoscopically via small incisions in the chest wall. There are technical challenges for the surgeon in the use of endoscopic techniques in any area of surgery but these surgeons were already fairly skilled in the new techniques; the real challenge was that the new technology required much greater coordination and communication between team members. Edmondson and colleagues examined how long teams took to develop these new skills, assessing progress by the length of the operation and other measures. Initially, operations using the new technique took two to three times as long as conventional open procedures.

Interestingly, many conventional assumptions about organizational and team change were not upheld. The support of senior management, which varied considerably from place to place, did not have much effect; nor did the status or seniority of the surgeon. Having regular briefings and debriefings was also not critical, although most teams did examine performance data retrospectively. Rather, the learning took place as the process unfolded in real time, and the more effective teams were able to take full advantage of the operation itself as a place of learning and training. How did they achieve this? There were three key factors. First, considerable thought was given to choosing the right people for the team to take on this new challenge; people were chosen not just for their seniority or technical skills but ability to work in a team. Second, and particularly important, was the way the task was framed to the team. In some institutions, the surgeons viewed the challenge as simply one of instructing the team what to do; these teams learned slowly. In others, the surgeon emphasized the challenge, the requirement of each person to contribute and the need for ongoing learning and communication throughout the process; these were the teams who progressed most rapidly (Box 12.9). Finally, in the rapidly learning teams the leaders and team members created an atmosphere of what Edmondson and colleagues call 'psychological safety'. In these teams, members were able to make suggestions, point out potential problems and admit mistakes when they occurred. By contrast, when people felt uneasy about acting this way, the learning process was stifled (Edmondson et al 2001).

Box 12.9 A tale of two cardiac surgery teams

(adapted from Edmondson et al 2001)

New technology as a plug-in component

The surgeon, senior and well-established in a major hospital, played no role in choosing the team, which was assembled according to seniority. He also didn't participate in the team's dry-run before the first case. He later explained that he did not see the new technique as particularly challenging technically. Consequently, he explained, it was 'not a matter of training myself but of training the team'. Such training would not require any change in his style of communicating with the team. 'Once I get the team set up, I never look up. It's they who have to make sure that everything is flowing'. Mastering the new technology proved slow and difficult for this team, with operations times remaining long even after 50 cases.

New technology as a team innovation project

Although this cardiac surgery department had no history of undertaking major research or innovation, it had recently hired a young surgeon who took an interest in the new approach. More than any of the surgeons in other hospitals, this surgeon realized that implementing the new technology would require the team to adopt a very different style. 'The ability of the surgeon to become a partner not a dictator is critical. You really do have to change what you're doing during an operation based on a suggestion from someone else in the team'. Team members noted that the hierarchy had changed, creating a free and open environment with input from everybody. This group was one of the two that learned the new technique most quickly, with operation times over an hour below the average after 20 procedures.

AND NOW BACK TO THE SYSTEM

In this chapter we have argued that both patients and staff have a key role to play in ensuring the safety of healthcare. In one sense this is obvious, in that people must obviously be competent in order to be safe. However, some specific qualities and behaviours are particularly important for safety: adherence to procedures and protocols, balanced by a willingness to think ahead, anticipate problems, respond to unusual circumstances and so on. It is clear, hopefully, that the system view must be balanced by examining the role individuals play. Yet, this interplay between people and systems is complex and we need to return to it once again, first because human performance is very much affected by the working environment and second because, counterintuitively, the positive contributions of individuals might impact adversely on the organization.

The influence of working conditions

> I have been awake for 30 hours and still have at least 5 more hours of work, not to mention three procedures. Every time I sit down to try and figure out why Mrs Long's kidney is deteriorating, I fall asleep.
> **(Volpp & Grande 2003 p 853)**

Anticipation, preparedness, the ability to think straight, personal drive and personal responsibility are all vulnerable to fatigue. All clinicians are hugely affected by their working environment and the demands, not only of the immediate task, but of the wider organization. Absurdly long hours, with consequent fatigue and stress, are one of the principal factors contributing to errors. The impact of a night's sleep deprivation on hand–eye coordination is comparable to that induced by a blood alcohol concentration of 0.10% (Dawson & Reid 1997). Being cared for by a doctor exhausted by the loss of a night's sleep is, at least in respect of hand–eye coordination, equivalent to being cared for by someone who is moderately drunk.

Reviews of the effects of sleep deprivation in other domains show substantial effects on a variety of mental tasks, sustained vigilance and motor skills. Studies in clinical settings have demonstrated a decrement in surgical skills after a night on call (Taffinder et al 1998), reduced ability to interpret electrocardiograms and slower responses in anaesthetic simulations with some sleep-deprived clinicians actually falling asleep during the anaesthetic simulations (Veasey et al 2002, Weinger & Ancoli-Israel 2002). Most of these studies have been addressing simulated clinical tasks not involving actual patients. However, two substantial recent studies (Landrigan et al 2004, Lockley et al 2004) examined the sleep schedules of doctors on different shift systems using continuous recording of eye movements, sleep schedules and rate of serious clinical errors. The rate of serious clinical errors, monitored by methods that included direct observation, was 22% higher on critical care units during the traditional shift schedule (extended shifts of 24 hours or more) compared with a revised schedule that eliminated long shifts and reduced the number of hours worked each week. Thankfully, several countries are now beginning to take action to reduce doctors' hours, although progress is slow and there are many issues, such as loss of clinical experience during training, to be addressed. We still, however, have the ludicrous situation in which it is illegal to drive a coach, lorry or train while exhausted but perfectly acceptable to look after an intensive care unit.

The purpose of raising this issue here, at the end of a chapter on personal contributions to safety, is to stress once again the limits and constraints on human performance. Fatigue and excessive working hours provide us with a particularly powerful example of the way in which individual capacity is constrained and influenced by the working environment and the wider organizational context. The system view neglects the individual, but the individual perspective must always be set in the wider organizational context and address the interplay between the many factors that contribute to the delivery of care.

Positive personal characteristics can inhibit organizational learning

The performance of individuals also affects the wider organization, sometimes in unexpected ways. One might think that individual effort would always enhance organizational performance and enhance safety. But as so often with safety, there is a twist. The very ingenuity and resourcefulness that are rightly admired in clinical staff, and that produce immediate benefits for patients, can inhibit more fundamental organizational change.

In a fascinating study, Anita Tucker and Amy Edmondson (2003) carried out over 200 hours of observation of 26 nurses at nine different hospitals in the US.

They examined two types of process failure in healthcare: errors and problems. Problems were defined as disruptions in the workers' ability to carry out a pre-scribed task either because something they needed was unavailable or because something else was interfering with the work. Examples of problems include missing supplies, missing medications or missing information, such as med-ical records or laboratory results. It is not uncommon for medical staff to spend a large amount of time looking for charts and equipment. Often, each ward and unit has its own rules about the placement of charts and equipment. In addition, the organization of charts and equipment might vary within the hos-pital, making expeditious use of information or tools difficult for house staff who care for patients on multiple wards, especially in emergencies (Volpp & Grande 2003).

Both nurses and doctors are extremely adept at dealing with these prob-lems; they have to be or the system would collapse:

> Where is Mrs Tilly's chart? I can't remember where they keep the charts on this floor. I am covering her care for the regular resident and don't know her well. I was called to see her for respiratory distress, but I can't find the pulse oximeter or an Ambu-bag.
> **(Volpp & Grande 2003 p 853)**

> Working around problems is just part of my job. By being able to get i.v. bags or whatever else I need, it enables me to do my job and to have a positive impact on a person's life – like being able to get them clean linen. And I am the kind of person who does not just get one set of linen, I will bring back several for the other nurses.
> **(Tucker & Edmondson 2003 p 60)**

Tucker & Edmondson (2003) call the approach this nurse describes first-order problem-solving; being adaptable, flexible, responding to changes in demand and fixing problems. Admirable, of course, and reminiscent of the qualities espoused in high-reliability organizations. The problem is that this very resourcefulness can mean that nothing ever changes, as usually no one is informed that there were no i.v. bags. The i.v. bags are meant to be there in the first place and, ideally, the nurses should not have to waste their time looking for them. First-order problem-solving is effective in the short term but pre-vents problems surfacing as learning opportunities. In addition, first-order problem-solving might create problems elsewhere in the organization, as supplies go missing from other areas of the hospital, leading to further organizational problems.

Second-order problem-solving involves patching the immediate problem but also letting the relevant people know that the problem has occurred. Tucker & Edmondson (2003) cite an example of a nurse from intensive care calling a ward who had mistakenly kept an ICU bed after moving a sick child to their ward; she simply let them know what happened to prevent future problems.

Tucker & Edmondson (2003) emphasize that all the nurses they observed worked well beyond their allotted hours and were dedicated to patient care, yet the problems persisted. They argue that, although these problems are entrenched, many are relatively straightforward to resolve, given some time and commitment. The answer, they suggest, lies in the counterintuitive notion that positive personal and organizational attributes are preventing organizational change. First, individual vigilance and resourcefulness, and the ability to solve problems, militate against change, as we have discussed. Second, this is compounded and reinforced by a system that makes sure that nurses are constantly used to the full, which means that they only have time to care for patients and not to resolve wider organizational issues. Third, they point out that many quality improvement methods rely on empowering front-line workers, such as nurses, to resolve problems. This is certainly important for resolving immediate difficulties. The downside, however, can be that the managers, who actually have the power to resolve these problems in the longer term, are not aware of them and not engaged to resolve them. It is clear, for instance, that each hospital should develop a single system for chart storage, placement of vital sign flow charts, location and type of equipment, storage and composition of procedure kits, and examination-room layout so that valuable time is not lost looking for equipment or determining how to use unfamiliar equipment (Volpp & Grande 2003). Instead, however, the system runs on adaptability and improvisation, papering over the cracks rather than sorting out the processes. The cardinal virtues and abilities of clinical staff are being squandered on administrative and organizational inefficiencies rather than put at the service of patients. In the longer term, wards and units that persistently have to battle against organizational inefficiency gradually cease to function effectively.

A LAST WORD

Looking back on the ideas, evidence and proposals that this book contains, drawn from across the patient-safety spectrum, allows us to reflect both on the extent to which the book has succeeded in its aims and on the view it has conveyed of patient safety. The book has hopefully, at the very least, convinced you that patient safety is vital for both patients and clinicians throughout the world. Working on patient safety offers, just as much as work on any of the major health problems we face, a chance to prevent unnecessary suffering and improve people's lives. Hopefully, too, something has been conveyed of the landscape of patient safety, the central concepts and what has been discovered about the nature, causes and prevention of error and harm. Perhaps you will also agree with the assertion in the preface that patient safety is a tough problem. My own view is that we have many good ideas and concepts, some solid evidence and many promising avenues to explore, but we are nevertheless still at the beginning. Many areas of healthcare have hardly been examined at all, understanding of the causes of error and harm is still relatively primitive, evidence for change is limited to a few key areas and we do not have a clear conceptual map of how to integrate the various safety interventions and components of safety into a coherent whole. In addition, there is much to be done in terms of cultural change, engaging clinicians and managers, and driving patient safety through regulatory pressure, policy and the political process.

Above all, for anyone who has read this book and who is working or associated with healthcare in whatever capacity, I would hope that you feel that patient safety is a subject worthy of your attention. Understanding and creating safety is a challenge equal to understanding any of the biological systems that medicine seeks to influence. Although the challenge is immense, it is clear that we are making some progress in awareness, in understanding and on action to prevent harm and care for those affected. Treating patients one at a time brings obvious and immediate benefits but working to change the processes and systems of healthcare can ultimately benefit many more.

REFERENCES

Amalberti R, Deblon F 1992 Cognitive modelling of fighter aircraft process control: a step towards an intelligent on-board assistance system. International Journal of Man Machine Studies 36: 639–671

Berwick DM 2003 Escape fire. Designs for the future of healthcare. Jossey Bass, San Francisco

Burke JP 2003 Infection control – a problem for patient safety. New England Journal of Medicine 348:651

Cooper JB, Taqueti VR 2004 A brief history of the development of mannequin simulators for clinical education and training. Quality & Safety in Health Care 13(suppl 1):i11–i18

Coulter A 1999 Paternalism or partnership? Patients have grown up – and there's no going back. British Medical Journal 319:719–720

Coulter A 2001 Quality of hospital care. Measuring patients' experiences. Proceedings of the Royal College Physicians Edinburgh 31 (suppl 9):34–36

Dawson D, Reid K 1997 Fatigue, alcohol and performance impairment. Nature 388:235

Dominguez C, Flach JM, McDermott PC et al 2004 The conversion decision in laparoscopic decision making. In: Smith K, Shanteau J, Johnson P (eds) Psychological investigations of competence in decision making. Cambridge: Cambridge University Press

Dorner D 1996 The logic of failure. Recognizing and avoiding error in complex situations. Perseus Books, Cambridge, Massachusetts.

Edmondson A, Bohner R, Pisano G 2001 Speeding up team learning. Harvard Business Review 79:125–132

Gawande A 2002 Complications: a surgeon's notes on an imperfect science. Picador, New York

Helmreich RL 2000 On error management: lessons from aviation. British Medical Journal 320:781–785

Helmreich RL, Merrit AC 1998 Culture at work in aviation and medicine: national, organisational and professional influences. Ashgate, Aldershot

Ilgen DR 1999 Teams embedded in organizations: some implications. American Psychologist 54:129–139

Joint Commission for Accreditation of Healthcare Organisations (JCAHO) 2004 Speaking up. Online. Available at: http://www.jcaho.org

Landrigan CP, Rothschild JM, Cronin JW et al 2004 Effect of reducing interns' work hours on serious medical errors in intensive care units [see comment]. New England Journal of Medicine 351:1838–1848

Langewitz W, Denz M, Keller A et al 2002 Spontaneous talking time at start of consultation in outpatient clinic: cohort study. British Medical Journal 325:682–683

Larson EL, Bryan JL, Adler LM et al 1997 A multifaceted approach to changing handwashing behavior. American Journal of Infection Control 25:3–10

Leonard M, Graham S, Bonacum D 2004 The human factor: the critical importance of effective teamwork and communication in providing safe care. Quality & Safety in Health Care 13(suppl 1):i85–i90

Lingard L, Espin S, Whyte S et al 2004 Communication failures in the operating room: an observational classification of recurrent types and effects. Quality & Safety in Health Care 13:330–334

Lockley SW, Cronin JW, Evans EE et al 2004 Effect of reducing interns' weekly work hours on sleep and attentional failures. New England Journal of Medicine 351(18):1829–1837

Marvel MK, Epstein RM, Flowers K et al 1999 Soliciting the patient's agenda: have we improved? Journal of the American Medical Association 281:283–287

Morey JC, Simon R, Jay GD et al 2002 Error reduction and performance improvement in the emergency department through formal teamwork training: evaluation results of the MedTeams project. Health Services Research 37:1553–1581

Moss F 2004 The clinician, the patient and the organisation: a crucial three sided relationship. Quality & Safety in Health Care 13:406–407

Neale G 2004 Systems failure. Clinical Risk 10:195–196

Paris CR, Salas E, Cannon-Bowers JA 2000 Teamwork in multi-person systems: a review and analysis. Ergonomics 43:1052–1075

Pittet D 2001 Compliance with hand disinfection and its impact on hospital-acquired infections. Journal of Hospital Infection 48 (suppl A):S40–S46

Pittet D, Hugonnet S, Harbarth S et al 2000 Effectiveness of a hospital-wide programme to improve compliance with hand hygiene. Infection Control Programme. Lancet 356:1307–1312

Polet P, Vanderhaegen F, Amalberti R 2003 Modelling border-line tolerated conditions of use (BTCU) and associated risks. Safety Science 41:111–136

Reason J 2004 Beyond the organisational accident: the need for 'error wisdom' on the frontline. Quality & Safety in Health Care 13(suppl 2):ii28–ii33

Risser DT, Rice MM, Salisbury ML et al 1999 The potential for improved teamwork to reduce medical errors in the emergency department. The MedTeams Research Consortium. Annals of Emergency Medicine 34:373–383

Taffinder NJ, McManus IC, Gul Y et al 1998 Effect of sleep deprivation on surgeons' dexterity on laparoscopy simulator. Lancet 352:1191

Tucker AL, Edmondson A 2003 Why hospitals don't learn from failures. Organisational and psychological dynamics that inhibit change. California Management Review 45:55–72

Veasey S, Rosen R, Barzansky B et al 2002 Sleep loss and fatigue in residency training: a reappraisal. Journal of the American Medical Association 288:1116–1124

Vincent CA, Coulter A 2002 Patient safety: what about the patient? Quality & Safety in Health Care 11:76–80

Volpp KG, Grande D 2003 Residents' suggestions for reducing errors in teaching hospitals. New England Journal of Medicine 348:851–855

Weinger MB, Ancoli-Israel S 2002 Sleep deprivation and clinical performance. Journal of the American Medical Association 287:955–957

People create safety

INDEX

Note: Suffixes on page numbers:–
'b' refers to Boxes.
'f' refers to Figures.
't' refers to Tables.

Absent-mindedness, 196, 197b
  forcing functions and, 202
Abuse of patients, pathological culture,
    154–155
Access maximization, safety *vs*, 22
Accident and emergency departments
  as high-reliability organizations, 163
  see also Emergency medicine
Accidents, 75–98
  bereavement from, 124
  James Reason on, 27
  organizational (Reason), 105–108
Accountability
  reporting systems and, 61–64
  see also Responsibility
Action plans, learning from incidents, 115t
Active participants, patients as, 214–216
Acute respiratory distress syndrome
    (ARDS), ventilation protocols, 205b
Adaptability of workers, 96
Adaptive mechanism, forgetting as,
    197–198
Administration *see* Management;
    Managers; System factors
Administrative data analysis, 35t
Adrenaline, 136
  half-life of safety compared to, 158
  intravenous infusion, 50b
Adverse drug events, 9, 49–51
  reduction at St Joseph' Medical Centre,
    189–191
  Yellow Card scheme, 59
Adverse events
  case record review, 40–45
  definition, 34, 40, 41b
  errors compared with, 82
  inadequacy of term, 128
  long-term aspects, 134–136
  mortality, 45–47

primary care, 48–49
psychological effects, 43, 123–124
reportable incidents compared with, 70
staff support after, 132, 135, 139–151, 150
surgery, 47–48
see also Utah–Colorado Medical Practice
    Study
Adverse outcomes, amelioration, 14
Advisory Committee on the Safety of
    Nuclear Installations, on safety cul-
    ture, 157
Advocates, family members as, 217b
Agency for Healthcare Research and
    Quality (AHRQ), report, 180,
    183–186
Agreed policy of open disclosure, 133, 149
AHRQ (Agency for Healthcare Research
    and Quality), report, 180, 183–186
Air embolism, 29b
Aircraft carriers, 162
Airliners
  Vincennes incident, 91b
  see also Aviation
Alcohol dependence, rates of correct care, 37
Alcohol rub, hand hygiene, 219–220
Alert systems, laboratory abnormalities, 204
Alexander, David, on suicide and psychia-
    try, 144–145, 147–148
All Changed, Changed Utterly (BMJ), on
    Bristol paediatric cardiac surgery
    affair, 18
Allergy
  adverse drug events, 51
  failure of communication on, 187
Amalberti, R.
  on airline pilots, 81
  aviation safety, 165
  error rates in aviation, 94–95
  and F. Deblon, fighter aircraft flying, 224,
    225
Amelioration of adverse outcomes, 14
American Society of Anesthesiologists
  Closed Claims Project, 39–40
  Ellison Pierce (president), 25

Index

Index

Index